Natural Forms of Defense
Against Biological, Chemical, & Nuclear Threats

A Clear Guide Linking Natural & Conventional
Forms of Emergency Health Care

John Brighton, N.D.

Trafford
PUBLISHING® www.trafford.com
North America & international
toll-free: 1 888 232 4444 (USA & Canada)
fax: 812 355 4082

Dedication

This book is dedicated to my grandchildren
Javier
Mariela
Jan Andres
Who represent for me the children of the world

Acknowledgements

I'm deeply grateful for all the help and love provided by my wife Christine. Without her this book could not have been written. I'm also very grateful for the emotional and spontaneous financial support towards this book by our dear friends Larry and Teri White. Many thanks go to Norman Kanter who provided much valuable advice on the design of the book. Thanks also go to Jeff Menges who helped to create and print the cover design, especially for his patience and good cheer.

J.B.

Contents

<u>DISCLAIMER</u>

PERSONAL RESPONSIBILITY STATEMENT

This book is a reference volume designed solely to provide education and information on selected natural substances and processes, and not as medical advice. It is not intended for diag-
nosing or treating ailments or for prescribing remedies in any way, and it is not meant to be a
substitute for professional medical help. Because individuals differ widely in their reactions to
various substances, and because there is always risk involved, the author and the publisher urge
you to consult a physician or other qualified health care provider prior to starting any new treatment or program, or if you have any questions regarding a medical condition. The author and
the publisher are neither responsible nor liable for any adverse consequences or effects resulting
from the use of any of the information or suggestions contained in this book. If you are not
willing to assume the risk and responsibility, please do not use this book.

NATURAL FORMS OF DEFENSE
AGAINST BIOLOGICAL, CHEMICAL, AND
NUCLEAR THREATS

INTRODUCTION

KNOWLEDGE IS THE ANTIDOTE FOR PANIC

Since the tragic events that took place in the United States on September 11, and the bioterrorist attacks that followed with anthrax, our level of vigilance has dramatically increased. Terrorists aim to break down the resources that sustain a social fabric—its food and water, its institutions, its treasured symbols, its psychological integrity—in order to disrupt the normal flow of life. By doing so they seek to instill fear and panic in the general public. Using the sophisticated technology of our times, they have the capability to fashion portable nuclear devices, and to turn germs or toxic chemicals into **weapons of mass destruction** (WMD).

Many of these weapons are relatively easy to make, easy to hide, and easy to use. As we have seen, it takes about 500 milligrams (a teaspoon or so) of anthrax spores made into a fine powder and delivered inside an envelope to cause unsuspected harm, death, and panic. With a hundred kilograms of anthrax (equivalent to a five pound bag of sugar) a catastrophic attack could be produced on thousands of people. If this amount were released over a large city it might very well kill between one and three million people!

While our daily routines may continue as before, no nation can sustain such attacks and remain thinking in the same way. Because of this, many are asking questions about topics they never thought would occupy their minds. Will other bioweapons be used against us? How would they be produced? How would they be launched, and where would be the most likely places? Is a nuclear attack possible? Are we prepared?

In my profession as a health consultant I have spent over 22 years advising people on how to deal in natural ways with common diseases. Following these events, I found myself searching for nature's answers to strange and complex problems. At first, it seemed unlikely that the gentle healing methods used by naturalistic practitioners could be used as a form of defense in warfare. It seemed that the medicinal products—antibiotics, vaccines, and antidotes—of a "harder" science would appear more appropriate.

As I examined the issues and the nature of the threats we face, I came to realize that the naturalistic approach could make a significant contribution, and, most importantly, could do so without competing against the conventional form of medicine. In fact, it could augment it. Moreover, all of the information led me to believe that in the kind of emergency situations that I am addressing a combined approach could work in a synergistic manner that would be more beneficial than if either were used alone. This would occur when the best of each method are combined.

For example, conventional medicine is renowned for its diagnostic procedures, surgery, and emergency medicine. It is probably second to none when it deals with physical traumas, burns, poisonings, and the like. It has developed some of the most focused methods to kill germs, particularly bacterial pathogens. Yet these achievements have a weak side when it comes to prevention.

Naturalistic forms of healing would complement it by adding a preventative dimension, which aims at strengthening the host with a variety of supportive interventions such as: nutrition, detoxification of major organ systems, rehabilitative strategies, and mind-body integrative measures that address the whole person within a particular social and environmental context.

While conventional medicine's reliance on antibiotics has had much success, its emphasis on antibiotic/bacteriostatic treatments has come under question. As valuable as it is to destroy bacterial growth with drugs, there are some serious problems that develop when this exists as a singular endeavor.

One major problem is the growing bacterial resistance to the most powerful drugs being used. Antibiotics are used not only by physicians, but also with farm animals, in over-the-counter pharmaceuticals, and other products. This overuse has weakened their potency. Doctors are stretching the limits while scientists are searching for new drugs.

Another problem that occurs with the use of antimicrobials (and drugs in general) is related to how they interfere with nutrients that are vital for the healing process. For example, these medicines interfere with the absorption or utilization of a number of B vitamins (especially B6), vitamin K, vitamin C, and magnesium. While this may not seem critical, the B's and magnesium are necessary for numerous metabolic processes in the body, notably the conversion of amino acids into proteins.

This not only involves all the tissue of the body but also the manufacture of immune cells in particular. Depletion of vitamin K can aggravate bleeding disorders. Vitamin C has been called the "stress vitamin" because the system relies on it so heavily during periods of stress (physical, chemical, emotional). Animals that produce their own vitamin C are known to increase its production ten to one hundred fold during periods of illness.

Holistically oriented physicians known to practice orthomolecular medicine have documented this fact with humans.[1] This dramatic increase is due to the fact that the small reserves are quickly used up as soon as a person comes under some form of stress. During such periods, vitamin C will be drawn from other less vital tissue in the body. As the illness progresses, the demand for vitamin C and other nutrients grows exponentially, which leads to a cascade of problems as the body is unable to deal with the assault without the resources it needs. So, with the concomitant use of antibiotics the loss of nutrients is compounded further to the point where the candle of life is burning at both ends.

It is not uncommon to notice a faster healing time with those who compensate with nutrients while undergoing antibiotic treatments. Almost any standard medical textbook alludes to those with conditions of compromised immunity (such as those with HIV or those suffering from poor nutrition) as being more vulnerable to the disease process. However, it ignores the research that reveals how the immune system also becomes compromised as the result of many other forms of stress (physical, chemical, emotional, lack of vital resources) and not only from chronic disease conditions, extreme malnutrition, or from immuno-suppressive medications. The immune system, being one of various systems in the body, is the arena where powerful dramas will play out during a terrorist event.

During such an event, the mounting numbers of sick people could quite easily overwhelm our emergency resources to the point where many would be waiting for diagnostic tests, treatment, and a hospital bed. Panic could further aggravate the situation such that those with ordinary infections like the flu would fear the worst and further tax the already overworked resources. The answer, it seems so obvious to me, is not a vaccine for every imaginable pathogen or to have the population on prophylactic drugs (so damaging to the system as this would be), but to start thinking in terms of prevention using the natural resources available today.

This kind of prevention needs to be designed to accomplish the overall goal of reducing the need for emergency medicine so that it may be used more effectively when ab-

---

[1] See: Carthcart, R. (M.D.). Vitamin C, Titrating to Bowel Tolerance, Anascorbemia, and Acute Induced Scurvy. (Derived from the Internet.)

solutely needed. This, from a naturalistic perspective, would need to be focused on a program that assists people to sustain and preserve a strong immune system based on the scientific knowledge we have today about how the immune system functions.

Factors Involved in Immune Strength

Our current method of health acknowledges two broad lines of defense: *innate (nonspecific) immunity*, and *acquired (specific) immunity*.

Innate immunity consists of the skin, the mucous membranes, the inflammatory response, phagocytosis (immune cells that destroy circulating bacteria, viruses, and foreign bodies), and the production of fever (since the growth of many bacteria and viruses is slowed down during a fever).

Acquired immunity occurs when the immune system develops antibodies when exposed to foreign organisms (or from immunization).

As valuable as this model is, it does not consider other factors to be of importance to the immune response (with the exception of those predisposed to illness). Yet the immune system is affected by a variety of forces in a holistic manner.

For over fifty years tremendous leaps have occurred in our understanding of what enhances or decreases immune function. Many areas of research regarding immunity agree that immune function is affected by the following six general areas: 1) genetics, 2) the mind (psychology), 3) the society, 4) physiological needs, 5) the environment, 6) and therapeutic interventions. As we can see, the immune system is holistically intertwined with at least six dimensions of influence. Of these, the genetic dimension seems the most static or fixed; the other five are open and flexible where influential energy and information exchanges move back and forth quite easily.

The field of psychoneuroimmunology has proven that the mind and the body are intimately connected so that thoughts and feelings affect immunity, and immunity affects how one thinks and feels.[2] Studies in this area have shown that social feelings and human interaction can also have positive or negative effects on the healing process.[3] For instance the feeling of loneliness dampens the immune response whereas the feeling of being loved increases its potency. Numerous studies have demonstrated how nutrients can have powerful effects on immune function, and how certain vitamins, minerals, oils, and amino acids contribute to optimal health.[4] Studies have shown how weather conditions affect immune response, and how the environmental conditions (e.g., pollution) may increase susceptibility to disease. There is a wealth of information on how various kinds of human interventions (treatments and therapies) can affect the immune function.[5] Each of these areas represents a modifiable and relevant supportive line of defense.

In considering the areas that affect immune response the supportive lines of defense would include:
- A psychological dimension
- A social dimension
- A preventative dimension
- An environmental dimension
- A specific dimension

It may seem surprising to look at these five lines and wonder how they could work in a crisis situation. The whole idea of this holistic strategy is to employ prevention and immune enhancing factors in order to reduce the level of crisis to begin with, so that the dependency on antimicrobials and other valuable medical resources can be considerably reduced, and, most importantly, preserved for when they would be needed most.

---

[2] See: Rossi, E. (1986). The Psychobiology of Mind-Body Healing: New Concepts of Therapeutic Hypnosis. W.W. Norton & Company, Inc.: New York, NY.
[3] See: Goleman, D. Emotional Intelligence.
[4] See: Segala, M., Ed. (2000). Disease Prevention and Treatment. Life Extension Foundation: Hollywood, FL.
[5] See: Balch, P.; Balch, J (M.D.). (2000). Prescriptions for Nutritional Healing. Avery Publishing Group: Garden City Park, NY.

Also, by integrating the medical and naturalistic systems, a level of what I perceive as *synergistic complexity* is added. This would be beneficial in dealing with the growing problems of microbial resistance and malicious bioengineering. These two problems make terrorism a unique health issue in our highly technologically advanced times. This becomes more critical when one considers the number of agents that can be used as weapons of mass destruction. To help clarify the nature of this threat, it would be useful to get an idea of:

- How many possible weapons of mass destruction are we dealing with?
- What are the factors involved in the creation of a weapon of mass destruction?
- How do microbes develop resistance to our most powerful medications?
- How can germs be bio-engineered to create super bugs?
- And, how can *synergistic complexity* provide a possible solution?

The Potential Number of Threats

While we have heard about anthrax, (and there is worry about the use of smallpox) there are many other kinds of bacteria and viruses, plus toxic chemicals that can be just as harmful, or rendered so through bioengineering. Concerned about our safety, the Centers for Disease Control and a number of bacteriologists have issued warnings that identify which kinds of bacteria, viruses and toxic chemicals would most likely be used by terrorists. All of these agents can kill or produce serious illness. To this list I have added nuclear threats, which of course are not biological or chemical in nature, but are harmful mainly through radiation.

Bacterial Weapons of Mass Destruction

- Anthrax is also known as "wool sorter's disease" because it is typically found among those who work with sheep and other farm animals and their products. It spreads by tiny spores, which can be made into fine powder that can become airborne (aerosolized) and infect the lungs with a trio of powerful and deadly toxins.
- Plague is also known as the "Black Death." During the Middle Ages it killed millions of people; its use as a bioweapon goes back to antiquity. It has already been made into a weapon by bioweapons programs in various countries.
- Tularemia is not commonly known, and it is not as deadly as the above-mentioned agents, but it takes only 10 to 50 organisms to cause a pneumonia-like disease. It can be spread as an aerosol and can cause serious incapacitation.
- Cholera is a diarrheal disease that severely dehydrates its victims, and if left untreated can be lethal 50% of the time. Various governments have already turned it into a bioweapon to affect water supplies.
- Melioidosis is a potentially fatal disease resistant to many antibiotics. It produces confusing symptoms (making it difficult to diagnose) and a long-term chronic illness that can affect many organ systems of the body. It can be made into a dangerous aerosol.
- Q fever is an acute disease that can severely affect many organs in the body, especially the lungs, the heart, and the brain. Transmission typically occurs through contact with materials contaminated with the blood, feces, etc., of infected animals. These contaminants can be made into a powder, which can be used as a weapon that targets the respiratory system.
- Brucellosis is an acute infection that is spread by the secretions and excretions of infected animals. While not often fatal, it can debilitate with severe multi-organ complications for months

or years. It can be aerosolized into a weapon.

- Glanders is a serious disease for which there is no vaccine or current reliable treatment. It has been developed as an aerosolized weapon.
- Multidrug Resistant Tuberculosis, as the name implies, is a highly resistant strain of tuberculosis that can cause a chronic and potentially fatal disorder that is affecting millions of people worldwide. It can also be turned into an aerosolized weapon that could affect huge portions of any population.

Biological Toxins as Weapons of Mass Destruction

- Botulism is a toxin produced by a bacteria and it is the most toxic substance known. It can be aerosolized.
- Ricin is a deadly toxin produced from castor beans, and it is widely available. It can be aerosolized and used to contaminate foods.
- Epsilon Toxin is derived from the bacteria *Clostridium perfringens* which produces a deadly disorder.
- Staphylococcus Enterotoxin B is produced by the common bacterium *Staphylococcus aureus*. It causes ordinary food poisoning; only a small amount can cause dire effects. It can be aerosolized.
- Saxitoxin develops in shellfish and produces a rapid, deadly disorder known as paralytic shellfish poisoning. It can be made into an aerosolized weapon.
- Trichothecene Mycotoxins are lethal toxins produced by fungus molds. These toxins have already been used as biowarfare weapons.

Viral Weapons of Mass Destruction

- Smallpox is a highly infectious disease once thought eradicated from the face of the planet. It is transmitted by res-

piratory droplets, infected lesions, or through contact with linens and other objects, and can be turned into airborne WMD.

- Viral Hemorrhagic Fever Viruses can spread to humans by exposure to rodents or aerosols derived from their droppings; they are characterized by widespread bleeding and multi-organ failures. Ebola and Marburg are examples of viruses of this variety. They can all be weaponized.
- Tickborne Encephalitis Viruses represent over 400 kinds of viruses that attack the nervous system, especially the brain. They can all be weaponized.

Chemical Weapons of Mass Destruction

- Blister/Vesicants like mustard gas have been used in war to cause burns and large blisters to incapacitate soldiers. They can affect the eyes, skin, and lungs. These agents are easy to produce and deliver.
- Blood Agents are made from arsenic into the highly toxic gas arsine that can quickly destroy red blood cells once inhaled. They are quite easy to produce and deliver.
- Cyanogens are cyanide-based chemicals that can disturb the body's cellular metabolism and rapidly cause death within 6-8 minutes after high exposure. They are easy to produce and deliver.
- Choking/Lung/Pulmonary Damaging Agents are a series of chemical formulas used to disrupt the respiratory system. These agents often incapacitate but some can be deadly. These chemicals are widely used in industry and can be the targets of sabotage.
- Vomiting Agents are a group of chemicals used during World War I to cause the troops to remove protective gear and be exposed to more lethal gases. They are mainly irritants that

could be used to cause confusion and panic.

Nuclear Threats

- Terrorists would more likely use a smaller nuclear device, or sabotage a nuclear reactor or the transport of nuclear materials. Each event has its particular harmful characteristics that involve radiation, fallout, blast effects, and thermal effects to the body.

Factors Involved in the Creation of WMD

Weapons of mass destruction (WMD) can vary from simple compounds of common chemicals and pathogenic organisms to complex nuclear fission bombs. While different kinds of education are required to effectively produce WMD they have become relatively easy to manufacture. Virtually all major terrorist attacks to date have mostly used explosives. However, with the anthrax episodes the degree of threat has expanded to the full spectrum of terrorist possibilities. Therefore, an assessment of what it takes to produce WMD would help us to prepare for the likelihood of some agents being used over others. What makes an agent attractive to a terrorist would involve the following:

- Available information about the agent that would not be difficult to learn. This information could be disseminated by a trained instructor, through correspondence courses, the Internet, and the like. With the dissolution of the Soviet Union many highly trained microbiologists involved with bioweaponry have become available on the world market for jobs. Also, any disgruntled scientist from any part of the industrialized world could assist any rogue nation or group to create a biowarfare program. Information on chemical agents is accessible worldwide. Information on how to manufacture nuclear weapons is becoming increasingly available to many nations.
- Easy to house. It should not take up too much room and not require sophisticated technology to store. Usually, the biological agents can be placed in a container in a refrigerator or stored in sealed containers at room temperature. Chemicals are very easy to house and store. Nuclear materials are significantly more difficult in this regard.
- Ease of performing research and bioengineering to create strains of germs resistant to medications, etc. This skill requires more technical knowhow of antibiotic medicines and bioengineering, but one highly trained person can train and supervise a fairly large group of non-technically trained people to perform such complex tasks.
- Ease of manufacture with minimal danger. Most of the chemical agents are fairly easy to manufacture, even with a minimal knowledge of chemistry. It has been shown that the manufacture of biological agents can be as easy as using a process similar to fermenting cheese. However, some of the agents are not so easy to work with.
- Availability of the ingredients. Almost all of the ingredients to create biological and chemical agents are easily obtained in the world markets. Nuclear weapons are in question.
- Low cost. Agents may be manufactured or purchased from other sources. Chemicals are relatively cheap. Biological agents are somewhat more expensive. Nuclear material is costly.
- Difficulty for being quickly detected. Ideally, it should be tasteless, odorless, colorless, and not be quickly detectable by instruments, laboratory procedures, or people.
- Has a quick rate of action or incubation time.

- Durability of the agent. It should be able to be stored for lengthy periods of time and not quickly degrade upon release when used as a weapon. Many biological agents can be transformed into a powder and stored under optimal conditions for many years. "When microbes are frozen in exactly the right way (surrounded by sugar and protein, cooled quickly, and put under high vacuum to remove ice in a process known as sublimation), they can enter a dormant state in which they behave like vegetative spores. This process is known as lyophilization, or freeze-drying. Once dormant, the germ remains asleep even when returned to room temperature, staying that way for years or even decades."[6]
- Ease of transport. One should be able to take it across borders in a concealed manner.
- Ease of delivery by various methods such as air (aerosol), water, soil, foods, mail, or in military warheads.
- Ability to inflict widespread harm through sheer exposure and/or contagion.
- No available treatment.

As easy as it all appears, the choice and use of WMD occurs within a context of counteracting social forces, which include:
- New developments in technology
- New medications.
- The development of portable, sensitive biochemical detectors capable of providing accurate onsite information.
- A more educated and alert population.
- Reduction in sharing technologies and information.
- Legal constraints in acquiring raw materials, equipment, and supplies.
- Military and law-enforcement counter measures.

---

[6] Miller, J.; Engeberg, S. (2001). Germs: Biological Weapons & America's Secret War. Simon & Schuster: New York, NY. (P. 59.)

Microbial Encounters of the Third Kind

Scientists have come to realize that many germs of medical significance have developed resistance to a growing number of our most powerful antibiotics. As I mentioned, these problems were caused by their overuse in treatment, in farming, in over-the-counter products, and in animal-based foods. Furthermore, antibiotics can destroy only bacteria; they are useless when it comes to viruses. Even so they are often prescribed for viral diseases. This unnecessary use has added to the problem not only as an impetus for microbial evolution but also by destabilizing the bacterial ecology in the host. Such destabilization paves the way for other more sinister opportunistic infections that require additional antibiotic treatments in an endless vicious cycle of punch and counter punch.

Dr. Cass Ingram expresses the severity of the problem of bacterial resistance in his book, *The Cure is in The Cupboard*. He writes: "Medicine is incapacitated by the rising incidence of infectious diseases, particularly drug resistant infections. Obviously, drugs have failed to protect humanity against the ravages of infectious diseases, since the death rate from infections has risen steadily every decade for the past thirty years."[7] Realizing the drawbacks of the conventional medical approach, Dr. Ingram strongly recommends the use of natural remedies when he states: "It is evident that only natural antibiotics and antiseptics can be relied upon for salvation. This is because there is no guarantee that if powerful diseases, such as flesh eating bacteria, cryptosporidium, ebola, dengue, Hantavirus, Lyme, E. coli, Salmonella, hepatitis, encephalitis, or tuberculosis strike that the individual will survive even with the help of modern medicine."

In a context of a biowarfare scenario, this problem of over use could become worse as people lean towards antibiotics in unprece-

---

[7] (P. 178.)

12

dented numbers. This crisis is just beginning to rear its head in the U.S., but it has been brewing for years in other parts of the world.

In 1994, Laurie Garrett wrote a book entitled *The Coming Plague* to warn us about this threat. In it she reports how the spread of *new* and potentially devastating diseases has been fostered in places around the world with unpurified drinking water, improper use of antibiotics, local warfare, massive refugee migrations, and changing social and environmental conditions. While the multiple causes behind these microbial adaptations have been recognized, the use of antibiotics has not become more judicious, and the actual dynamics of how germs adapt is just beginning to be understood. As our knowledge increases of how microbes evolve, we're starting to realize the strangeness of the challenge that lies ahead.

Our so-called "war on germs" is an activity in which scientists are in battle with creatures that exist in another dimension. Their time is incredibly faster than ours. Their space is so minute. We can only see them through microscopes. To some scientists, viruses (only visible through an electron microscope) do not appear to possess all the characteristics of living organisms. Of the microbes, viruses occupy a unique position in biology. Unlike bacteria, they are unable to capture and store free energy, or to be functionally active outside their hosts, yet these half-living critters seem to have a formidable intelligence!

We don't exactly know the purpose of microbes in the universal scheme of things or why they aim to destroy us. It seems odd to us that these tiny organisms or pieces of viral nucleic acid can think and give us a run for our money; and the money and time spent on trying to outwit them is enormous.

Yet they are intelligent in a collective way just as we are intelligent in a collective way; what makes them so difficult is the speed of their reaction time and their exponential capacity to multiply. They seem to know about biochemistry, gene splicing, how to transform their molecular make up, how to defend themselves and, how to disrupt our cellular

structures and metabolic functions. Each time I think about these abilities I truly believe that microbes are creatures from another dimensional reality.

As bacteriologists learn new ways to attack germs, germs are also displaying some counteracting creativity at a learning-rate that is quite frankly staggering. For example, the immune system must respond in a matter of days to the fast minute-by-minute pace of microbial replication and mutations. "A typical bacterial strain may divide once every 20 minutes, producing over 1 billion descendants in just 10 hours! Given the fact that mutations arise only about once every 100,000 to 1,000,000 with human cells and that the mutation rate of microorganisms such as HIV and its variants approaches 1 million times that of human cells, evolutionary change in some pathogens can be extraordinarily rapid, making them moving targets for an attacking immune system."[8]

The most important strategy underlying our antimicrobial therapy is to disrupt the structure and function of microorganisms while not damaging the host. It uses *selective toxicity* to inhibit the germ from carrying out cell wall synthesis, protein synthesis, synthesis of nucleic acid, and alteration of membrane functions.

Microorganisms respond to antimicrobial drugs by: 1) producing enzymes that inactivate the drug; 2) mutating their gene structure (the most common form of resistance); 3) decreasing the permeability of their outer surfaces; 4) excreting them (using a mechanism known as the "multidrug resistance pump").

An article by Christine Soares entitled *Staph Killers* (January 2002 issue of *Discover* magazine) might help us appreciate the nature of this ongoing duel. This example involves the ubiquitous bacterium *Staphylococcus aureas* (staph), which "causes a variety of swift and deadly infections including toxic

---

[8] Lappé, M., (1997). The Tao of Immunology: A Revolutionary New Understanding Of Our Body's Defenses. Plenum Trade Plenum Press: New York, NY. (P. 33.)

shock syndrome and sepsis—and rapidly develops resistance to antibiotics. ... Amongst the bugs' best defenses is the ability to share information with other bacteria by swapping genes." Keiichi Hiramatsu, a bacteriologist at the Juntendo University in Tokyo, published the genome of *S. aureas*. He proved that staph had swapped strategic genetic information not only from a wide variety of organisms but also from humans! "This capacity, Hiramatsu warned, means that even strains which are now harmless could quickly turn nasty." It is mind boggling to realize the tremendous technology that is being employed to deal with these pestiferous one-celled creatures! However, *S. aureas* has other survival tricks up its sleeve.

In the same article, Soares mentions another study in which James Musser, at the National Institute of Allergy and Infectious Disease, showed how different strains of staph could steal genes and transform themselves simultaneously in different places around the world. "He analyzed genes in 36 strains of staph to determine that many had picked up the same virulence and resistance genes independently. The gene for methicillin resistance, for example, had been acquired by five separate strains in five different places." Staph resistance to methicillin represents about half of all the life-threatening infections in U.S. hospitals today. Because of the tremendous speed at which microbes learn to adapt to our biochemical medications they keep whittling away at our antibiotic options. It may take twenty minutes for a germ population to adjust to a new antibiotic and develop resistance to it.

In his book, *Herbal Antibiotics: Natural Alternatives for Treating Drug-Resistant Bacteria*, Stephen Harrod Buhner reports how this swapping of information takes place. "Bacteria are single-cell organisms containing, among other things, special loops of their DNA called plasmids. ... During an information exchange, a resistant bacterium extrudes a filament of itself, a plasmid, to the nonresistant bacterium, which opens a door in its cell wall. Within the filament is a copy of the portion of the resistant bacterium's DNA. Specifically, it contains the encoded information on resistance to one or more antibiotics."[9] Thusly, the learned resistance is passed on to future generations of bacteria. Viruses also transfer plasmids in this manner. However, this is not the only way it happens.

"Bacteria that have the ability to resist antibiotics are now known to emit unique pheromones to attract bacteria to themselves in order to exchange resistance information. It is almost as if they put up a sign that says 'bacterial resistance information here'. The seminal discoveries of genetic researcher Barbara McClintock are also at work. Bacteria, like corn, also possess 'jumping genes', or transposons, that are able to jump from bacterium to bacterium independently of plasmid exchange. These transposons also have the ability to 'teach' antibiotic resistance. Furthermore, bacteria also have diseases: bacterial viruses (called bacteriophages). These viruses, as they infect other bacteria, pass on the information for resistance. Finally, bacteria release free-roving pieces of their DNA, which carry resistance information. Other bacteria that encounter it ingest it, thereby learning how to survive antibiotics."

An even more interesting conundrum is the way bacteria learn resistance to multiple antibiotics after encountering only one antibiotic. "Medical researchers have placed bacteria into solutions containing only tetracycline in such a way that the bacteria are not killed; they live in a tetracycline-heavy environment. In short order the bacteria develop resistance to tetracycline, but they also develop resistance to other antibiotics that they have never encountered."[10]

One might wonder if bacteria and other germs are capable of broadcasting their information through electromagnetic waves, or via the immaterial morphic fields proposed by

---

[9] (P. 8.)
[10] (P. 9.)

14

Rupert Sheldrake[11]; for how could such gene swapping or so-called "jumping genes" traverse such great distances? In any case, this uncanny ability appears close to the supernatural.

The article by Soares is actually a report on how scientists are confronting bacterial resistance by disrupting the signals germs use to trigger drug-blocking genes. They have already deciphered the signal system germs use to carry out this feat.

Soares also mentions other research that is underway for an even more effective germicidal approach. She writes, "Better still, of course, would be a medication that kills all staph strains so quickly and effectively that they never have time to develop resistance. Such a new type of antibiotic is in the works at the Scripps Research Institute, where Reza Ghadiri and colleagues have created peptide molecules that home in on bacterial cells, leaving mammalian cells alone. Once these peptides find a bacterium, they nestle into its outer membrane, then shape-shift themselves into nanotubes, which act as spigots, draining the cells and killing them within minutes." Yet, even with this, the staph might find a way out. If such becomes the case, the duel will continue, and the scientists would need to reconfigure the synthetic molecules to outwit the bugs.

This brief foray into the interconnectedness of the microbial world exemplifies how these creatures communicate and learn, and, at the same time, alerts us as to the challenges the human immune system faces.

Germs and Terrorists in Collusion

What further complicates the issue of biological WMD is the fact that they are being *designed* to resist the most effective medications. With some training, a terrorist can accelerate and amplify the level of resistance in a matter of weeks. In short, we're not just dealing with the evolutionary capabilities of microbes but also with the added effect of malicious bioengineering. Germs and terrorists are colluding against humanity!

With the discovery in 1953 of how DNA, or dioxyribonuleic acid, governs our heredity we learned that the genetic code was a language shared by all living creatures on earth. "In the early 1970s, scientists took advantage of this commonality to found the field of gene engineering, also known as bioengineering or gene splicing. Now scientists could edit, rewrite, and rearrange life's script, moving a line or whole chapter from one creature to another. It was biological cut and paste. With growing ease, genes were recombined and rearranged."[12] This capability opened the doors to medical possibilities that could benefit the human race and, at the same time, it also pried open the lid to Pandora's box.

Therefore, it's not simply a matter of knowing the accidental or natural occurrence of pathologies of these agents, but to realize that their most insidious characteristics are being strengthened through technologies that are becoming increasingly available and easy to employ. Some of these agents are easier to produce than others. There are hundreds of different kinds of germs that could be used in this manner.

Nevertheless, genetic engineers can only transfer genes that contain information the organism has already learned. They could help microbes learn to adapt to antibiotics or other medications by immersing them in dilute amounts of the medicinal agent and gradually increasing the concentration, causing them to adapt by gradual steps. This process has been possible with antimicrobials that perform a singular lethal event such as blocking the synthesis of a particular protein necessary for the germ to replicate. But, it would not appear to work when the antimicrobial event is multidimensional, for there would be too many variables to control.

[11] See: ... (1989). The Presence of the Past: Morphic Resonance And The Habits Of Nature. Random House, Inc.: New York, NY.

[12] Miller, J.; Engeberg, S., previously cited, p. 66.

Synergistic Complexity

A naturalistic form of healing would attempt to overcome an infectious disease in a holistic manner by employing at least five of the afore-mentioned supportive lines of defense. This complex yet synergistic approach would not only befuddle the microbe but also the colluding bioengineer, for there is no way that the immune strength of the host plus an array of complex therapeutic substances can be mimicked in a biological culture. However, some aspects of this strategy are not new to conventional medicine.

To combat resistance in hospital settings, the epicenter of learning for the microbial world, physicians have learned to combine two or more antibiotics to confuse the germs. While they cope and develop resistance to one of the drugs they succumb to the others. In other words, the Achilles heel of the microbial world is *complexity*. They can deal with the singularity of a "magic bullet" but not very well with two or three at a time.

Nature has been tempering the microbe world with a similar strategy, for we find in a number of herbs with antibiotic activity a variety of substances that contribute to this effect. For example, a clove of garlic is known to contain 33 active sulfur compounds, 17 amino acids, plus 35 other unknown constituents. Buhner views the complexity of garlic as being responsible for its success as a broad-spectrum antimicrobial. He points out that the active ingredient in penicillin is penicillin.

In addition to antimicrobial activity, garlic also has beneficial immune modulating effects. Therefore, nature's answer to resistance lies in complexity. By combining the naturalistic and conventional methods into a single synergistic strategy we could augment this complexity. We would at least critically slow down microbial resistance and the terrorist's capacity to create superbugs.

Synergistic Complexity and the Healing Process

The practice of synergistic complexity is not only aimed against germs. It is also an approach that seeks to support the mind-body complex so that it can perform more effectively against the assault of toxic chemicals and radiation.

The description of the healing process by conventional medicine is essentially crisis oriented. It focuses on singular obvious causes of disease and rarely addresses psychological aspects. What is lacking is a more comprehensive description of other mind-body functions that occur simultaneously as the organism begins to protect itself from disease.

The immune system not only needs to be nurtured, it also needs the support of positive mental attitudes and the detoxifiction processes that occur throughout the body (especially in the liver). The use of substances, such as antioxidants and natural sulphur compounds, are synergistic components of this complexity that play a crucial role in ridding the body of the toxins produced by germs, chemicals, and radiation.

Once the immune system becomes mobilized it is like an army that needs more supplies and ammunition and other forms of support than when it is at peace. The typical medical method attacks the most obvious issues but it does not re-supply the soldiers at the front.

Moreover, as the nutrients that support this complexity become scarce, the inflammatory stage of the process can become excessive. When out of control, the inflammatory response generated by the immune system can cause as much damage as the toxic assault.

Most of the conditions addressed in this book cause serious harm by: triggering excessive inflammation, disrupting certain metabolic pathways, disrupting blood flow and volume, and thereby causing shock.

Holistic practitioners (like orthomolecular physicians) have shown how the availability of certain nutrients can avert many of the problems that typically occur during the disease process by supporting the mind-body system to do what it knows how to do best.

The Nature of This Book

In the pages that follow, I begin by discussing **The Five Supportive Lines of Defense:**
1. The Psychological,
2. The Social,
3. The Preventative,
4. The Environmental, and
5. The Specific.

This will help to acquaint the reader with details of a more coordinated form of defense in general, and how these various lines support the immune system.

In the following section I have provided a closer look at **The Specific Nature of Potential Weapons of Mass Destruction.** Here one would have a handy reference that:
- Describes each agent,
- How it causes disease,
- Lists its typical symptoms,
- Evaluates how it might be used as a weapon,
- Summarizes the conventional methods of treatment,

- And shows how the supportive lines of defense could be used synergistically to improve our health options against these diseases.

To the best of my ability, I have aimed to include all age groups, certain predisposing medical conditions, and, of course, pets (dogs and cats).

A more detailed explanation for the recommendations can be found in the chapter **The Five Supportive Lines of Natural Defense.** This chapter contains the rationale of my suggestions.

The final chapter is dedicated to new ideas and some of the **Emerging Technologies** that show promise to assist us in averting or surviving these potential threats. All of the suggested items of use and services mentioned in the book are listed under **Resources**. Finally, I've included a complete list of **References**, should anyone have an interest in delving deeper into certain topics.

It seems important to mention that while the emphasis is on natural forms of defense against WMD, many of these suggestions are also applicable with other kinds of infectious diseases and toxicities from chemical or other sources.

THE FIVE SUPPORTIVE LINES OF
NATURAL DEFENSE

The Psychological Line

The use of the mind to foster physical wellness has a long and culturally diverse history. Throughout the ancient world it was known that symbolism in the form of words, images, and ritual could have profound effects on the physical nature of the body. For example, the Biblical aphorism "As a man thinketh in his heart so is he" is indicative of this knowledge.

To the ancient world, the soul was analogous to what we today understand as the mind. According to Socrates: "All good and evil originates in the soul, and overflows from thence, as if from the head into the eyes. And therefore if the head and the body are to be well, you must begin by curing the soul; that is the first thing."[13] How then did the people of this era go about curing the soul or the mind in order to heal the body?

For the healers of the pre-modern world (ancient and Medieval periods) it was necessary to have a deep level of *trust* in the meaning of the symbols conveyed through words and other practices as a prerequisite to the healing process. To trust meant that one *believed* it to be true, that is, unconditionally possible. They understood that without this precondition little in the way of healing would occur.

Many of the healing methods used in this era were essentially repetitive rituals—prayer, mantra, chanting, movements, etc.—as a way to create belief or bypass the unbelieving or negative aspects of the mind. The repetitive rituals engrained the message by sheer rote, but the repetition itself was able to also create a very influential trance state. However, while the effects of belief on the body were well known, it was not known how this actu-

ally occurred. Nevertheless, the healers of old were intuitively onto something, which took the scientific methods of the modern era to figure out.

Scientific Understanding of the Mind-Body Relationship

In the last fifty years the scientific understanding of the mind-body relationship has increased tremendously. The idea of a psychological line of defense emerges from research done to study the effects of *stress* on the body and, in particular, on the immune system. The seminal research was done by medical scientists, of which the most outstanding were Claude Bernard, Walter B. Cannon, and Hans Selye.

Bernard developed the concept of *homeostasis* as the major process by which the body maintains a relative inner constancy to compensate for the changes occurring in the outer environment. Homeostasis is sustained by a vast network of feedback loops regulated by centers in the brain and the endocrine glands.

Building on the work of Bernard, Cannon described in his book, *The Wisdom of the Body,* the innate reaction the body produces when it is confronted by stress. He named this reaction the "fight-or-flight" response.

Selye refined the homeostatic model developed by Bernard and Cannon with research that showed how various forms of stress produce a rather standard series of reactions which he named the General Adaptive Syndrome (GAS). What makes Selye's work unique is the emphasis he placed on the idea that mental forms of stress were just as important as the physical and chemical forms in triggering the GAS. The nature of the GAS was also another major contribution because it described in detail how excessive amounts

---

[13] Murphy, M. (1993). The Future Of The Body: Exploration into the Further Evolution of Human Nature. The Putman Publishing Group: New York, NY. (P. 259.)

of stress had a suppressive effect on the immune system.

The syndrome occurs when mental information passes through a regulatory system located in the brain (known as the limbic-hypothalamic system) where it is converted (or transduced) into messenger molecules. These molecules cause the pituitary gland to stimulate the adrenal gland to release stress hormones (e.g., adrenaline, norepinephrine, cortisol).

Selye's work set the stage for future research to explore how mental states (positive and negative) passing through the regulatory centers in the brain are transformed into physiological realities. This spawned more research in a diversity of disciplines—psychobiology, biochemistry, neuropsychiatry, biofeedback—that converged into the field known as psychoneuroimmunology (PNI), which studies the relationship between psychological states and the immune response.

Convergence of the Ancient and Modern Worlds

The scientific findings on the mind-body relationship helped to form a conceptual bridge between the ancient and modern eras. Because of the reciprocal relationship between the brain (or neurological system) and the body, it was now possible to explain how belief could render a non-medicinal substance, such as a sugar pill, into a powerful healing agent (also known as the "placebo effect"). It also explained how information transmitted via a hypnotic state could influence many organ systems in the body, or how meditation and prayer could heal illness, and so on. These findings also helped to understand how certain physical exercises such as yoga or Tai Chi, or how bodywork such as from chiropractic or massage therapy could have an influence on one's thoughts and feelings.

The ability to intentionally access this system afforded a profound level of control over once-thought "involuntary" physiological functions such as the autonomic nervous system. As the ancient world knew, trust, unconditional belief, and a relaxed body are the preconditions to put one in touch with mind-body interactions. However, the scientific understanding of what constituted a relaxed, trusting mind-body state began to occur when biofeedback entered the picture.

Biofeedback

Feedback is a term that was adopted from information theory (cybernetics). The theory sought to understand how a mechanical or living system recycles information in order to control its interactions with the environment or itself. A simple example of feedback occurs when we look in a mirror to comb our hair in order to control our movements.

Biofeedback incorporates the feedback process as a way to amplify ordinarily undetectable activities going on in the systems of the body. A simple bio-amplifier is the stethoscope a doctor uses to listen to your heart. It causes the ordinarily imperceptible heartbeat to be heard. Bio-amplification devices are like a microscope in that they "magnify" activity going on at an imperceptible level so it can be experienced by the senses.

Using the principles of feedback, engineers were able to develop electronic bio-amplifiers (essentially, the technology that amplifies the sounds in a stereo system) that could pick up subtle activities of the body. Electronic bio-amplification equipment combines with computer technology to convert the signals into measurements. For instance, it is this technology that is used today to track and measure blood pressure, pulse rate, breathing rate, muscle tension, temperature, and metabolic rate. What was so special about it was that it allowed researchers to detect physiological changes that occurred during periods of stress, and to compare them with data acquired during periods of calmness.

For example, during periods of stress the blood pressure rises, the heartbeat accelerates, breathing becomes quicker, metabolic rate increases, the sympathetic nervous system becomes more active, the adrenal glands secrete stress hormones, sweating increases, digestive juices diminish, and brainwaves are less synchronized and become faster, and immunity diminishes.

A major breakthrough occurred when studies revealed that biofeedback could be used to increase self-awareness of these physiological indicators and voluntarily reverse them. Biofeedback, as a therapeutic method, became a reality for many people suffering from a wide range of disorders such as headaches, hypertension, attention-deficit and hyper activity (especially with children), urinary incontinence, physical rehabilitation, and alcoholism.[14] It was also found useful for spiritual development.[15] It turned out to be another modality, very similar to various forms of meditation, to quiet the mind and calm the body. As a psychological form of defense it has positive immune modulating effects.

Biofeedback is similar to meditation because both methods turn awareness inward, forming a feedback cycle between the observer and the mind-body interactions. The repetitive nature of the feedback process (information recycling back into itself) is what causes it to be amplified into the conscious field of the observer. Once this occurs the negative thoughts, feelings, and sensations are released from the subconscious state allowing the mind-body relationship to enter into the optimal level of homeostasis. The observer simply clears the impediments to healing and allows the mind-body complex to heal itself.

This process is quite in keeping with the naturalistic concept that the mind-body complex knows, from eons of evolutionary experience, how to mend itself when mental, physical, and chemical toxins are cleared away. Furthermore, each individual is in some measure like everyone else and, is also uniquely constituted.

Mind-Body-Feedback

Thus far, the discussion has been about the biological form of self-awareness where physiological aspects are fed back to the observer. Self-awareness also has a mental aspect, where thoughts and feelings are fed back to the observer before they are converted by the limbic-hypothalamic system into messenger molecules and subsequent physical states.

Therefore, biofeedback is a term that does not fully encompass the scope of self-awareness. As the practice of meditation advances, the scope of subtle information becomes increasingly more evident, and one becomes aware of mind activity seeking to become physical action. It is at this level that one would be able to more effectively modify the cause behind the physical effect. Negative thoughts and feelings would be caught in their seed stage, and one would be able to replace them with positive seeds conducive to the physical experience of happiness and wellness. One important area that needs to be watched for is the mental attitude that sabotages mind-body harmony.

The Healing Power of Acceptance

Much of our negativity comes from conditioning and biochemical imbalance. These negative programs keep the mind and the body in a shaky relationship, not allowing the full unity that is possible and the potential healing that could occur. Optimal healing occurs through the power of wholeness when mind and body are in sync.

Various forms of meditation move the mind away from stressful mental states by simply observing the conflicts and accepting things as they are, and letting them go. While one may not be fully aware of the exact nature of the inner conflict, acceptance has the power to neutralize the negative force. Neutralization occurs because a counter force

[14] See: Schwartz, M., Ed. (1995). Biofeedback: A Practitioner's Guide. The Guilford Press: New York, NY.

[15] See: Evans, J.; Abarbanel, A.; Eds. (1999). Introduction To Quantitative EEG And Neurofeedback (especially Chapter 13 by Nancy E. White). Academic Press: San Diego, CA.

must be present for any force to exist. Take the counter force away and the negative force dissipates. This is why forgiveness is such a powerful principle.

Methods That Calm the Mind and Heal the Body

The methods presented here are selections that I have made based on my own experience and from the supportive research; they are not the only methods. The selections were made with simplicity, convenience, and effectiveness in mind. They are not substitutes for professional mental therapy.

The Relaxation Response is a method that was developed by Dr. Herbert Benson as a result of his research with meditators and mystics. He is one of the pioneers who realized that many forms of meditation and prayer produced a beneficial relaxed state in the body. While Selye discovered the dynamics of mental stress on the body, Benson scientifically verified the physiological benefits that occur when one repeats a soothing sound, word, or phrase to oneself. He dubbed it The Relaxation Response. The method is quite simple.[16]

- Choose a sonorous word, phrase, or sound as the mental tool that one will use to elicit the relaxation response. It should be simple and short. It may or may not be derived from one's religious belief system. It need not have any meaning at all. But, it should not be harsh.
- Find a quiet place anywhere. However, after some practice it could be performed in a moving train or airplane or even in a noisy waiting room.

- One should sit in an upright yet comfortable position. Breathe in deeply and release slowly 2 – 5 times to relax the body. Close the eyes. Gently repeat in one's mind the chosen sound, word, or phrase.
- The repetition will evoke many thoughts, feelings, and sensations that will initially be distracting. It may even lull you to sleep. Persist in returning to the practice and ignore what has occurred.
- The objective is to learn how to observe without being caught up in what comes before your mind.
- It is not a method for creating indifference, but mental clarity and calmness in the most challenging situations. Moreover, it preserves and improves your health.
- Perform twice daily for 15 – 30 minutes or more. Find what suits you best.
- Eventually, the Relaxation Response will become part of you and will arise automatically in trying moments.

Thought Field Therapy, a technique developed by Dr. Roger Callahan,[17] combines eastern and western modalities for tapping the subtle (quantum) field of the mind. It involves learning a series of steps in which certain meridian points on the body are tapped, the eyes are moved in a certain way, and a phrase of acceptance is repeated to oneself. The phrase is focused on a particular problem or issue. For example, if I want to work with issue X, then I would repeat: "Even though I have issue X, I deeply and completely accept myself." The technique has had much success with fears, anxiety, phobias, etc. However, it must be taught by a certified practitioner. Once you learn it you can practice on your own

---

[16] For more details see: Benson, H.; Stuart, E. The Wellness Book: The Comprehensive Guide To Maintaining Health And Treating Stress-Related Illness. Simon & Schuster: New York, NY. Also: Benson, H.; Proctor, W. (1984). Beyond the Relaxation Response. Times Books: New York, NY.

[17] Callahan, R.; Callahan, J. (1996). Thought Field Therapy™ (TFT)™ and Trauma: Treatment and Theory. Private Publication.

Hypnotherapy. Most of the processes that control body functions occur below our awareness. These processes occur in brain areas that are below the cortex (the uppermost layer of the brain). In normal waking consciousness, they are inaccessible; therefore, it's not possible to establish a feedback relationship with them to alter unhealthy mental attitudes and blocked energy pathways. Hypnosis is a method that can provide a pathway to these deeper layers of the mind-body relationship. The scientific literature on hypnotherapy has shown how effective it can be to alter physiological states such as blood pressure or immune response (and inflammation).[18] One can seek a qualified hypnotherapist or take courses to learn how to perform it on oneself (autosuggestion).

CranioSacral Therapy, developed by Dr. John Upledger, D.O., is an important modality that uses light touch techniques to work with many physical issues, including falls and other forms of trauma.

In the October 2002 *Massage Today*, Dr. Upledger writes:
"...practitioners are trained to gently monitor the cranio-sacral rhythm to detect and release imbalances and restrictions in the membranes that could potentially cause sensory, motor or neurological dysfunctions. As such, Cranio-Sacral Therapy is never intended to cure disease, but simply to facilitate the body's ability to self-correct. It offers a comprehensive, whole-body structural and functional evaluation protocol." An advanced level of training, called SomatoEmotional Release, addresses emotional trauma.

Qualified practitioners can be located by contacting the Upledger Institute in Palm Beach Gardens, FL (see resources.)

Reiki is a healing technique that has become quite popular today around the world. It is a kind of meditative laying on of the hands from a trained practitioner to a recipient. Practitioners are seen as conduits for this healing energy. Reiki can also be transmitted from a distance. It works well for those who need to calm themselves and to augment their healing potentials. It is also used with children and pets. Classes are widely available that teach how to perform Reiki on oneself and on others.

Tai Chi is a form of moving meditation that incorporates many gentle positions and postures that help to calm the body and expand the mind. This form of creating inner tranquility is advised for those who have difficulty meditating or praying in a sitting position. One has to learn the movements from a trained and certified practitioner.

Flower Essences are a form of natural treatments using dilute essences of plants to create emotional health. Its founder, Dr. Edward Bach (1897-1936), believed that physical problems were preceded by negative emotional states. These flower essences act on the subtle energy fields of the body in a way similar to homeopathy. The remedies are chosen based on certain personality characteristics and the nature of one's emotional states. For example, the *Rescue Remedy*—a combination of cherry plum, clematis, impatiens, rock rose, and Star of Bethlehem—is taken for any pattern that presents with fear, panic, apprehension, inconsolable crying, anxiety, tension, and night terrors.

While there are a variety of other remedies, *Rescue Remedy* seems appropriate for the kinds of emotions that could arise from the negative energy pattern fueled by hatred and weapons of mass destruction. It has been found to be excellent for alleviating any crisis-caused form of stress. It doesn't matter if the cause is an accident, bad news, or anxiety about a possible event. It is especially useful when one feels emotionally overwhelmed by anxiety, powerlessness, and frustration.

---

[18] See: LeCron, L., Ed. (1968). Experimental Hypnosis. The Citadel Press: New York, NY.

Biochemical Imbalance And the Mind

In looking at both sides of the mind-body equation, scientists have discovered that a lack of or overabundance of certain bio-chemicals can also be a cause of mind-body disharmony. While all vitamins (especially the B-Complex), minerals, amino acids, etc., are needed for psychological integrity, many of these biochemical needs will be addressed through The Preventative Line of Defense. Here attention will be given to those that have a direct influence on mental function such as the neurotransmitters dopamine, seratonin, and GABA (gamma- aminobutyric acid), melatonin, and epinephrine.

Dopamine

Dopamine works with the sympathetic nervous system and is the precursor of epinephrine (adrenalin). It has an inhibitory effect on movement. When levels in the brain are diminished, symptoms of rigidity, tremors, and uncontrolled movement characteristic of Parkinson's disease can occur. Dopamine rises in the brain to facilitate attention or alertness. Physicians use it to reverse the effects of hypotension and shock. Dopamine is naturally found in the herb:

- Velvet Bean (*Mucuna pruriens*), with about 50 mg or 15% of L-dopa per 333 mg of the herb; by Solray®.
- **Note:** caution and physician's advice needed if being treated for hypertension, cardiac or pulmonary disease, or if taking medications with L-dopa.

Follow directions on the container.

Seratonin

Seratonin is a major neurotransmitter in the brain made from the amino acid tryptophan. Seratonin plays an important role in mood, sleep, and appetite. Low levels can lead to sleep disorders, depression, anxiety, and a craving for sweets (concentrated carbohydrates). It produces a calming effect on the mind. The following natural substances contribute to the production of seratonin.

- 5-H-TP (5 Hydroxy L Tryptophan).

- St. John's Wort
- SAMe

To keep things simple, I prefer to use 5-H-TP instead of the others. One can take 100-200 mg 1-3 times a day between meals with a glass of water or juice. However, all can be used (follow the directions on the containers).

GABA

Gamma-aminobutyric acid (GABA) is an amino acid that functions as an inhibitory neurotransmitter in the brain and the spinal cord. It prevents excessive nerve activity, and as a result helps to calm the central nervous system. It works synergistically with two B vitamins, niacinamide and inositol, to prevent stress related messages from reaching the motor cortex of the brain. "GABA can be taken to calm the body in much the same way as diazepam (Valium), chlordiazepoxide (Librium), and other tranquilizers, but without fear of addiction."[19] Overuse of GABA can cause the very symptoms it can relieve when used in appropriate amounts. It is available in health-food stores. The recommended dose is: 500-700 mg, 1-3 times daily, between meals or at least 30 minutes before food with a 10 ounce glass of water only.

Melatonin

Melatonin is a hormone produced in the pineal gland to regulate the sleep-wake cycle. The pineal gland is a small cone-shaped structure found in the center of the brain that is sensitive to light. Darkness stimulates the gland to excrete melatonin to bring on sleep. Its production tends to decline with age. Research has shown that during deep sleep the immune system is at a peak of healing activity. Lack of sound sleep not only can lower the resistance of the body but also can negatively affect mental states. Melatonin has also been found to be a powerful antioxidant and cancer fighter. Dosages can range from 1-20 mg taken with a glass of water near bedtime. Therapeutic dosages have reached 50 mg daily (and more with cancer patients).

---

[19] Balch, P., Balch, J., previously cited, p. 47.

With a bit of mind-stretch, it is possible to expand our concept of defense beyond the body and into the social sphere that surrounds us. This dimension provides an interactive form of care, creating powerful effects on the healing process. The social aspect of care is so ingrained in most societies that it often goes unnoticed, except when we need someone else to help us with a health problem. Perhaps the most obvious example is the emotional and physical care parents typically provide for their children; they could not survive without it.

In addition to the familial support there are also friends, institutions, and, as is now being acknowledged in many hospitals, the positive healing emotion from pets. Often this line spontaneously emerges from the collective soul, if you will, during moments of crisis. During such moments our deepest commonalities are evoked and we express the cooperative and compassionate elements that make us human.

A poignant example was the outpouring of care that manifested, and continues to do so, from the events that took place on September 11. It cannot be ignored how close the social and the psychological lines of defense are. The additive influence creates a sense of security that helps to neutralize those negative mental states and their dire effects on the immune response. Medical research has come to realize the importance of this healing influence that rises collectively from the heart as a kind of non-linear form of intelligence.

Daniel Goleman, the author of *Emotional Intelligence*[20], has written about how this c o-hesive social force affects the doctor-patient relationship. "Beyond the humanitarian argument for physicians to offer care along with cure, there are other compelling reasons to consider the psychological and social reality of patients as being within the medical realm rather than separate from it. By now the sci-entific case can be made that there is a margin of *medical* effectiveness, both in prevention and treatment that can be gained by treating people's emotional state along with their medical conditions. Not in every case or every condition, of course. But looking at data from hundreds and hundreds of cases, there is on average enough increment of medical benefit to suggest that an emotional intervention should be a standard part of medical care for the range of serious disease."[21]

In their book *The Healing Brain*, Robert Ornstein and David Sobel[22] comment on the physical effects that social interactions have on the body. "Social connectedness is so basic and vital to human health that it affects blood pressure, the incidence of heart disease, and the intimate workings of the immune system." Studies have shown that when this connectedness is challenged people will experience a level of stress based on how valuable this connection was for them.

The research done by Thomas Holmes, Richard Rahe, and colleagues during the 1960s, studied the nature and importance of these relationships in terms of positive and negative events occurring in a person's life. The positive social events included marriage, vacations, social achievements, and the like. The negative ones included such events as separation from family and friends, the loss of those close to one, loss of a job, illness, and so on. They found fifteen key events, which they ranked by degree of importance based on the response to two questionnaires. Using this data, they devised the following scale to measure the stress level each event might produce based on the values from people representing three different cultures.

[20] ... (1995). Bantam Doubleday Dell Publishing Group, Inc.: New York, NY.

[21] ...(P. 165.)

[22] ... (1987). The Healing Brain: Breakthrough Discoveries About How the Brain Keeps Us Healthy. Simon & Schuster Inc.: New York, NY.

Ratings of Stressful Life Events[23]
Life Change Values Ranked By Ethnicity

Event	American	European	Japanese
Death of spouse	1	1	1
Divorce	2	3	3
Separation	3	5	7
Jail term	4	2	2
Death of close family member	5	18	4
Personal injury or Illness	6	8	5
Marriage	7	4	6
Fired from Job	8	9	8
Marital Reconciliation	9	7	15
Retirement	10	17	11
Change in health of family member	11	20	9
Pregnancy	12	6	13
Sexual issues.	13	15	10
Addition of new Family member	14	13	23
Major business Readjustment	15	11	12
	American	**European**	**Japanese**

Scoring of the test resulted in significant differences in values from one culture to another. This, of course, is a reflection of the belief system. Based on their scoring system of Life Change Units (LCU), scores of 150-199 were considered to produce a mild form of stress. Scores of 200-299 were moderate in terms of stress, while scores over 300 represented a high level of stress.

It is interesting to note that "People who scored highly on the number of life changes had more traffic accidents than those who scored lower; and children whose parents moved, divorced, or got a large raise had all sorts of complications including higher suicide rates. And, as in (the) studies of bereavement, people who experienced numerous major life events were more likely to suffer from a staggering variety of medical conditions such as influenza, heart disease, diabetes, leukemia, rheumatoid arthritis, schizophrenia, psychosomatic symptoms, and de-

pression, as well as difficulties in pregnancy."[24]

As can be seen, the psychological, social, and physiological dimensions are closely related. Stressful social events can also trigger the fight-or-flight response or the stress adaptive syndrome. However, Selye's research revealed that stress is not in-and-of-itself a negative factor. It depends on the degree of stress. Mild to moderate levels of stress (which, of course is relative from person-to-person) produce what he called "*eustress*" or good stress, which can become a beneficial motivating factor, including immune response. Excessive amounts of *perceived* stress lead to what Selye called "*distress*" or bad stress.

How an individual perceives an event is a very important factor. As we have seen, it can vary from culture-to-culture, but it can also vary from person-to-person. Therefore, it's not just that specific events are negative or stress producing; it depends on how each individual *interprets* the event.

Most people tend to blame the event as the cause of stress rather than their interpretation of it. (This is also true of so-called positive events.) A certain level of emotional maturity and intellectual understanding is required in order to absorb external shocks and not allow them to overly disturb one's internal tranquility or mental-and-physical equilibrium (homeostasis).

Emotional connectedness to other people need not be a source for worry (distress) but can be transformed by the mind into compassion, care, concern, and useful action (if necessary). The event, however powerful it may appear, can be turned into eustress.

Obviously, the interpretation of the event will depend on the context in which it occurs. In a potential biowarfare or nuclear scenario one will tend to think of the worst that could happen to them. This kind of thinking can lead to panic, which, of course, is a distressful interpretation. While it's important to under-

---

[23] Adapted from The Healing Brain, cited above.

[24] ...The Healing Brain, P. 209.

stand the potential consequences, "futurizing" about what may happen is not helpful. Instead of worrying one could transform the perception into proactive steps to protect one's self and others. However, this proactive thinking and acting needs to be couched in the neutralizing attitude of acceptance: change what is possible to change and leave the impossible alone.

Some of the common ways we can help one another are by offering:
- Emotional support.
- Helpful information.
- Shelter.
- Clothing.
- Transportation and ambulatory assistance.
- Financial assistance.
- Food, and other forms of nutrients.
- Family support.
- Political pro-activity for creating and/or improving the quality of institutional emergency, private, and hospital health care.
- Therapeutic interventions in the form of pre-emergency-medical care.

Neighborhood Defense Support Group

Consider starting a Neighborhood Defense Support Group in your community. Feeling the concern and camaraderie of people provides that inner sustenance that helps people cope with the most pressing issues of our time. Find a place to meet (home, apartment, church, school, public meeting hall, etc.) Set up an agenda based on the topics in this book, as a start. Invite speakers from various relevant organizations. Pick a starting date. Find a simple way to broadcast the event. Let the news media know. Keep a record of the meetings. This is one of the best examples of using the social line. (**The American Civil Defense Association** is an excellent source of information.)

Emergency Telephone Numbers

It's important to know the emergency numbers in your area. Write them down and keep them near the telephone, in your wallet, etc.

Learn Basic First Aid and Home Care

The main objectives of training individuals in first aid and home care are: to preserve life, to minimize the effects of injury or illness, to relieve suffering or distress, and to provide continuing care and assist in rehabilitation. Learning the basics of first aid and home care skills prepares individuals to serve effectively in a national emergency. If such an emergency occurs, the emergency medical systems may become overwhelmed, and doctors and nurses may not be readily available to assist you. Thus the importance of these skills takes on a new dimension. The survival of the sick and injured may become your responsibility.

Natural & Conventional First Aid Supplies
A simple first aid kit kept in a convenient place (e.g., in home, your shelter, or in your evacuation kit) should contain:

❑ **Check List**
Applications
❑ 1 bottle mild antiseptic solution (use to clean cuts): 3 % Hydrogen Peroxide, or Grapefruit Seed Extract Solution (40 drops per pint or 475 ml of water, in a spray bottle)
❑ Sealed alcohol swab packets
❑ Tincture of Yarrow (*Achillea millefolium*) applied to gauze to cover a clean wound to help stop bleeding
❑ 1 small bottle toothache drops (for temporary treatment of toothache) such as Oil of Clove applied with a cotton swab to tooth and gum
❑ Mild soap
❑ 1 tube of petroleum jelly (natural non-petroleum forms are available)
❑ Antibacterial ointments such as Neosporin, Bacitracin and/or Colloidal Silver/Aloe Salve to use topically
❑ 2 tubes of Aloe Vera Gel (not requiring refrigeration) for burns
Bandages, Applicators, Fasteners
❑ Cotton swabs
❑ Elastic (Ace) bandages 2-3 inches wide (for wrapping sprains, for applying pressure to

large wound)

- Several Triangular cloths 40 X 40 X 55 inches (to use as a sling, to hold splints in place for broken ankle, etc.)
- Liquid bandage (for minor cuts and scrapes)
- Butterfly bandages to hold together the edges of cuts
- 5 yards 2-inch gauze bandage
- 12 4" x 4" sterile pads (use to cover cuts, wounds and burns)
- 12 assorted individual adhesive dressings (use for minor cuts)
- 2 large dressing pads 8" x 8"
- 5 yards 1/2 inch adhesive tape
- 12 assorted safety pins
- 1 packet paper tissues and towels
- Eye patch

Assessment Tools

- 1 thermometer (mercury and/or digital); ear thermometer is best to get readings from unconscious victims
- Stethoscope to hear heartbeat and breathing
- Blood pressure monitor (manual or digital) to determine hypotension (shock)
- Small flashlight to look into eyes, throat, ears, etc. and/or wound in poor light
- Small mirror to detect moisture from breathing
- Watch or small clock with second hand or digital readout

Miscellaneous Items

- Wooden and/or plastic tongue depressors (to check mouth and throat, and to use to scrape toxic materials off skin); also, can be used as splints for fingers
- 1 pair small scissors (blunt ended)
- Measuring cup
- Measuring spoons
- Eye droppers
- 1 medicine glass
- 1 pair tweezers
- Space blanket to keep person warm
- Plastic or glass spray bottles
- Plastic spoons to stir, scoop, and apply

Remedies[25]

- 1 small bottle aspirin tablets for aches and pains and/or Bromelain (500 mg.) with Papain (100-300 mg) as anti-inflammatory, or Fever-few (200-500 mg) with Magnesium Citrate (200 mg) for headaches
- Valerian Root tea or capsules to relax tense muscles
- 4 oz baking soda and 8 oz table salt (make a drinking solution by adding: 1 tsp salt and 1/2 tsp baking soda to 1 qt. of water to quell acid stomach)
- Activated Charcoal powder, capsules, or tablets taken in or with water to quell acid stomach or absorb toxins or for diarrhea; can also be used as a drawing poultice
- Charco-Zyme (activated charcoal + digestive enzymes) for acid-indigestion, flatulence, bloating after ingestion of food
- Allergy pills or antihistamines and/or Quercetin (500 mg) for allergies
- Walley's Ear Oil for ear aches and infection (place few drops in affected ear and plug with cotton overnight)
- Herbal laxative capsules such as Aloe Vera Powder (use 1-4 with glass of water near bedtime)
- Melatonin (0.5-21 mg) to help with insomnia, for adults **only**; with children (especially infants) use scent of lavender; with older children use scent of lavender and/or skullcap tea
- Grapefruit Seed Extract (liquid concentrate, must be diluted) used as an antiseptic, decontaminant, and antimicrobial.
- Syrup of Ipecac to induce vomiting (don't use after administration of activated charcoal)

Special Needs

Individuals requiring special medication such as insulin should maintain at least 100-day supplies.

---

[25] Other possibilities are available under the Specific Line of Defense for each agent. See this line for more detailed information on how to use the natural substances.

Instruction[26]

- ❑ Nuclear War Survival Skills, by Cresson Kearny. Available from: **KI4U**, 212 Oil Patch Lane, Gonzales, TX 78629. Tel: (830) 540-4188. Can be printed from the Internet: www.KI4U.com. An excellent source of detailed information regarding potential nuclear incidents.
- ❑ Weapons of Mass Destruction: Emergency Care, by Robert De Lorenzo, and Robert Porter. Published by Prentice Hall, Inc. A very useful book in lay language for first responders. Available in bookstores.
- ❑ The Natural Health First-Aid Guide: The Definitive Handbook of Natural Remedies for Treating Minor Emergencies, by Mark Mayell and the editors of Natural Health Magazine. A clear and comprehensive source of valuable information. Available in bookstores.
- ❑ The American Medical Association Handbook of First Aid and Emergency Care. Published by Random House. Available in bookstores.
- ❑ Emergency Medical Procedures: For the Home, Auto, and Workplace. Published by Prentice Hall Press. Available in bookstores.
- ❑ Homeopathy 911: What to Do in an Emergency Before Help Arrives, in bookstores.
- ❑ Natural Remedies for Dogs and Cats, by CJ Puotinen. An excellent book for how to help these pets with natural health products. Also consider her: The Encyclopedia of Natural Pet Care. Keats Publishing. Available in bookstores.

First Aid Hints

Keep calm. Do not be hurried unless you are in a situation of extreme danger.

Assessment

- When possible determine the cause of danger to victim and/or to yourself
- Determine the extent of danger to victim and/or yourself
- Keep the injured person lying down in a comfortable position, his head level with his body until you determine whether his injuries are serious.
- Check for vital signs: **Airway, Breathing,** and **Circulation, (ABC).**

Also, examine for:

- Serious bleeding
- Broken bones.
- These must be treated immediately before any attempt is made to move the injured person.
- Keep him comfortably warm with blankets or other coverings, (under the patient as well, if possible)
- Never attempt to give a semi-conscious or unconscious person anything by mouth.

Unconsciousness

- An unconscious patient lying on his back may be strangled by his own tongue, which will tend to fall back and obstruct the airway.
- All unconscious persons should be placed lying half over on their sides, supported by their bent leg and arm, leaning towards their faces, (three-quarter-prone position).
- If the patient is breathing quietly and easily and his lips are pink and have no froth on them, breathing is not obstructed.
- If the patient is breathing noisily and with difficulty, if his lips are blue and frothing, or if his chest is sucked inwards when he breathes in, his airway is obstructed and he needs immediate attention to clear it. If the airway is clear, place the casualty on his back; supporting his shoulders on a pad of any suitable material available; tilting the head back with one hand on the forehead, the other lifting the neck.

When Breathing Stops

- If his breathing stops you can breathe for the patient by blowing air into his lungs.
- If the airway is clear, place the casualty on his back; supporting his shoulders on a pad of any suitable material available; tilting the head back with

---

[26] I'm indebted to these publications for the information provided on first aid and home care. See Bibliography for publisher specifics.

one hand on the forehead, the other lifting the neck.

- Take a deep breath. Pinch the casualty's nostrils. Place mouth to mouth tightly. Blow into the casualty's lungs strongly enough to cause his chest to rise.
- The cycle should be repeated every 3 to 5 seconds for an adult and a little more frequently for a child.
- Blow more gently for a child or a baby, but strongly enough to make the chest rise.
- If there is no heartbeat, manual chest compression may be required (learn from first aid manual), alternating with assisted breathing. (With some agents caution needs to be exercised that the toxin is not exhaled into the lungs of the helper.)

Wounds

You Must:

- Stop bleeding (hemorrhage): If a wound is bleeding profusely, hold it firmly with your hand until you can secure an emergency dressing. Any thick pad of clean, soft, compressible material large enough to cover the wound will make a good dressing. Clean handkerchiefs, towels, sanitary pads, handkerchiefs or sheets make good emergency dressings.
- Keep out germs (infection): Cover the wound with a clean dressing to keep out dirt and germs. Bandage it firmly to stop the bleeding.

Burns

- Cover the burned area with large, thick, dry dressing and bandage it on firmly.
- Encourage the casualty to drink plenty of fluids. A solution of salt and soda is useful to give to casualties with burns and to those who have suffered from serious bleeding.

Broken Bones/Fractures

- If a limb is very painful and cannot be used, appears to be bent in the wrong place or the casualty says he heard or felt the bone snap, it is likely that a bone is broken.
- Sharp ends of a broken bone may damage important structures such as blood vessels and nerves.
- A broken limb should be steadied and supported to prevent movement of the broken ends before attempting to move the patient.
- If a person's back or neck is so severely injured that he is afraid to move because of pain, or cannot move or feel his limbs, you should assume that he has a spinal fracture.
- He should be moved on a hard, firm stretcher taking great care not to "jack-knife" him by picking up his feet and shoulders. Improvised stretchers can be made from a door, wide board, window shutter, etc. Fill in the natural hollows of the back and neck with padding and support the head on both sides to prevent movement.
- **DO NOT:** Put strong antiseptics into a wound.
- **DO NOT:** Remove clothing that is stuck to a burn.
- **DO NOT:** Break any blisters or apply creams or grease to a large burn.
- **DO NOT:** Give anything by mouth to a semi-conscious patient, or to a patient with internal abdominal wounds.

Infant Care

Before medical or nursing help becomes available you may also encounter infant care problems.

- Breastfeeding is preferable but, if not possible, then a formula using powdered or evaporated milk should be prepared under clean conditions.

- If vomiting or diarrhea occurs infants and children become dehydrated very quickly. To avoid this from occurring give frequent sips of decontaminated water.
- If a rash or fever develops, keep others away from the sick child.

Emotional Problems

Persons who become emotionally disturbed following a disaster should be treated calmly but firmly. They should be kept in small groups, preferably with persons whom they know, and be encouraged to "talk out" their problem. If they are not otherwise injured they should be given something to do. It may be necessary to enlist the aid of one other calm person to help subdue the overexcited patient. If a stunned or dazed reaction persists over 6 to 8 hours this should be reported to a doctor or nurse immediately.

To help children reduce fears: let them talk about their fears and worries. Stick to family routines. Supervise what they hear and see on the media (radio, TV). Reassure them that parents, teachers, doctors, etc. are doing everything possible to ensure their safety and health. Arm yourself with facts, and respond to them in a calm manner. Children are especially affected by fears expressed by those who care for them.

Radiation Sickness

The following suggestions might be useful for those who become sick from nuclear radiation.

- Treatment includes rest, the provision of whatever nutritional food and drink is available, and personal encouragement to get well.
- Swab the mouth gently with mild, warm salt and water if it becomes sore.
- As these patients are susceptible to infection, keep wounds clean and cov-

ered with a sterile dressing. Separate these patients from persons with colds, rash or fever.

Improvised Equipment

The following suggestions may help you care for your patient when proper equipment is not available.

- Bed: A couch, mattress or any well padded, firm surface; if too low raise on bricks, boxes or wooden blocks.
- Bedding Protection: Old crib pads cut into a convenient size and placed over a waterproof sheeting; or several layers of newspaper and heavy brown paper covered with old soft cotton. (Never use thin plastic if patient is a child.)
- Backrest: A straight-backed chair turned upside down at head of bed and securely tied to bed; a triangular bolster or cushions from a chair.
- Pressure Pads: Soft cushion or foam or sponge rubber pads will protect heels, elbows, back of head or any other body pressure point.
- Bedpan or Urinal: For bedpan use a padded dish or pan; for urinal any wide-necked bottle or jar
- Hot Water Bottle: A heated brick wrapped in several layers of newspaper.

Information/Instructions for Helpers

Keep the following suggested form in a conspicuous place as a way to advise first responders or others that come to help. Change it to meet your/family particular needs.

PLEASE READ BEFORE HELPING ME/US

Name

Address

Phone   **Date of Birth**

Relative(s)/Friend(s) to Contact:

Employer(s):

Medical Information

Conditions: **Meds/Dosage/Times/Kept in:**

Known allergies:

                                                              Blood Type:

My Physicians: **Phone #'s:**

Supplement I need take: **Amount**   **When**   **With/Without Food**   **Kept in:**

Foods I need to eat: **Where to find/Preparation:**

Location of Emergency Kit:

Emergency Telelphone Number(s) in this Area:

Special Instructions:

31

So far I have discussed how immunity is a holistic convergence of psychological and social dimensions. Here I address the use of preventative care as a way to maintain a strong immune response. This is the wise person's way of thinking ahead instead of waiting to deal with a crisis. Our medical norm for health is a crisis oriented one that waits for a problem and then proceeds to fix it. There's a saying that reflects this attitude, "If it's not broken don't fix it." However, a system, (whether it be a car or the human body) when not maintained properly will most likely require more "fixing" than one that has been maintained.

As I researched the nature of the WMD listed by the CDC it was obvious that those who are predisposed—by age, illness, life-style, immune-suppressive medications—would be more likely to succumb to even a mild exposure of these potentially lethal agents. In such cases, prevention can make the difference between life and death.

Even those who would qualify as healthy under the current symptom-free norms could quite likely have suppressed immunity, and they could be just as vulnerable as the clinically diagnosed. A crucial factor in survival, as we have seen with anthrax cases, is early treatment. Those with stronger immune systems would certainly have an advantage because their healthy immune system would overcome or delay the onset of the disease.

The experience of feeling at the peak of health has become a memory of youth for many people. Perhaps this is due to the fact that we're rarely taught by our educational system how to maintain our health. This has led to a huge number of illnesses, and the false acceptance of the inevitability of periodically occurring infections. If prevention were practiced on a wider scale the incidence of colds, influenza, and other infectious diseases would decline dramatically. Inadequate nutrition and life-style have much to do with the incidence of periodically recurring illness.

I'm not talking about becoming a health fanatic. What I propose as a preventative program is quite easy, although it does require developing a few healthy habits, like taking a few minutes several times daily to mix a few nutrient-rich powders in water or juice, and taking a few capsules. Other factors that would augment the level of health are:

Exercise

Perform some daily exercise like taking a brisk walk, or take the stairs instead of the elevator (ok to stop a few floors from your destination and walk up a few flights of stairs), dance, light runs, clean your house, or car, etc. The more enjoyable it is the better. There's no need to become a high performance athlete. Avoid too much exercise since research has shown that excessive exercise can have a negative effect on immune function.[27] A good measure is to stop when breathing through the mouth begins and/or sweat breaks out on the brow. Gradually come to a rest.

It's important to remember that the expenditure of energy should be followed by an adequate amount of quality rest and recuperation (on the level of the Relaxation Response). An excellent book on the subject is John Douillard's *Body, Mind, and Sport*.[28] His rich background as a trainer plus his knowledge of nutrition, body types, and the mind-body relationship brings common sense to the question of exercise.

Avoid Smoking

If you can't stop, consider hypnotherapy. While the habit still has you in its grips make sure to take plenty of antioxidants (see the recommendations in the Preventative Program).

---

[27] See: Lappé, M., (1997). The Tao of Immunology: A Revolutionary New Understanding of Our Body's Defenses. Plenum Trade Plenum Press: New York, NY.
[28] ... (1994). Crown Trade Paperbacks: New York, NY.

Avoid/Reduce Alcohol

Alcoholic beverages should be kept at a minimum, such as an occasional glass of wine or beer with dinner.

Stop/Manage Caffeine

Avoid ingesting excessive amounts of caffeine as too much caffeine dampens the immune system, although a cup of coffee per day may be fine. During periods of stress and fatigue stop all caffeine products.

Good Digestion

Make sure you digest foods well and have at least 2 satisfactory bowel movements daily. If not, consume more fibrous foods, and drink plenty of water.

Deep Sleep

Develop regularity in you life by getting to sleep within a certain range of time (preferably before 11 pm) and arising 7-8 hours later. Studies have revealed that peak immune activity occurs during deep sleep.

Detox

At least twice yearly give yourself a one or two week detoxification of the bowels, liver, kidneys, and the gallbladder.

Wholeness

According to the current reductive way of thinking, much if not all of the ability to heal is attributed to the immune system. While the immune system is miraculous in its own right, it relies on every other organ system to carry out its role. It needs the heart. It needs the liver. It needs the kidneys. It needs the lungs. It needs the brain, and so on. It cannot work optimally without them. Immunity is a holistic process.

Natural foods and substances—vitamins, minerals, proteins, carbohydrates, essential fatty acids, and pure water—are needed to sustain the physiological aspects of healing. They provide the molecules and atoms that are converted into the miracle of life.

Research on the holistic use of micronutrients and a variety of other substances has become well established, especially with regards to bolstering immune function. Many informative books have been written on this subject (see Bibliography for recommendations),

so I won't proceed to reinvent the wheel. However, I will briefly touch on the key characteristics of the substances that I recommend for sustaining optimal health.

Vitamins

Vitamins are micronutrients essential for sustaining all the metabolic processes in the body. Metabolism involves the breakdown of substances (catabolism), and the subsequent release of energy, and constructive processes (anabolism) that build and restore all the tissues of the body. The body is constantly breaking down and reconstructing itself in a balanced manner.

Vitamins work in a harmonious manner with enzymes and minerals to carry out numerous metabolic functions. That is why vitamins are also referred to as co-enzymes. Enzymes are catalysts that activate all the biochemical reactions that continuously occur within the body.

Vitamins are classified into two groups: fat-soluble and water-soluble. The fat-soluble vitamins are: A, D, E, and K. The water-soluble vitamins include C and the B complex. Fat-soluble vitamins can be stored in the body in the fatty tissue and in the liver. Water-soluble vitamins cannot be stored, with one exception, B_{12}. The body uses what it needs and excretes the remainder in the urine on a daily basis.

Nevertheless, all vitamins are consumed as they perform their metabolic activities and must be replenished on a regular basis. During periods of stress and illness the water-soluble vitamins are the first to go, especially vitamin C.

Also, there are other vitamin-like substances that play important roles in the metabolic processes of the body.

There's no need to go into the details of these nutrients because all of them contribute synergistically to the overall health of the mind-body complex and especially to immune function. Moreover, there are numerous books that describe how these nutrients work and provide considerable references of scientific studies.[29] A representative formula is found in the following product.

Daily Nutrients for General Health and Immune Strength

Representative Product: All ONE™ (Rice Base Formula)[30] By Nutritech

Amount Per Serving of 1 Heaping Tablespoon
Vitamins

Vitamin A (palmitate)	8,000 IU
Beta Carotene (pro-vitamin A)	7,000 IU
Vitamin B-1 (thiamine)	25 mg
Vitamin B-2 (riboflavin)	25 mg
Vitamin B-3 (niacinimide)	100 mg
Vitamin B-5 (pantothenic acid)	100 mg
Vitamin B-6 (pyroxidine)	25 mg
Vitamin B-12 (cyanocobalamin)	25 mcg
Biotin (d-biotin)	25 mcg
Choline	100 mg
Folic Acid (folate)	400 mcg
Inositol	100 mg
PABA (para-aminobenzoic acid)	25 mg
Vitamin C (ascorbic acid)	400 mg
Bioflavonoids (lemon)	400 mg
Hesperidin	25 mg
Rutin	25 mg
Vitamin D3 (cholecalciferol)	500 IU
Vitamin E (d-alpha-tocopherol succinate)	400 IU
Vitamin K	5 mcg

Minerals

Calcium (citrate, carbonate, dicalcium phosphate, amino acid chelate)	500 mg
Copper (amino acid chelate)	0.2 mg
Chromium (amino acid chelate)	50 mcg
Iodine (potassium iodide)	180 mcg
Magnesium (carbonate)	200 mg
Manganese (carbonate)	4 mg
Molybdenum (amino acid chelate)	50 mcg
Phosphorous (dicalcium phosphate)	200 mg
Potassium (citrate, alginate)	99 mg
Selenium (proteinate)	50 mcg
Zinc (oxide)	15 mg

Amino Acids

Alanine	210 mg
Arginine	300 mg
Aspartic Acid	337 mg
Cystine/Cysteine	97 mg
Glutamic Acid	682 mg
Glycine	165 mg
Histadine*	90 mg
Isoleucine*	157 mg
Lysine*	90 mg
Leucine*	322 mg
Methionine*	82 mg
Phenylalanine*	210 mg
Proline	172 mg
Threonine*	135 mg
Tryptophan*	45 mg
Tyrosine	187 mg
Valine*	240 mg

Vegetarian and lactose intolerant formula.

Provides: Calories 32; Total Carbohydrates 4 g; Dietary Fiber 2 g; Protein (from organic rice) 4 g. In a base of papain, betaine (digestive enzymes), kelp 3 mg, and high-fiber rice protein from rice that's been enzymatically digested by purified plant enzymes.

Does not contain: yeast; gluten; sugar; sweeteners; flavors; colors; binders; excipients; fillers; iron.

Note: Although **iron** is a vital nutrient, I recommend that it be taken separately as an herbal liquid form (e.g., <u>Floradix</u> is a good liquid herbal formula, and there are others) because one can control the dosage. Menopausal women may need less. Men may not need to supplement with iron at all (it can cause increase of free radicals in the prostate). Since iron is also vital for bacterial growth I recommend that it be suspended during bacterial infections.   It is better to get iron from food if there is no serious deficiency (e.g., iron-deficiency anemia). With infectious diseases avoid supplementing with iron beyond what is available from foods.

Alternative Liquid High Potency Multi Vitamin Formula
Representative Product: Vita Quick By Twin Lab

One tbsp Contains:

---

[29] See Bibliography: Balch & Balch, Prescriptions for Nutritional Healing; PDR For Herbal Supplements; PDR for Nutritional Supplements; Herbal Medicines Comprehensive Data Base.

[30] Or, any other comparable formula.

* Essential Amino Acids.

Vitamin A (Beta Carotene)	10,000 IU
Vitamin C	150 mg
Vitamin D	400 IU
Vitamin E	30 IU
Thiamin (B1)	25 mg
Riboflavin (B2)	25 mg
Niacin (B3)	150 mg
Vitamin B6	30 mg
Folic Acid	400 mcg
Vitamin B-12	50 mcg
Biotin	50 mcg
Pantothenic Acid	150 mg
PABA	10 mg
Choline	200 mg
Inositol	100 mg

Note: This product is suitable for vegetarians. It has all-natural pineapple and orange flavors with fructose. No artificial colors, salt and sodium free. Recommended dose: 1 tbsp daily. May also be mixed with favorite juice or non-heated beverage.

Complementary Liquid Trace Mineral Formula
Representative Product: Liquid Multiple-Minerals
By Innovative Natural Products

Contains a full-spectrum of ionic (trace) minerals to complement the above multi-vitamin formula. This product is 100 % lead free. Recommended dosage: 1 tbsp daily. May be combined in juice with the above.

Liquid Multi Vitamins and Trace Minerals for Children
Representative Product: Mighty Vita-Kids
By Tropical Oasis

One tbsp contains:	
Vitamin A (Palmitate)	5000 IU
Vitamin C	60 mg
Vitamin D	400 IU
Vitamin E	30 IU
Vitamin K	.25 mg
Vitamin B-1	1.5 mg
Vitamin B-2	1.7 mg
Vitamin B-3	20 mg
Vitamin B-6	2 mg
Vitamin B-12	6 mcg
Folic Acid	400 mcg
Biotin	300 mcg
Pantothenic Acid	10 mg
Bioflavonoids	1.25 mg
Quercetin	2.50 mg
Ionized Minerals	1.12 ml
Amino Acids	10 mg

Note: Serving size 1/2 fl. Oz (15 ml) = 1 tbsp. Dosage per weight of child: 10-50 lbs, 1tsp; 51-75 lbs, 1 1/2 tsp; 76 + lbs, 1 tbsp daily with food. Refrigerate, and avoid storing in direct sunlight. Has a natural cranberry- aloe-vera flavor.

The above formulas would be fully complemented by a green-food formula that would add to the spectrum of support. This additional boost would include powerful antioxidants, tissue and blood cleansers, liver support, blood builders, digestive enzymes, and probiotic factors (derived from fruits, vegetables, grains, herbs, and bee products). A representative example is found in the following product.

Green Food Supplement
Representative Product: Magma Plus™ [31]
By Green Foods

Ingredients Per 3 Teaspoons

Powdered juice from:

- Organically-grown young <u>Barley Grass</u>
- <u>Mixed Vegetables</u> (carrot, wheat grass, alfalfa, lettuce, cabbage, daikon radish, bean sprouts, celery, tomato, spinach, kale)
- <u>Maltodextrin</u>: a complex natural sweetener that won't drastically affect blood sugar
- <u>Lecithin</u>, emulsifies fats in the liver, helps lower cholesterol
- <u>Bee Products</u> (honey, bee pollen, royal jelly)
- <u>Mixed Fruits</u> (apple, banana, pineapple, papaya, mango, raspberry): rich in enzymes and OPCs (oligomeric proanthocyanadins)
- <u>Chicory Root Extract (FOS)</u>, excellent source of beta carotene with anti-inflammatory properties; providing fructo-oligosacharides as a probiotic factor
- <u>Wheat Germ Extract</u>: rich in vitamin E and energy producing octocosanol
- <u>Probiotic Culture</u> (L. bifidus, L. acidophilus, L. planatarum),
- <u>Spirulina</u>, blue-green algae rich in vitamins, minerals, GLA, and proteins.
- <u>Chlorella</u>: rich in vitamins, minerals, amino acids, enzymes, and tissue detoxifying substances
- <u>Licorice Root Extract</u>: an adrenal stimulant for healing and energy
- <u>Pearl Barley Extract</u>, rich in essential nutrients
- <u>Vitamin E</u>, (See vitamin E above).
- <u>Acerola Extract</u>, rich source of vitamin C.
- <u>Brown Rice</u>: rich in B vitamins and fiber

---

[31] Or comparable product.

- Red Beet Extract, stimulates production of red blood cells
- Milk Thistle Extract, protects liver cells.
- Echinacea Purpurea Extract, immune stimulant and cell-membrane protector.
- Siberian Ginseng Extract, a powerful general adaptogenic tonic.
- American Ginseng Extract, a powerful general adaptogenic tonic.
- Astragalus Extract, immune stimulant and broad-spectrum antimicrobial.
- Aloe Vera, liver tonic and detoxifier.
- Green Tea Extract, antioxidant that protects against tumor formation in colon, and is a useful iron-chelator against infections
- Ginger Root Extract: disgestive aid, tonic, anti-inflammatory
- Stevia Extract, non-caloric herbal sweetener.
- Reishi Mushroom Extract: immune stimulant, and antimicrobial
- Cayenne Pepper: hemostatic, metabolic stimulant, pain reliever
- Garlic: broad-spectrum antimicrobial, cardiotonic
- Cat's Claw Extract: potent antimicrobial, anti-inflammatory
- Yucca Root Extract, decreases aborption of bacterial toxins
- Ginkgo Biloba Extract dilates capillaries and increases delivery of oxygen to the tissue
- Garcinia Cambogia Extract blocks the conversion of sugars into fat.
- Glucomannan, a water-soluble fiber that forms bulk and a feeling of satiety, somewhat curbing the appetite.
- Bilberry Extract, a powerful antioxidant, protects the eyes
- Grapeseed Extract is a powerful antioxidant, rich in OPCs that strengthen capillaries
- Digestive Enzymes (lipase, amylase, protease).

Supplement Information: Total Calories 36; Calories from fat 9; Total Carbohydrates 7 g; Dietary Fiber 3 g; Sugars 1 g; Protein 1 g; Vitamin A (beta carotene) 9,500 IU; Vitamin C 70 mg; Vitamin E 135 IU; Thiamine (B-1) 0.6 mg; Vitamin B-6 300 mcg; Pantothenic Acid 2.5 mg; Calcium 25 mg; Iron 4.5 mg; Magnesium 40 mg; Sodium 27 mg; Phosphorus 110 mg; Chlorophyll 15 mg.
Note: This formula is rich in cold-processed active enzymes, food-based micronutrients, amino acids, bioflavonoids, chlorophyll, and antioxidants. It can be used as a full- spectrum food, and also as a detoxifier.

Alternative Green Supplement for Children
Representative Product: Yummy Greens (Chewable)
By Solar Green®

One tablet contains:

Vitamin A (Beta Carotene)	156 IU
Vitamin C (Ascorbic acid)	38 mg
Organic Wheat Grass Powder	31 mg
Organic Barley Grass Powder	31 mg
Organic Alfalfa Leaf	31 mg
Chlorella Broken Cell Algae	31 mg
Organic Hawaiian Spirulina	31 mg
Kelp	19 mg

Note: This product is fruit-punch flavored. Contains all essential vitamins and trace minerals, protein, and fiber. Xylitol is the natural sweetener, which is not prone to cause tooth decay. It is **not recommended** for children under the age of 2. Recommended dosage: 1 tablet up to 4 times a day.

Essential Fatty Acids

Essential fatty acids (EFA's) are popularly known as the "good oils". Technically, they are referred to as *vitamin F* or *polyunsaturates*. They provide the basic molecules from which all fats in the body are made and, as the name implies, they must be acquired through the diet since the body cannot make them. All cells need EFA's to function and to support the structure of their membranes. High concentrations are found in brain cells. They also take part in the messenger molecules of the body, especially as precursors to substances known as *prostaglandins*. Acting like hormones, protaglandins control the mechanisms that trigger and turn off inflammation. While EFA's play numerous roles in the biochemistry of the body, it is their connection to inflammation that is of major concern here.

All infectious and traumatic incidents discussed in this book will be complicated by inflammation of the tissue. As was mentioned earlier, inflammation is produced as part of the process to launch an immune response. All too often, the response gets started but cannot easily stop. Unable to stop, the excessive inflammatory response may be more damaging to the system than the pathogen or agent of trauma. Inflammation may be acute, lasting for a relatively brief period of time, or chronic, lasting for months or years. Chronic inflammation has recently been implicated in a wide variety of degenerative diseases.[32]

Udo's Choice (to be taken with the above recommendations) 3000 mg (of essential fatty acids) 2-3 times daily.[33] The blend consists of: flax oil, sesame oil, medium chain triglycerides from coconut or palm oil, evening primrose oil (13mg GLA/15ml), soy lecithin (GMO free), rice bran and germ oils, oat bran and germ oils, tocotrienols.

Foods

Foods are another interesting source for natural defense. Find an eating style that you are comfortable with. Having negative emotions about eating the "right" foods is more damaging than eating the "wrong" foods. However, if you're emotional about the right foods, the power of the food will increase ten fold. Two books that might be of help to guide you to a healthy dietary are: Annemarie Colbin's *Food And Healing*[34], and R ebecca Wood's *The New Whole Foods Encyclopedia*[35] To these I would add Amadea Morningstar's *Ayurvedic Cooking for Westerners.*[36] Ayurveda is an ancient yet evolving system of medicine from India. It incorporates constitutional types in its method of healing. Morningstar's book explains the nature of this system, and provides many recipes based on one's constitutional nature.

Do your best to eat whole (unrefined or processed) foods that are organically grown. If this is not possible, clean all foods extra well to wash off pesticides, etc. Avoid re-

fined sugar, soft drinks (make your own with natural sparkling water and juice), and saturated fats (from animals, butter, etc.). Reduce flesh foods (especially meats of hoofed animals). Increase fruits and vegetables. Drink plenty of water: (periodically rather than much at one time is best), for it keeps the system flowing. Decaffeinated teas are fine. Dilute fruit juices. Low-calories meals have been shown to correlate with excellent health and longevity, especially during the healing process (soups are excellent).

Lung Kichadi

Kichadis are at the core of Ayurvedic nutritional healing. They are simple stews consisting of rice and split mung beans to which a variety of herbs and spices can be added based on the health needs of the person. I have chosen this recipe because with most of the WMD the lungs will be critically challenged. Kichadis also help to detoxify the body of harmful substances, plus they are gentle on the digestive system. Here's the recipe:

Preparation time: 2 hours. Serves: 2 – 3 people.
1/2 cup of basmati rice
1/4 cup split mung beans
6 cups water
1 tablespoon of ghee (clarified butter)
1 teaspoon cumin seeds
1/8 teaspoon hing (asafoetida)
1 teaspoon coriander seeds
1/4 teaspoon cardamom seeds
1 teaspoon black peppercorns
1/2 teaspoon of ajwan
1 tablespoon ghee
1 more teaspoon of ghee
3/4 teaspoons of cinnamon
1/4 teaspoon of ground cloves
1 teaspoon of turmeric
3/4 teaspoon of salt (or rock salt)
1/4 teaspoon of dry ginger
1/2 small onion, chopped
4 cloves of garlic
1/2 tsp of ground cumin
2-4 cups of fresh vegetables: carrots, greens, string beans or zucchini, chopped
2 medium sweet potatoes
1 stick of kombu
2 more cups water, as needed

Wash the rice and split mung until the rinse water is clear. Warm a tablespoon of ghee in a medium sauce-

[32] See: Segala, M., Ed. (2000), previously cited. Also: Newmark, T.; Schulick, P., previously cited.
[33] Or similar product.
[34] …(1986)….Ballantine Books: New York, NY.
[35] …(1999)….Penguin Books: New York, NY.
[36] …(1995). Lotus Press. Twin Lakes, WI.

pan and add the whole cumin seeds, ajwan, and hing. Lightly brown them. Wash sweet potatoes and dice into 1/2" pieces. Add the sweet potatoes, rice, mung, kombu and water and bring to a boil. Warm 1tablespoon ghee in a small skillet; add cardamom, coriander, peppercorns and dry ginger, and sauté for 2 to 3 minutes. Stir in the rest of the spices with the onion and garlic. Put the sautéed spices in a blender with 1/2 cup or less of water and grind well. Pour this spice mixture into the rice and mung. Rinse out the blender with the last 2 cups water and add it to the kichadi. Add the vegetables; cook 20 minutes or more. Optional: add 1tablespoon flaxseed in the last 15 minutes of cooking to enhance clearing of the lungs. Simply mix it into the kichadi as it is cooking.

Digestive Aids

These aids help the body to digest foods and absorb nutrients. When these functions are not working well all that one is taking to bolster the first line of defense would be wasted. Therefore, they have specific use for those who have frequent indigestion such as bloating, stomach acidity, cramping, excessive flatulence, belching, and the like. Digestive aids can be used with any stage of the disease process. However, with some conditions (see specific agent) some may be contraindicated, for they may aggravate the condition.

Enzymes

Enzymes perform numerous metabolic functions in the body. They are also involved in digestive processes where they breakdown protein, starches, and fats into smaller molecules that the body can process. Here the focus is on digestive enzymes because they are involved in the initial stages of making nutrients available to the body.

Digestive enzymes are found in the digestive tract. They consist of protease, amylase, and lipase. Protease breaks down protein. Amylase breaks down carbohydrates (starches, sugars). Lipase breaks down fats. The pancreas (exocrine) also produces these enzymes and secretes them into the duodenum (the first six inches of the small intestine) as pancreatin.

If you experience frequent bloating or excessive production of gas it is quite likely due to a lack of enzymes. [It is also possible that the reason for this might be due to a structural blockage of the pancreas. It may be due to pancreatic insufficiency from pancreatitis, removal of the pancreas, and other pancreatic obstructive disorders. It's always good to confer with your physician to check this out.] When such is the case, consider taking a pancreatic enzyme formula available in most health food stores. These formulas typically contain: (Nat Med Comp Data Base.)

- 25 USP (US Pharmacopeia) units of Amylase activity
- 25 USP units of Protease activity
- 02 USP units of Lipase activity

A more potent formula is labeled as a multiple of these three minimum activities, e.g., pancreatin 4X.

There are enterically coated pancreatic formulas designed to dissolve in the duodenum.

There are formulations that contain higher amounts of Lipase activity for those who have specific difficulty digesting fats. (This is often the case with people who have had the gallbladder removed or who have some form of gallbladder dysfunction. The gallbladder delivers bile into the duodenum to help with the break down of fats.) Amongst a variety of other brands in the market, the one product that has an impressive amount of digestive enzymes (including high levels of lipase) is **OmegaZyme**. (This product contains: protease, amylase, lipase, cellulase, lactase, alpha-G, glucoamylase, invertase, malt diastase, pectinase, xylanase, bromelain, papain, probiotics, and botanicals.)

KidZYME (Renew Life) is designed for children. It contains plant enzymes, pepsin, bromelaine, probiotics (e.g., acidophilus, bifidus, F.O.S.), L-glutamine, and N-acetyl-glucosamine to support digestive lining integrity.

Stomach Acid

Betaine Hydrochloride (HCL) is a supplemental form of hydrochloric acid (hydrogen chloride, an acid secreted by the cells lining the stomach). This acid creates the stomach environment that allows the substance pepsinogen to be converted into the enzyme pepsin, which is involved in the breakdown of protein. People who don't secrete sufficient HCL will have difficulty digesting proteins, and they often experience that food "sits" in the stomach for an inordinate amount of time. The incomplete break down of foods can lead to allergic reactions.

Important: HCL kills pathogens that enter through the digestive tract. Low levels of HCL are conducive to gastrointestinal infections that can disturb the natural bacterial ecology (flora) of the system and lead to opportunistic overgrowth of, for instance, candida, overburdening the immune system. If needed, one should consider supplementing with Betaine HCL.

Typical dose can range from 325-650 mg after a meal that contains protein. Do not take on an empty stomach, only after food.

Those who have been diagnosed with acid reflux, hiatal hernia, or ulcers ought to avoid use of this supplement.

There are digestive aids with pancreatic enzymes and HCL for those who have signs of these combined needs.

Stimulants

Sometimes the digestive process is hampered by certain foods, or through wrong food combinations. For instance, the excessive use of raw foods can slow down the digestive "fire" (gastric juices), or the excessive use of mucous-forming foods (dairy) can dowse the digestive "fire" so that food just sits there and ferments in the stomach. One may also experience the loss of appetite. Stimulants can be used to activate the natural production of gastric juices and enzymes in order to foster proper digestion. A sprinkling of salt, or the use of pickled vegetables can be taken before meals to stimulate the digestive system.

Ginger (Root) is a common spice possessing many therapeutic qualities. As a digestive aid ginger counteracts nausea, vomiting, and loss of appetite by stimulating digestive enzymes and modulating a substance known as 5-HT (5-hydroxytryptamine). "Studies suggest that

the daily consumption of ginger might enhance digestive absorption by as much as 200 per cent."[37]

To improve digestion of a meal or to increase absorption of dietary supplements take ginger 10-15 minutes before a meal. Dosages can be given as follows:
- Dried root 1000 mg
- Fresh root 1 tsp grated
- Liquid extract 2 droppers (2 milliliters)
- Syrup 2 tsp (10 milliliters)
- Maximum daily dose is about 4 grams

As a general tonic drink a cup of ginger tea or a glass of homemade ginger ale 1-3 times daily.

As an anti-emetic (vomiting, and for nausea) use 2 grams of powdered ginger taken with a glass of room temperature or warm water.

With children reduce dose to 1/4 to 1/2 of the adult dose.

Avoid using large or therapeutic amounts during pregnancy. For morning sickness it would be best to use red raspberry tea and supplemental vitamin B-6.

Trikatu is a product based on a traditional Ayurvedic formula from India that I have found useful in this regard. It is produced by Planetary Formulas (Three Spices Sinus Complex) and one tablet contains a proprietary blend of 1000 mg of ginger root, long pepper fruit, black pepper seed, and dehydrated honey.

Dosage: 1-2 tablets can be taken just before or with meals as a digestive aid, to increase nutrient absorption, and/or as a stimulant between meals to reduce high levels of mucous.

Calming Agent

Fennel seed is a spicy, sweet, aromatic herb that has been traditionally used for stomach discomfort such as indigestion, gas and flatu-

---

[37] Schulick, P. (1994). Ginger: Common Spice & Wonder Drug. Herbal Free Press, Ltd.: Brattleboro, VT. (P. 45.)

lence, and for spasms of the gastrointestinal tract.

Dosage: it is typically taken as a tea with or between meals as needed. Use 1 tsp per cup of heated water. It can also be taken as a cool tea. The encapsulated powder can be taken from 3-9 grams per day. Usually, dosage starts with 1-2 (1000 mg) capsule(s) at a time.

Laxatives

Excessive bowel dryness or the inability to have regular daily bowel movements can not only clog the system but also increase the toxic load on the body. The gastrointestinal system is populated with a variety of flora (friendly and unfriendly bacteria) that process nutrients and provide antimicrobial activity. When the system is not flowing properly these advantages can be diminished, and when they are, the bowel ecology is disturbed; additional colonies of bacteria may flare up and complicate an ongoing infection with another pathogen. While we have probably heard about using prunes, and perhaps the herb cascara sagrada, there are a few others that I would recommend.

Aloe Vera Powder (not the juice or gel) is made from the skin of the aloe plant, and it is a very effective laxative. Take 1-4 (300-500 mg) capsules with 8 ounces of water near bedtime to ensure bowel movements in the morning.

Magnesium is also very helpful for supporting proper bowel movements. Use between 200-300 mg of magnesium citrate 2-3 times daily with food. The last dose should be as close to bedtime as possible.

KidLAX™ (Renew Life) is a gentle, natural laxative formula for children who experience occasional constipation. Comes in tiny capsule for easy swallowing. Contains: flax seed, prune, fig, rhubarb root, peach leaf, lactobacillus acidophilus, bifidobacterium bifidum and bifidobacterium infantis.

PETS

In addition to their dietary, dogs and cats can benefit from the following preventative formulas.

Vet's 2000
(Multi Vitamin/Mineral for Dogs)[38]
By Nutradontics, Inc.

One tablet contains

Vitamin A (Acetate)	87 IU
Vitamin D3	8.7 IU
Vitamin B1	170 mcg
Vitamin B2	1 mcg
Protein	340 mg
Phosphorous	18 mg
Iron	3 mg
Wheat Germ Oil	5 mg
Lecithin	50 mg
Inositol	4 mg
Soy Bean Concentrate	151 mg
Choline	5 mg
Niacin	60 mcg
Vitamin E	664 mcg

In a base of: meat and bone meal, animal and vegetable fat, iron oxide, and stearic acid.
Dosage: 1 tab for puppies; 2 tabs for small dogs; 3 tabs for medium size dogs; 5 tabs or large dogs; 6 tabs for extra-large dogs. Pregnant/lactating add 50% more. Tablets are chewable or can be crushed and mixed into food.

Vet's 2000
(Multi Vitamin/Mineral for Cats)[39]
By Nutradontics, Inc.

One tablet contains:

Vitamin A (Acetate)	750 IU
Vitamin D3	75 IU
Vitamin B1	0.5 mg
Vitamin B2	0.5 mg
Vitamin B6	0.05 mg
Vitamin B12	0.10 mcg
Protein	250 mg
Dried Brewer's Yeast	250 mg
Dibasic Calcium Phosphate	125 mg
Ferrous Gluconate	8.1 mg
Wheat Germ Oil	1.5 mg
Lecithin	7.5 mg
Cephalin	7.5 mg
Inositol	7.5 mg

[38] Or comparable product.
[39] Or comparable product.

Soy Bean Concentrate	12.5 mg
Choline	1.25 mg
Niacinamide	5.0 mg
Folic Acid	25 mcg

In a base of fish meal, desiccated liver, gelatin, whey, silicon dioxide, iron oxide, magnesium stearate, and stearic acid.

Dosage: Cats 1-2 tabs per day. Kittens 1 tab daily. For pregnant/lactating cats increase dosage by 50% or as directed by a vet. Tablets are chewable or can be crushed and mixed into food.

Green Food for Pets

There are green food supplements for dogs and cats such as **Barley Dog**, and **Barley Cat** produced by **Green Foods**.

The Environmental Line

The environment is one of the most powerful lines of influence because we are inevitably immersed within it. The seasons, the chemical makeup of the atmosphere, the terrain, its water supply, the food sources, its devised objects, and its impressions are factors that deeply affect us holistically in many ways. They combine to create an energy field that can psychologically lift us up or bring us down. They may also add to the toxic load of the mind-body relationship. These ups and downs have a powerful relationship to the immune system.

Environmental Factors Affecting Immunity

Light

There is often talk about the weather, and, for some, a series of cloudy days can cause feelings of depression. This has been studied in countries where cloudy days predominate, and it has been called "seasonal affective disorder" (SAD). People with SAD develop clinical depression and may feel so down as to commit suicide. It was discovered that the depression was brought on by the lack of full-spectrum light emanating from the sun. When those prone to SAD were exposed to (artificially produced) **full-spectrum light** on a regular basis they were relieved of their depression. While they could not alter the weather conditions to remove the clouds, they were able to compensate in their homes to alter their immediate environment as a line of defense. They not only were able to free themselves from depression but they also supported their immune systems in the process of doing so.

Impressions

Many are familiar with the influence chemicals in the atmosphere have on health, but the effect impressions have on our moods, and hence on our physical health, is not so well known. Impressions are the environmental patterns we take in through the senses. These patterns can produce negative or positive effects, and consequently can, as we have seen with the psychological line, affect our health and level of immunity. Persisting foul odors, horrible sights, gray days, and harsh sounds can be just as polluting as a noxious chemical in the air. However, just as the victim of SAD can compensate for the unalterable natural reality, it is possible to expose oneself to positive impressions to achieve the same effect.

Find ways during the day to experience a dose of beauty. Take in the flowers, enjoy the architecture, take some time to read poetry, listen to your favorite music, and so on. Some people apply perfume or a soothing and uplifting essential oil to a handkerchief and periodically take a whiff. In one's home or office (if possible) one can change the energy pattern of the air by vaporizing an essential oil of choice. I use a small ultrasonic humidifier to deliver essential oil scents and decontaminants into the air. (5-10 drops per pint of water.) These environmental measures are especially important during an illness, for they add a vital supportive line of defense.

Air Quality

Today there are few populated areas in the world that are not subject to the effects of industrial, farming, and motor vehicle pollutants. People living in areas known to score high on the pollution index ought to consider compensating with **antioxidant nutrients** that protect the lungs. An air filtration system is another consideration. Additionally, one may also look into getting an <u>Ozone and Negative Ion Generator</u> to clean the air. Such measures help to reduce the toxic load and give the immune system a rest.

Water

Where does the water you drink come from? Is it heavily chlorinated? Many naturalistic practitioners have doubts about the health benefits of chlorinated water. Chlorine is toxic to the body. In small amounts it is not so evident, but over time the incremental effects may add to the toxic load of the system. Water passed through an effective filtration system or high quality bottled water is best.

Physical Factors

Do you live in the "wide open spaces", or in a small town, or in a crowded environment full of concrete, asphalt, and steel? Are there hills? Does the wind blow freely, frequently, or hardly ever at all? Does sunlight shine through into the area or is it often blocked? Do you work in a tight stuffy building? Is it dusty, old, and moldy? How is the air circulated? Is it a high rise? How do you feel about it? These factors can affect your health.

Social Factors

The physical presence of people can have immune consequences. Areas of high population density tend to spread diseases more quickly than sparsely populated areas. Terrorists have focused on highly populated areas where the outcome of an event can have high numbers of physical and emotional casualties. Factors that need to be considered are:

- Places where people congregate to eat, shop, travel;
- The work place;
- Holidays with special symbolic significance;
- Special events of mass attraction (sports, parades, entertainment, political, etc.).

Environmental Signs of Subversive Activity

- Unusual amount of dead or sick animals/birds/fish.
- The lack of activity or absence of animal/birds/fish.
- Unusual amount of dead insects, absence of, or lack of activity.
- Large areas of dead or withered vegetation that cannot be explained naturally.
- Unusual numbers of people experiencing unexplained rashes, blisters, or other skin condition.
- Unusual numbers of sick or dying people with similar symptoms, occurring in a rather short period of time.
- Mass casualties.
- Low lying fog-like clouds.
- Unscheduled aerial spraying, especially at night.
- Strange abandoned packages or spray equipment.
- Sticky and/or oily film on surfaces.
- Loose powdery substances in the atmosphere.
- Packages or mail with no return address or with an unfamiliar return address.

Environmental Protection

As we have seen in the disease process, this stage is where transmission occurs and it is where preventative measures can be implemented. For instance, with mosquito carriers (vectors) of infectious diseases a program to destroy their natural breeding habitats is a commonly used approach. Furthermore, one could increase defense against these creatures with repellents and/or physical barriers such as with clothing or screens.

Diseases caused by WMD would not follow their natural processes but would be introduced into the environment in unpredictable circumstances. However, what can we do as ordinary citizens to protect ourselves from these noxious agents from an environmental perspective? Several important deterrents come to mind, namely, detection, protective items, and decontamination.

Biological Detection

Biosensors are used to identify pathogens released into the environment. The armed forces are surely the leader in the use and development of these instruments. Since 9/11 a flurry of creative activity, spurred by governmental fast track funding, has taken place. The detection industry has improved on the range, sensitivity, accuracy, and portability of these instruments. These devices can be used to test samples on site, or some can be placed in strategic places in a building, etc. The biological detection industry is on the verge of launching some major advances. However, these possibilities are just hitting the market place, and there is great promise that the products will be continually refined. Here are some promising developments to date.

Bio Threat Alert™ Test Strip

The biotech lab, Tetracore, Inc., has produced the BTA™ Test Strip, which provides onsite screening (by first responders) for a series of biological agents. They have test strips for: anthrax (bacterium and spores), ricin toxin, botulism, Staphylococcal enterotoxin B, plague, tularemia, and smallpox. The literature lists the following benefits:

- Rapid hand-held on-site screening test
- Recognizes both vegetative and spore forms
- Anthrax BTA is highly specific: no cross reaction with common bacteria
- Visual results in 1-15 minutes
- Economical and compact
- Can be used with individuals and for feedback with decontamination

To do the test, a sample is gathered and placed into a tiny well on the strip, which is about the size of a credit card. Next to the

well is a small window that will provide feedback as to whether the sample is positive or negative for the agent being measured. A highly concentrated sample will take about 1 minute to get the result whereas a more diluted one may take up to 15 minutes. The BTA™ Test Strip employs a technology similar to that used in many laboratory medical screening tests.

The technique used is known as lateral flow immunochromatography. The actual chemistry involved uses unique biological substances or "antibodies" that are specifically attracted to the target substance. When the level of the target substance is present above a certain amount or concentration, the antibodies and the target substance combine in the strip and form a reddish band that appears in the "S" Window. Even though this is considered a very accurate screening device, results from the Beta Strip still need to be confirmed by a qualified reference laboratory. This is required of all screening tests.

Handheld Advanced Nucleic Acid Analyzer (HANAA)

This detection system is being developed by the Lawrence Livermore National Laboratory, which is operated by the University of California for the U.S. Department of Energy. According to the literature on the HANAA system:

- Uses a technique known as *polymerase chain reaction* (PCR), which amplifies the DNA of the agent to a detectable level
- A probe is inserted into the unit to identify the signature DNA of the agent.
- It is about the size of a brick and weighs less than a kilogram (approximately 2 1/2 lbs.)
- Was designed for emergency response groups such as fire fighters, police, etc.
- Each system can test four samples at once
- Produce results within 30 minutes

- The system doesn't test for all unknowns
- The operator must have an idea of what germ is being tested for

This system, in my opinion, would work well with the BTA™ test strip as a way to roughly determine the pathogen, and quickly confirm the finding. However, the system could in principle detect as few as 10 individual bacteria in a sample in less than 30 minutes.

Autonomous Pathogen Detection System (APDS)

Again, the Lawrence Livermore National Laboratories has developed the APDS, which is a system capable of 24-hour monitoring for pathogens. This system:

- Is about the size and shape of a lectern or mailbox
- Would be situated in one strategic spot
- Functions like a "smoke detector", picking up aerosol particulate
- Analyzes the samples using PCR and flow cytometry, which uses antibodies to identify the pathogens
- Delivers quite accurate results within 30 minutes
- Is being expanded to detect hundreds of pathogens simultaneously in one sample.

Detection of Chemical Agents

Again, the detection of chemical WMD has been a concern for the armed forces; most of what exists is for military purposes, although there is some industrial use of the technology. HAZMAT teams are also using this kind of equipment, but not to the degree that they need to be. Cost of the devices and funding has much to do with this. New developments have emerged that make these possibilities more affordable. Several seem outstanding.

SAW MINICAD mk II

This is one kind of detector that seems practical for use by first-responders, certain interested groups, or even individuals. It is a portable, lightweight, and battery operated surface acoustic wave (SAW) chemical detector.

These kinds of detectors are able to identify and measure many chemical agents simultaneously. The SAW MINICAD mk II detects Nerve and Blister Agents (GA, GB, GD, GF, & HD), and it can be used remotely to define areas of exposure and to determine degree of decontamination. It is inexpensive and available commercially.

Dräger Civil Defense System

Headquartered in Germany, where it is known as Draegerwerk, Dräger is one of the leaders in the manufacture of toxic chemical and explosive detectors. It produces a device known as the Dräger CDS Agent Testing System, which utilizes colorimetric detector tubes to test up to 5 different chemical agents simultaneously, including nerve, blood, lung, and nose and throat irritating agents. This is a portable system that is sold commercially to the public.

MAXxess

MAXxess is a company that specializes in the design and manufacture of high-level security electronics and management systems. It is owned by Odetics, Inc., based in Anaheim, CA, and provides products and systems that employ information technology in the security business. MAXxess now has the exclusive capability of integrating the Dräger Gas Detection Systems with its security management software. The Dräger sensor system can detect all principal chemical WMD, plus over 1000 more. Most U.S. Fire Departments use Dräger equipment.

These sensors can be placed strategically in any facility, around the perimeter, at vehicle entrances and loading docks, or wherever a threat is expected. Hand held devices could be used to monitor personnel and vehicles.

The sensor stations are small, portable and mobile. The detectors can continuously sample multiple remote locations. When a toxic chemical is detected, a particular alarm is automatically displayed at the designated security control room along with the corresponding video display, indicating where the threat is present. The automated response also alerts the operator to open or close doors in order to evacuate areas, isolate areas, and aid emergency responders. This is perhaps one of the most sophisticated detection systems available commercially to the public.

Radiation Detectors

Because radiation cannot be detected by the senses, measuring devices are needed to become aware of its presence and potential harmful levels. There are two kinds of radiation detectors: **Survey meters** such as a Geiger counter, and **dosimeters**. Survey meters measure the amount of radiation in the environment whereas the dosimeter measures the amount of radiation exposure to tissue incurred over a certain period of time.

There are many radiation detectors on the market since these devices have a variety of medical and industrial applications. Prices and claims of effectiveness will vary. Perhaps the most informative source and supplier of such equipment can be found on the Internet at **radmeters4U.com.**

This company provides a variety of survey meters (both new and refurbished), dosimeters, and service. They also provide valuable information on how to evaluate and protect oneself from nuclear incidents (mainly from a large megaton bomb). Before venturing into purchasing a radiation detection device, I would strongly recommend learning as much as possible about what these detectors do and how they work.

For those who like to tinker and learn and not spend too much money, there is the **1 KFM Kit** (the Kearney Fallout Radiation Meter), available from **radmeters4U.com**. It has everything needed to make and use a radiation measuring device. It accurately measures dose rates from 30 Mr/hr (0.30 R/hr) up to 43 R/hr.[40] The KFM was developed by Cresson H. Kearney[41] at the Oak Ridge National Laboratory, and it has undergone rigor-

ous scientific testing in several laboratories to confirm its accuracy and dependability. The unit comes with very detailed construction, operating and testing instructions. This would make an excellent project for a Neighborhood Defense Support Group!

For the slightly more technically inclined, a practical detector is the **Gamma-Scout®** (GS). It is a light, compact, hand held unit that fits comfortably in hand or pocket. It has the following features:

- Remains on all the time to check for alpha, beta, gamma, and x-rays in the environment.
- Determines potential exposure time of tissue in terms of *microsievert* units of measurement[42].
- It is supplied with a long life 10 year V-Max® battery.
- It is shock resistant.
- Has a large digital display.
- An easy-to-read multi-function 9-button keypad with numerous options for data display including date, time.
- GS Comes with User Guide, CD-ROM, Computer Cable to connect to a PC for evaluation, and a Carrying Case. It can be used in the home and/or work place.

Bio-Chemical Shelter

To reduce exposure to biological and chemical agents released in the outer environment, go indoors and turn on the radio or television for information on the status of the problem. Inside, put on protective mask (if available), close all doors, seal all windows with packaging or comparable tape. Seal off air passage ways and ducts such as fire places, chimney flues, air conditioners, and the like. Some tips for creating a bio-chemically safe room or area are:

- Choose an area with the least amount of windows or no windows at all (if available)

---

[40] See chapter Potential Nuclear Threats for more information on these measures.

[41] Author of a book I highly recommend: *Nuclear War Survival Skills.*

[42] For definition see section on Potential Nuclear Agents.

- Seal it off from the outer environment with packaging or duct tape
- Use large plastic clear sheets (e.g., paint drop cloths) with no holes or tears in them, to seal the windows, etc.
- A rolled up damp towel(s) can be used to seal the gap at the base of the door(s)
- The room would ideally be close to a bathroom, most of which could also be sealed off
- A portable toilet could also be made available if bathroom is not nearby
- A 3 week storage of emergency food, water, and supplies should be prepared
- Portable or makeshift beds (air mattresses, sleeping bags, etc.) could also be added
- Emergency first aid kit, masks, gloves, and plastic bags for waste
- Supply of decontaminant solution (e.g., GSE, or ASAP) in large spray bottle
- Electric heater, blankets, might be useful depending on the area and climate
- Add other items that meet your special needs such as for children, size of family, those with special medical needs, housemates, friends, pets, etc.
- This room could also be used to quarantine victims of contagious diseases
- Two rooms might be used or turned into emergency safety quarters

Positive/Negative Overpressure Bio-Safe Room(s)

The *American Civil Defense Association* recommends preparing an area that would filter out harmful pathogens using a vacuum cleaner or a HEPA filter. The following outline is gleaned from their recommendations:

Vacuum Cleaner Method:
- A common vacuum cleaner can be used (as was publicized by the late Dr. Conrad Chester of the Oak Ridge National Lab) to create a bio-safe room in your home or apartment

- Use a HEPA filter or a very dirty filter bag (a clean one will not work) in **only** one room with a window or opening to the outside
- Place the sucking wand halfway outside the window, and close the window on the wand and seal around it with plastic sheet, pillows, etc., using tape to secure (A precut piece of plywood to fit the window with a hole for the wand would be a good choice)
- After completion of set up, turn the unit on and let it run
- The filtered air enters the room and exits through cracks in the door and walls, etc, forming a bio-safe positively pressurized environment
- **Drawback:** the air entering will have the temperature of the air outside, and one would need to compensate for that in the room with a heater, fan, or cooling device. Moreover, this is not a long-term solution since the motor of the vacuum cleaner could burn out.

HEPA Filter Method:
- Use a small HEPA filter forced-air purifier to pull air from one room into another enclosed room. Choose a unit with a "system" HEPA rating, not just for the filter element, capable of killing bacteria, viruses via an electronically-charged ionizing filter.
- This will maintain the ambient temperature in the house or apartment
- There will be no need to open a window
- However, it may require opening a space through a wall to place the unit
- Another possibility would be to build out of ply wood, or even sturdy cardboard, an air-tight box that fits snugly (and sealed with tape) around the exhaust end of the HEPA unit with a 5 inch hole cut at the other side, where one would attach a flexible plastic duct tube used in woodworking shops to filter out dust into a huge vacuum cleaner (you won't need this). This

tube would empty out in the other room, or even out a window. These tubes and all the fittings are available from woodworker retail stores such as Woodworker's Warehouse.

Entire House/Apartment Bio-Filtration:
(See the **Sanuvox** units mentioned below under Ultra Violet Light to decontaminate.)

Important: Bio-Chemical Safety Rooms **are not** suitable to protect against **radioactive fallout**. However, a shelter designed to shield radioactive particles could also be designed as a bio-chemical safety area.

Decontamination

In clinical settings certain environmental measures are used to prevent further transmission of contaminating disease. One is physical isolation of patients that have been exposed, and the use of masks and gowns. Another involves the use of decontaminants where germs tend to gather such as hypochlorite solutions (chlorine and water) and iodine.

- Formula for 0.5% hypochlorite solution to decontaminate skin: 1 part of regular **Clorox** for every 10 parts of water.
- Or: 1 part of **Ultra Strength Bleach** products for every 12 parts of water.
- Wash whole body or affected area with soap and water. (Not on eyes.)
- Use the hypochlorite solution as needed. (**Not on eyes.**)
- Don't use on open wounds.
- After applying wash off **no later than 5 minutes** with soap and water.

In terms of the environment hypochlorite solutions are the conventional decontaminant of choice. The problem with these solutions is that they are highly irritating to human tissue. They are also corrosive to many materials. Yet most agents can be neutralized with hypochlorite solution. What follows are some natural substitutes that are not harmful to human tissue and they are safe to the environment.

Vinegar
Vinegar diluted with water in varying concentrations can serve as a useful disinfectant. The ratio of vinegar to water that I have used as a surface disinfectant is 1-part vinegar to 2-parts water. It is an inexpensive way to clean shower stalls, toilets, etc., and to clean fruits and vegetables.

Tea Tree Oil
Tea tree oil is a powerful topical antiseptic that can be used in place of iodine. However, environmentally, I prefer to use it in an ultrasonic humidifier or mister to reduce the germ load in the air indoors.

Grapefruit Seed Extract
In my opinion, grapefruit seed extract (GSE) is the "gold standard" for natural disinfectants. According to the master herbalist Louise Tenney: "GSE is very powerful and effective, even when greatly diluted. In fact in a recent study at the Bio Research Laboratories of Redmond, Washington, GSE was compared to iodine, clorox bleach, tea tree oil and colloidal silver in order to determine which subsance worked best against certain microbes. GSE came out on top against all five microbes tested: *Candida albicans, Staphylococcus aureus, Salmonella typhi, Streptococcus faecium and E. coli.*"[43] GSE must always be diluted before being used. As a disinfectant add 40 drops to 1 quart (1 liter) of water. **Never use on eyes.** Can be used to clean hands, surfaces, eating utensils, toothbrushes, fruits and vegetables, rooms, linens, etc. It is one of the few disinfectants that can be ingested to work as a broad-spectrum antimicrobial.

Aerosolizers
A variety of these devices (misters, ultrasonic humidifiers, vaporizers, etc.) can be used with several essential oils (see Specific Line) to keep an environmental space fairly clean of pathogens.

---

[43] (2000). Grapefruit Seed Extract. Woodland Publishing. Pleasant Grove, UT. (P. 6.)

Ozone

In my office I use an ozone (03) generator to disinfect the area between clients. Ozone is a potent germicide. Ozone generators are being used to reduce the microbe load in agricultural settings. It can also be used to decontaminate water. What's useful about ozone is that it doesn't present any negative side effects to people or the environment.

Water Supply

Water purifiers are another way to protect against contaminated water. An effective water purification system that will provide decontamination of pathogens and toxic particulates is made by **EcoQuest**. This unit treats the water with ultraviolet rays and ozone, prior to passing it through a carbon filter. Ultraviolet light has been a standard method of water purification for well over 50 years for municipalities, water bottling plants, and hospitals.

As an extra precaution, all filtered water should be boiled for at least 10 minutes to ensure biological safety, and/or be decontaminated (see below). Pour back-and-forth into two containers to increase the oxygen content of the water to make it taste better.

The **Steri-Pen** (Hydro Photon) is a small (8 oz, 7 inches, fits in a coat pocket, pocket book, or brief case, etc.) and highly sophisticated battery powered, water purification system, using ultraviolet light. It is designed to treat up to 16 oz of clear water at a time. To operate, Steri-Pen is activated with a simple button sequence. After less than 1 minute of gentle stirring, the treated water is disinfected and ready to drink. University testing has shown it to cause a 99.9999% reduction of bacteria and greater than 99.99% reduction of viruses. The benefit of using ultraviolet light as the decontaminant is that it avoids the use of potentially toxic chemicals such as chlorine and iodine.

Should the water supply in one's area become contaminated beyond use, one would need to rely on bottled or stored water.

It may also be possible to draw water out of the air using a water-generating machine called **Vapaire**. This unit:

- Works like a dehumidifier
- Purifies the water through a 5-stage filtration process using replaceable filters available from the local hardware store
- Produces between 5-15 gallons per day depending on the humidity (2 gallons in very dry climates)
- Is economical in that the approximate cost per gallon is 25 cents
- Needs no plumbing or assembly
- Uses 110V or 220V power outlet
- Is about the size of an office water cooler
- Has a built in antimicrobial system

Personally, I would add some trace minerals (like **Concentrace**) to the water to compensate for the distillation process. Distilled water has no minerals and will leach minerals from the body. This would not be necessary when it is used for washing.

A regular dehumidifier could be used as a makeshift water source. The water-collecting pan would need to be cleaned and sterilized with GSE solution (see above). The collected water would then need to be passed through a filtering device, with some decontamination solution added, and then be stored in containers. Add trace minerals to the finished product. It could also be reserved for washing needs.

In a pinch, lacking these devices, one could disinfect bacterially contaminated water using 3 drops of grapefruit seed extract per 8 ounces (237 ml) of water. The taste would be a bit bitter, but drinkable. To reduce the slightly bitter taste, consider passing the water through a pitcher filter system (like the Britta™) after letting it sit for 30 minutes.

Another water decontaminant is a 96% elemental silver solution, known as **ASAP Solution®**, developed by American Biotech Labs, in Alpine, Utah. It is one of the most powerful antibacterial decontaminants on the market today. Research has shown that it can kill all the bacteria in raw river water in less than 20 minutes.

It is currently being tested by the FDA for approval for use on both humans and animals. It is very safe. Even when tested at 200 times the normal adult dosage, ASAP Solution® was found to be completely non-toxic. To decontaminate water, add 8 oz to 6.25 (and wait 2 minutes) or 12.5 gallons (and wait 20 minutes) of water. Tastes much better than water decontaminated with chlorine.

If none of these natural options are available, water can be made drinkable by adding **4 drops** of <u>pure</u> **liquid bleach (<u>with only sodium hypochlorite as the active ingredient, not the colorfast brands nor those with additives like scents or phosphate</u>**s) into **1 quart of water**. Let the solution sit for 30-60 minutes. Note: potency of liquid bleach begins to diminish after 6 months on the shelf.

In an emergency nuclear situation, where electricity is unavailable, one could devise a **water filtration container**. This can be done by punching small holes around the center of a large can or bucket. Then place 1 inch of washed pebbles at the bottom, and cover with a layer of porous cloth (towel, etc.). Gather enough uncontaminated soil from the ground (by scraping 5 inches off the surface) to pack 8 inches as the next layer in the can. Cover this layer with cloth, and add another inch or so of pebbles. Hang it over a collecting vessel. This water, while quite cleared of radiation, still needs to be decontaminated by any of the methods recommended above.

Water may be stored in thoroughly washed plastic, glass, fiberglass or enamel-lined metal containers. Never use a container that has held toxic substances. Sound plastic containers, such as soft water or soft-drink bottles are good. There are a variety of containers of food-grade containers of all sizes available on the market.

Emergency Daily Water Needs Per Adult

1.5-2 Quarts: Minimal amount for drinking in cool-cold climate. Double for nursing mothers, and during hot weather. None will be available for cooking or washing.

1 Gallon: Minimal amount for drinking, some cooking, and washing in cool-cold weather. Double for nursing mothers, and during hot weather.

2 Gallons: Ideal amount, allowing for cooking dry foods, washing utensils and the body, and nursing mothers. For all weather conditions. Allowing for some mild physical exertion.

Clothing/Linens/Towels

Whenever possible, wear a protective mask (or a makeshift handkerchief, dampened with <u>GSE solution</u>) to protect from harmful aerosols.

- Avoid touching eyes, nose, or mouth.
- Don't try to brush or shake off powders, etc. (See chapter on Potential Nuclear Threats for how to deal with radioactive fallout on clothing.)
- Ideally, spray clothing with GSE solution to keep aerosols down to provide an initial decontaminant. Keep from spraying the eyes.
- All contaminated clothing should be removed (unless not recommended for a particular agent under the Supportive Lines of Defense) and placed in a plastic bag, sealed, and marked as "hazardous material".
- Clothing (if necessary to reuse), linens, towels of the exposed or sick need to be washed (or discarded) with detergent containing bleach or GSE solution.
- Shoes should be sprayed (or washed) with hypochlorite or GSE solution and wiped clean.
- Whenever possible, wear rubber gloves when decontaminating, then wash gloves with soap and water before taking them off. Take off and hang to dry.

People/Pets

Soap and water, wash-and-rinse is the best way to decontaminate exposed skin areas or the whole body. <u>Tea Tree Oil Soap</u> would be ideal. Showering is best, but if a shower, or running, or clean water are not available use a large spray bottle with <u>GSE Solution</u> or <u>ASAP Solution®</u> initially followed by a copious spraying with large bottle filled with plain clean water (may need to be decontaminated if not clean). Use only plain water on eyes. Wipe down with paper towels, and discard in plastic bag for hazardous materials. Use protective gear if biological or chemical aerosols pose a hazard in the area.

Caution: Skin exposure to **Mustard Chemical agents** should **not** be washed down with water since it will spread the reaction. Water, in this instance, should only be used on the eyes. (See chapter on Potential Chemical Weapons for more information.) The **CENTECH GROUP, Inc.,** offers several professional decontamination kits for mustard agents. They also provide kits **for when the toxic substance is unknown**.

Biodegradable soap, GSE solution, or ASAP Solution® would be best for pets since they would have a tendency to lick themselves. These formulas would not be toxic. ASAP Solution® might be best with cats since they use their paws to clean themselves near their eyes. These solutions are nontoxic for children as well.

Common Sources of Contamination
Biological, chemical, and nuclear agents (see Potential Nuclear Threats for specifics) may settle on objects—door handles, levers, buttons, hand rails, telephones, switches, and the like—that are likely to be touched, causing a potential source of contamination. For biological agents spray with GSE solution (since it is non-corrosive) or hypochlorite solution. For chemical agents use hypochlorite solution since I have no knowledge that GSE solution would work in this regard.

Caution: Certain forms of **Mustard Gas** (which is actually a liquid), and especially **Lewisite**, are not very soluble in water and **cannot** be easily cleaned off surfaces.

Ultraviolet Light
Ultraviolet light (UVL) is also another decontaminant, but the intensity of the light (in terms of angstrom units[44]) is an important variable for it to be effective against different strains of bacteria. Ultraviolet light is used by the heating and air conditioning industry to protect these systems from being damaged by bacteria that eat the wires and the lubricants.

The problem with UVL is that it emits in straight lines that don't go around curved surfaces. So they are used in combination with synergistic chemical decontaminants. Nevertheless, these devices could be used in air ducts quite effectively, as long as the flow time of air is taken into consideration, because if it is too fast it will not allow enough light exposure to kill the pathogens.

Sanuvox are residential and light-commercial in-duct units that use a patented process involving ultraviolet light of germicidal intensities to purify the air. These units destroy viruses, bacteria, and mold, and neutralize chemical and biological contaminants. (However, I would not rely on them to detoxify chemical WMD.)

Protective Items
Disposable Medical Grade Respiratory Masks/Gloves
To provide protection against contact with or inhalation of biological agents, one should use a medical-grade mask capable of filtering organisms of 0.1 microns (or smaller) in size. These masks are available from the **MD Depot** and other sources.

Use latex (or comparable non-allergenic type for those who are sensitive to latex) gloves in an exposed area and whenever helping an exposed or sick person.

Caution: Any kind of mask should fit snugly against the face, forming an airtight seal. Men with beards need to take this into consideration, and they may need special masks. Replace used masks when they become clogged (resistance to breathing in-

---

[44] Angstrom is a unit for measuring the wavelength of radiant energy.

creases), damaged, or compromised in some way.

Protecting the Eyes

With diseases and chemical agents that can affect the delicate mucous membranes of the eyes, one would need to wear some form of protection. Some of the gas masks mentioned below provide this protection. However, one could complement masks that only cover the nose and mouth with swimmer's or scuba goggles. Small swimmer's goggles would be easier to carry and leave in various locations.

Protective Clothing

Perhaps the most practical gear to wear during biological, chemical, or nuclear incidents (after major fallout has cleared some 48 hours later), in addition to a mask and rubber gloves, are a waterproof rain poncho and high rubber boots. They should be decontaminated after use in an exposed area.

For those people who would like to go the extra mile, I would recommend that they look into acquiring professional gear, consisting of boots, gloves, and cover-all outfits, providing a higher range of NBC (nuclear, biological, and chemical) protection. These products should be bio-chemically absorbent, durable, air permeable (to support evaporative cooling), possibly fire resistant, and comfortable. To ensure absorbability, the fabric and construction should contain a *polymerically encapsulated carbon*. Some of these outfits include hood protection. If not, mask and hood protection would be required as separate items.

Sources for such gear are army surplus outlets (locally and on the Internet), and companies specializing in the manufacture and/or distribution of these products. A few examples are:

- **Xymid, LLC**, which provides chemical protective under-and-over garments to the military and first-responder organizations. They carry the LANX fabric systems that meet all the above-mentioned requirements.

- **ProtectiveSuits.com** is another source that provides 3M Emergency Response kits such as the one that includes: coveralls with attached hood and boots, Hazmat booties, Nitrile or Butyl gloves, and carrying bags.

Protective Containers for Food, Water, Etc.

During and/or before a biological, chemical, or nuclear attack all food and water should be stored in tightly sealed hard (non-leaching) plastic or glass containers. Non-refrigerated items should be stored in a dry, cool, place away from direct sunlight. Before opening the containers, they should be wiped with a paper towel (moistened with hypochlorite or GSE solution, and discarded).

Food and water stored for emergency situations should be periodically used and replaced to avoid spoilage.

Portable Emergency Gas Mask

While it is impractical to wear a gas mask all the time, it may be lifesaving to have one to traverse a site known to be contaminated with chemical WMD. Of all the choices that are available in the market, the one that seemed the most practical is the one manufactured in Israel. One of the U.S. distributors, **Joseph Prep** describes it as follows:

"EMERGENCY MASK is a Respiratory Protective Escape Device (RPED) designed to reduce the health risks and mortality rates associated with inhalation of toxic air. Pocket size (5 1/2" x 4 1/4" x 3/4") and lightweight (7 oz), EMERGENCY MASK is designed to be instantly available at all times. It can be carried discreetly or stored just about anywhere. It is maintenance free and has a five (5) year shelf life. In a toxic emergency, when each breath may carry illness or death, EMERGENCY MASK can be donned in seconds. To use simply tear open the sealed foil pouch, remove, unfold and pull the mask over your head. EMERGENCY MASK is comprised of a seamless hood with integrated visor and filter sections. The fire-resistant hood protects the entire head and seals at the neck. A fire-resistant visor protects the eyes and provides a wide field of view. The filter contain layers of charcoal cloth to absorb toxic gases and a particulate element to remove harmful particles including: Acrolein, Ammonia, Carbon Tetrachloride, Chlorine, DMMP (Sarin Nerve Gas Simulant), Hexane, Hydrogen Chloride, Hydrogen Cyanide, Hydrogen Sulphide, Nitrogen Dioxide, Sulfur Dioxide, Tear Gas (CS & CN), Pepper Spray (OC), Smoke Particles and Soot. **Notice:** This devices does not filter carbon monoxide—a lethal gas associated with fire." One size fits all adults. It has a passive design ideal for victim rescue. The mask is disposable.

EVAC-U8® Emergency
Escape Smoke Hood

This mask was designed to escape the noxious fumes of a fire. However, it is also an excellent portable gas mask providing up to 20 minutes of safety. The information on this equipment is as follows:

EVAC-U8® is currently in use by agencies and departments of the U.S. Federal and the Canadian governments worldwide. EVAC-U8® is effective against Carbon Monoxide. Built into the canister, slightly larger than a beverage can, is a multi-stage, air-purifying, chemical catalytic filter that removes carbon monoxide and other deadly gases present in fire. It requires little training or maintenance, and no fit testing is required. One size fits all. Its superior mouthpiece design combined with a positive pressure hood makes it highly resistant to edge leakage. It is effective against chemical agents such as Phosphene, Sarin, Tabun, and VX nerve gas! It is an affordable, essential piece of equipment for travel, providing peace of mind at home or office.

The Specific Line of Defense

The specific supportive line of defense would be considered after one has been, or is suspected to have been, exposed to a WMD. So in a sense there is some prevention involved, but for the most part it would be a way of caring for oneself (and/or others) after general or more advanced symptoms have appeared.

It is important to remember that these recommendations do not necessarily exclude conventional forms of medical treatment. They were designed to help someone who has no immediate access to the emergency health care system. They can also be used together with conventional care. This of course would be a decision that would be made by you and your physician.

For the sake of economy and expediency, I've selected what I consider to be the most effective products based on my personal experience as a naturopath and from extensive research. I've also sought to recommend supplements with multiple uses so that a relatively small repertoire can be employed in various ways.

Common Conditions
Related To WMD

In studying the mechanisms of disease presented by the agents, a number of recurring conditions emerged that I felt were the most important to address.

Initial

These are what physicians refer to as *prodromal* signs. They often resemble the coming on of a cold or the flu. During a crisis event, they may be evaluated more severely.

- Headache
- Fever
- Sweating
- Chills
- Cough (productive/nonproductive)
- Rashes

- Pimples
- Muscle aches
- Bone-joint discomfort/pain
- Tiredness, fatigue
- Nausea/Vomiting
- Dizziness

These symptoms actually point to the side effects, so to speak, of the general immune response getting into gear. Treating the symptoms might not have any bearing on the progression of the disease (e.g., relieving the headache, stopping the fever). Nevertheless, early diagnosis and medical treatment provide distinct advantages.

Nutripenia

During this period, the system is undergoing a drain on its nutrient stores, creating a condition that I have called *mild or localized nutripenia*. This condition is similar to what orthomolecular physicians have referred to as *anascorbemia*, the disease-evoked deficiency of vitamin C (ascorbic acid).[45] Nutripenia encompasses a larger range of vital nutrients that are lost to the disease process. Consumption of these vital nutrients will be taken from the tissue at or near the site of exposure. As the disorder progresses, nutrients will be drawn from other tissues around the body. According to this naturalistic point of view, the nutritional status of a person at the time of exposure will determine how long these prodromal symptoms may last and how intense they may be. It may also determine the extent to which the medical treatments may succeed.

In my view, it would be advantageous to replace the important nutrients as soon as these early signs appear. At the same time one can challenge the nature of the disease in both the conventional and natural manners.

---

[45] See: Cathcart, (MD), R., Vitamin C, Titrating To Bowel Tolerance, Anascorbemia, And Acute Induced Scurvy.

More Serious

As the disease or condition progresses, more serious developments emerge that may include any of the following general patterns.

Systemic Infection

Infection is a bacterial and/or viral invasion of tissue. Pathogens often use the lymphatic system and the blood stream to transport themselves around the body and spread their effects.

The lymphatic system consists of a vast network of thin vessels (capillaries), valves, ducts, nodes, and organs (tonsils, thymus, and spleen) involved in protecting and maintaining the fluid environment of the entire body. It also produces various blood cells. The lymphatic network transports nutrients and other substances to the blood system. It detoxifies and nurtures. Lymphocytes circulate in the lymphatic system and comprise about 25% of the white blood cell count. This percentage increases during infection. At certain areas in the body the lymphatic system intersects with the circulatory system to exchange fluids.

Lymphatic nodes distributed in certain key areas around the body (such as in the mouth, neck, arm pits, and the groin) trap and destroy pathogens, and, in doing so become swollen. The flow of the lymphatic fluid depends on physical movement of voluntary and involuntary muscles, and consequently, this is a slower moving system than the blood. Invasion of the blood spreads the disease more quickly, and it can lead to sepsis and shock, which often is life threatening.

Toxicity

Toxicity is the degree to which a noxious chemical or radiological element has invaded the tissue and caused damage, especially to the cell's nucleus (DNA).

Inflammation

Inflammation is characterized by redness, heat, swelling, tenderness, and pain, and can affect any organ system. It can produce conditions such as bronchitis or encephalitis (all the terms ending in ...*itis*), and pneumonia.

Edema

Edema often accompanies inflammation. It is an excessive accumulation of fluid that has been released from the small blood or lymphatic vessels (capillaries) into the tissues.

Cardiovascular/Blood Complications

Shock is a life-threatening situation that can be brought on by exposure to almost any of the WMD. It is essentially a physical condition in which the circulation becomes so compromised that the blood cannot reach the tissue of the vital organ systems. It is characterized by hypotension (very low blood pressure). Shock may be brought on by a variety of causes such as: blood loss, dehydration, serious infection, sudden expansion of blood vessels, allergic reactions, sudden decrease in blood sugar, and strong emotional events. The cause either lowers the vascular tension needed to maintain the blood pressure, or reduces the volume of blood needed to fill the blood vessels. Consequently, the lack of blood circulation causes the tissue to lose warmth and nutrients. Signs of shock include: cold moist skin, pallor, rapid breathing and heart rate, weakness, nausea, vomiting, and reduced consciousness. Treatment for shock involves the maintaining of body fluids (through IV drip), and, with loss of blood, the infusion of red blood cells. To help a person undergoing shock:

- Seek medical help immediately.
- Keep the person warm by covering the entire body with a blanket or coat. Use any kind of insulation such as leaves, paper, etc. if other items are not available.
- Check for a Medic Alert necklace or bracelet that might provide clues of the condition.
- Keep person in a horizontal position; find something to keep legs raised about 1 foot above the heart. Injured arms or legs should also be raised as well. All this reduces the load on the heart.
- If person is bleeding attempt to stop the blood flow by:

- Covering the wound with clean cloth or gauze or, if these are lacking, apply firm pressure with your hand.

Altered heart beat: too fast or too slow.

Hemorrhage: blood leakage into surrounding tissue.

Thrombocytopenia: blood leakage due to lack of the blood clotting factors of thrombocytes (platelets).

Hemolysis: rupture of red blood cells.

Immune Cells

Leukopenia: a lower than normal amount of white blood cells in the blood.

Gastrointestinal

Diarrhea (severe): a massive loss of fluids through the colon.

Respiratory

Dyspnea: shortness of breath.

Apnea: temporary stopping of breathing.

Inflammation, of the upper and lower respiratory system.

Skin

Burns: first degree, involving the superficial layers of skin; second degree, involving all but the deepest layers of skin; third degree, involving all the layers of skin and possibly the tissue beneath the skin. Inflamed and/or destroyed tissue.

Blisters: a pooling of serum or blood just under the superficial layer of the skin.

Neurological/Psychological

Paralysis: stoppage of neuromuscular activity.

Confusion: the inability to make decisions/disorientation.

Seizures/Convulsions: chaotic neuromuscular reactions.

Coma: loss of consciousness.

Distorted vision: blurriness, double vision.

Depression: no hope for the future.

Lack of Oxygen to the Tissue

Many of the disorders become serious due to (for one reason or another) the lack of oxygen to the tissue, a condition known as *anoxia*. A sign that anoxia is on the rise occurs when the heartbeat and breathing rates increase.

With severe anoxia, the mechanisms that regulate breathing fail. If at all possible, the body compensates by producing energy by the less efficient method of *anaerobic* (without oxygen) respiration. The tissue most sensitive to lack of oxygen are the brain, heart, pulmonary vessels, and liver.

Medical treatments to alleviate the anoxic burden include: the use of cardiovascular and respiratory stimulant drugs, mechanical ventilation, and oxygen therapy, accompanied by the monitoring of blood gases. People can increase the chances for survival with many of the WMD by using a portable supply of oxygen.

Nutritional

Severe Nutripenia: an acute or chronic massive loss of vital nutrients. As can be surmised, the most important nutrients are those that protect the various mechanisms of oxygen delivery to the tissue.

Seven Healing Strategies

Many of these conditions are caused by toxic chemicals, which are produced by germs or by human beings. The antitoxin strategy behind most conventional and naturalistic therapies encompasses seven healing strategies. These healing strategies are common to both conventional and natural forms of healing. They involve: *replacement, activation, antimicrobials, protective resistance, detoxification, regulation*, and *homeopathy*.

Let's take a look at how natural modalities for healing fulfill these objectives. Viewing naturalistic forms of healing from this perspective might help us to see the synergy that can exist between conventional and naturalistic therapies to support emergency health care.

Replacement

This strategy aims to sustain the mind-body complex by replacing vital substances lost to the toxic assault. It could use IV drips, blood transfusions, nutrients, or oxygen. The naturalistic approach extends the conventional one by adding the compensatory measures for nutripenia. The following nutrients are considered to be vital in this regard.

Oxygen

Naturalistic practitioners may refer to oxygen as vitamin O. We don't produce it, and it's vital for life. An available source of oxygen during an emergency can mean the difference between life and death. Emergency medical responders will usually have it on hand. It can also be made available through Hyperbaric Oxygen therapy.

Hyperbaric oxygenation involves the use of specially designed chambers that permit the delivery of 100% oxygen, by a professionally trained person, at an atmospheric pressure that is three times the normal level. This causes more oxygen to be absorbed by the blood.

Most WMD are likely to have a damaging effect on the respiratory system. A rehabilitation program might seriously consider using breathing exercises, such as the yoga *pranayama*, to restore respiratory health.

Vitamin C

Vitamin C (ascorbate) performs many healthful functions in the body. It is involved in tissue growth and repair, immune function, and it helps to metabolize other nutrients. It is a major nutrient for the adrenal glands, supporting the production of anti-stress hormones. As an antioxidant it binds to and excretes toxins from the body. It works inside cells (intracellularly) as well as in the spaces around them (extracellularly). While studies show that the intracellular needs may not exceed 200 mg the extracellular needs are many times more.

Vitamin C and E work synergistically to augment their effects more so than when taken alone. Because they can increase the absorption of iron they should not be taken together with bacterial infections (since iron supports bacterial growth).

The need for vitamin C can range between 500-2000 mg with relatively healthy individuals. Some may need considerably more. Because it is excreted in the urine, stores need to be replenished on a daily basis. With illness (or any form of stress) the need for C increases dramatically.

Many serious infectious diseases have been treated successfully by orthomolecular physicians by using oral or intravenously administered ascorbate. Because the symptoms of many of these disorders are quite similar to scurvy, the lack of vitamin C, or *anascorbemia*, is seen as the underlying cause.[46] The relationship between scurvy and the lack of vitamin C has been well established.

The symptoms of scurvy are quite similar to those produced by infectious diseases and to the toxic overload from noxious chemicals and radiation. Scurvy is characterized by: lassitude, malaise, bleeding gums, loss of teeth, nosebleeds, bruising, hemorrhages in any part of the body, easily acquired infections, poor healing of wounds, deterioration of joints, brittle and painful bones. Scurvy can cause death.

These physicians have also noticed that the supplementation with large doses of ascorbate has an augmenting effect on the concomitant use of antibiotics. This most likely is so because the antibiotics also contribute to the depletion of vitamin C stores. Phyllis A. Balch, C.N.C. and James F. Balch, M.D., report that "...the absorption of vitamin C is greatly reduced by antibiotic drugs, so a person taking antibiotics requires a higher than normal intake of this vitamin."[47]

Because of biochemical individualities, the amount of ascorbate that is absorbed by the body varies from person to person. The level of stress (physical, chemical, emotional) is also a factor to determine the amount a person will be able to use. To determine what your system needs, take 500-1000 mg of vitamin C 3-4 times daily with meals until the body begins to excrete what it cannot use. This is known as *body tolerance*, which is the largest dose a person can absorb without experiencing excessive gas, loose stools, or diarrhea.

During periods of wellness some people may find that their daily need may range between 1000 to 10,000 mg and more. During illness this may increase from 12,000-30,000 + mg daily. This amount will taper down as health returns. Vitamin C comes as ascorbate or as a mineral (buffered) ascorbate, which will not disturb the digestive system as much.

Some people may find vitamin C derived from corn to be intolerable (allergenic). If so, try another non-corn derivative of C.

Bioflavonoids

In the natural state vitamin C is often found in the plant kingdom together with bioflavonoids. Nature has coupled these two substances to work in a balanced and synergistic manner. Although bioflavonoids are not actual vitamins (sometimes referred to as vitamin P) they are necessary for the absorption of vitamin C, and therefore should be taken together.

There are a wide variety of bioflavonoids such as: citrin, flavones, hesperidin, quercetin, and rutin. Bioflavonoids and vitamin C work together to strengthen and protect capillaries. This is very important because the scurvy-like symptoms—bleeding, bruising, and edema, etc.—that occur during periods of cellular stress are the result of weakened capillaries, producing fluid loss and hemorrhaging.

When bioflavonoids are taken with the herb Horse Chestnut the tissue-tightening effects are augmented.

Vitamin E

During periods of the biochemical stress produced by free radicals, the antioxidant vitamin E is another highly challenged nutrient. While vitamin C protects against the water-soluble oxidants, vitamin E neutralizes the fat-soluble ones. This represents all the lipid (oil) membranes of cells. The free-radical activity going on during a microbial, chemical, or radiation assault to the tissue eats away at these lipid membranes, further weakening them to the disease process.

Co-Enzyme-Q-10

This vitamin-like substance is found in all cells of the body, where it plays a vital role inside the mitochondria to produce the energy of the body. It also acts as a very effective

---

[46] See: Dr. Cathcart cited above.

[47] ...(2000). Prescriptions for Nutritional Healing. Avery, a member of Penguin Putman, Inc.: New York, NY. (P. 13.)

antioxidant to protect cellular integrity. Its depletion essentially affects the extra level of energy the body needs to deal with the burden of the disease process. During an assault, it needs to be restored.

Dosage: 30-100 mg 3 times daily with food. Avoid taking more than 300 mg daily.

Concerns: Those who take medications that reduce the levels of Co-Q-10—such as HMG CoA Reductase Inhibitors (statins), Beta-blockers, Chlorpromazine, Tricyclic antidepressants, and Oral Hypoglycemic Agents (Micronase, Dymelor, Tolinase, etc.)—may need to consider increasing the daily amount. In such cases, advice from a physician may be useful.

Interactions: May decrease the action of anticoagulants (heparin, warfarin)

Vitamin A and Beta Carotene

Vitamin A is a well-known nutrient that prevents night blindness and skin disorders. It also enhances immunity (protecting against colds, flu, and other forms of infection), and it is involved in the repair of mucous membranes (so affected by many WMD). Vitamin A also acts as an antioxidant to protect cells from free radical damage.

Beta Carotene belongs to class of plant compounds known as *carotenoids*. It is converted into vitamin A in the liver.

The negative effects of taking large amounts of vitamin A can vary amongst individuals. The toxic dosage can range between 25,000 and 100, 000 international units (IU). Beta carotene does not pose such a risk since the body converts what it needs. During exposure to a WMD this nutrient would be critically challenged.

People who have difficulty digesting fats might benefit from taking beta carotene instead of the fat-soluble vitamin A. The emulsified or mycelized forms are better absorbed and place less stress on the liver.

Zinc

Amongst its many other bodily functions, zinc contributes to the health of the immune system and aids in wound healing. Diminished ability to taste or smell is indicative of zinc deficiency.

Dosage: Coffee diminishes absorption of zinc by 50%. The dose for adults should mimic that for treating the common cold with a zinc lozenge (containing 13.3-23 mg of zinc) dissolved in the mouth every 2 hours while awake. During an acute infectious disease up to 200 mg of zinc in divided doses can be given daily in tablet form for adults. Children can have 1/4 to 1/2 of these amounts when sick. Do not exceed recommended daily dosages as this may cause nausea. It is best taken with food.

Selenium

In miniscule amounts, selenium makes major contributions to the health of the body. One of its key roles is as a component of a major free-radical scavenger, glutathione peroxidase. Working with vitamin E, selenium also aids in the production of antibodies (so important for specific immunity), which may be one reason why its deficiency can result in increased infections. During viral diseases (such as AIDS), it assists to increase the production of both red and white blood cells.

Dosage: Not to exceed 400 mcg (micrograms) per day. Pregnant women should not exceed 200 mcg per day.

Vulnerable Enzymes

During many of these conditions, fever occurs as part of the immune response. Fever is considered to raise the heat of the body to a point that is inhospitable to microbes. However, high fevers not only destroy germs but they also can destroy vital enzymes. In this regard, Dr. Anthony Cichoke writes: "Slight elevations in body temperature increase the activity of the body's enzymes critical in combating the health crisis. However, if the temperature increases too much (exceeding the optimal temperature by even a small amount), enzymes are destroyed and an enzyme imbalance can result, leading to serious consequences. This loss of enzyme activity can lead to illness and ultimately death."[48] This loss especially occurs with enzymes responsible for regulating the inflammatory process.

Probiotics

Probiotics help to replace and maintain the bacterial ecology (flora) in the intestinal tract. This floral ecology is vital for keeping other potentially harmful bacteria in check, thereby preventing opportunistic infections such as *candidiasis*. Probiotic factors include: "friendly bacteria" such as *lactobacillus acidophilus*, floral nutrients such as *fructooligosaccharides* (FOS), and *lacto ferrin*, a substance that prevents harmful bacteria from attaching to the intestinal walls.

ACTIVATION

There are a number of natural and synthetic substances that are used to activate certain biological functions in the body. Some stimulate immune activity, others might aid in the production of red blood cells, while others might assist in the increase of energy.

AKG Shark Liver Oil

Shark liver oil contains substances known as *alkylglycerols* (AKG) that, according to studies[49], are able to stimulate the production of platelets, and to enhance immune function. There are diseases caused by biological agents that cause a rapid loss of blood platelets (thrombocytopenia), and shark liver oil with AKGs might prove beneficial.

Dosage: 5 capsules daily of 200 mg of AKG Shark Liver Oil.

Caution: Should not be taken in such high doses for over 30 days since it might over stimulate the production of platelets.

Co-Enzyme-Q-10

Studies have shown that Co-Q-10 (ubiquinone), in addition to its antioxidant properties, plays a key role in the production of energy in the energy factory of the cell known as the mitochondria. Consequently, it aids the circulation and oxygenation of tissue, and it also stimulates immune response. Because of this, it has a history of being used with cardiovascular problems.

Dosage: 30-100 mg 1-3 times a day with food.

L-Tyrosine

L-Tyrosine is an amino acid that plays an important role in the production of thyroxin, a hormone produced by the thyroid gland. When L-Tyrosine is taken with kelp (a seaweed rich in organic iodine) thyroid function can be improved. A simple test using the underarm temperature, to evaluate thyroid output was developed by Dr. Broda Barns.[50]

The test involves taking the underarm temperature first thing in the morning (without getting out of bed, talking, or any other form of activity in order to measure the *resting metabolic* rate) for at least five days in a row, and recording the results. Normal thyroid output should average between 97.6° F to 98.2° F. If the results are lower than 97.6° F, it indicates a sluggish (hypo) thyroid, and L-Tyrosine and Kelp would be indicated. If it is higher than 98.2° F, thyroid function may be too fast (hyper), and these nutrients would not be used.

Dosage: 500-1000 mg 2-3 times a day, between meals at least 45 minutes before eating, with a glass of water only.

Licorice Root

Licorice root is an herb that has been used for centuries as constituent of various formulas to activate other herbs. It works by stimulating the adrenal glands to produce hormones involved in the healing process. Licorice root is considered an active herb that can elevate blood pressure. It may be useful to use with mild degrees of hypotension (low blood pressure) caused by low adrenal output (hypoadrenalism).

---

[48] … (1999). The Complete Book Of Enzyme Therapy: A Complete and Up-To-Date Reference to Effective Remedies Using Enzymes, Vitamins, and Minerals. Avery Publishing Group: Garden City Park, NY. (P. 40.)

[49] As reported in: Segala, M. Ed., previously cited, p. 45.

[50] …. Hypothyroidism: The Unsuspected Illness.

Dosage: The crushed or powdered herb (100-500 mg) can be taken directly or to make tea.

Caution: Those who have high blood pressure (hypertension) should avoid using this herb.

Velvet Bean

Velvet bean (*Mucana pruriens,* the seed extract) is an active herb containing the neurotransmitter L-dopa, a precursor to epinephrine, an adrenal hormone involved in maintaining blood pressure. Naturalistic practitioners have used this herb to help with Parkinson's disease and to stimulate adrenal output to help relieve hypotension. **Solaray®** produces a Velvet Bean product with 15% L-dopa from 333 mg (per capsule) of the seed extract.

Dosage: as a dietary supplement, take one capsule in the morning and one capsule in the afternoon, with meals or a glass of water.

Caution: Consult your physician before use if being treated for hypertension or cardiac or pulmonary disease or if taking medications containing L-dopa. Not recommended for use with prescription MAO-inhibiting antidepressants.

Ginseng

Ginseng root is considered to be an *adaptogen*, an herb that increases the body's resistance to stress. It does this by helping to regulate the various organ systems of the body. It has been used for centuries (especially in the far East) primarily as a tonic for fatigue, weakness, and nutritional deficiencies. It is particularly nourishing to the male reproductive system, the blood and circulatory systems.

There are varieties of ginseng—Chinese and American, red and white species (*Panax Qinquefolium*); Korean (*Panax Ginseng*), and others—varying in potency, but all are essentially adaptogenic tonics that stimulate the healing process.

Dosage: capsules, liquid, powder forms: follow directions on the container.

Caution: women with estrogen-related tumors should avoid this herb.

ANTIMICROBIAL

This approach seeks to neutralize or destroy pathogens using: synthetic and/or natural antimicrobials and environmental measures. Here we are looking at agents that have specific antimicrobial properties, and not just general immune enhancing activity. They were selected because research has demonstrated their potential activity against many of the microbes deemed possible as WMD. They have also been shown to be effective against strains that have developed resistance to antibacterial and antiviral treatments.

The Herxheimmer Effect

Therapeutic amounts of any kind of antimicrobial (synthetic or natural) can produce what is known as the *Herxheimmer reaction*, discovered by the German dermatologist Karl Herxheimmer (1861-1944), who found there could be an increase in symptoms after the administration of a drug. The naturalistic interpretation attributes this reaction to the unusual release of chemical, bacterial, or viral toxins into the general circulation, causing a toxic overload. This is known as the "die off effect" or "healing crisis", and it is looked on favorably as a sign that the healing process is underway. During this phase it is important to help flush out the toxins by drinking plenty of water.

Garlic

Garlic has been shown through extensive research to improve general health, especially for the cardiovascular system and immune response. It is remarkable for its broad range of antimicrobial activity, especially with drug-resistant strains of bacteria.[51] It is also a powerful antioxidant capable of offering protection against the effects of radiation.[52] While it can be used more specifically as an antimicrobial it is listed here because it is also amenable as a food (and not as powerful as

---

[51] See: Buhner, S. (1999). Herbal Antibiotics: Natural Alternatives for Treating Drug-Resistant Bacteria. Story Books: Pownal, VT.
[52] Lau, B. (1997). Garlic And You: The Modern Medicine. Apple Publishing Co., Ltd.: Vancouver, BC, Canada. (P.40.)

Grapefruit Extract or GSE, which is not a substance that can be used in the daily dietary). Therefore, it can be used to boost the general health of the system and to augment the effects of GSE.

As a preventative take 3 capsules daily. Buhner recommends that one can eat 1 clove up to 3 times daily for prevention. "The cloves may be diced and mixed with honey for palatability and to reduce a possible nauseating effect. ... Care should be taken in consuming it in quantity. Though an entire bulb produces little juice, it is exceptionally potent and is, actually, quite a strong emetic even in small quantities. The best approach is to start with 1/4 teaspoon (1 ml) in a full glass of something like tomato juice or carrot juice and work up from there. ... During acute episodes, 3 to 9 *bulbs* a day are reportedly being used by some clinicians."[53]

For acute episodes one can take the powdered form, up to 30 capsules, divided into smaller doses, daily. When parsley is added to the garlic it helps reduce the strong odor in the breath. There are deodorized garlic products such as the Kyolic brand[54] that are less intense, yet quite as effective as the raw form. "With Kyolic aged garlic people have taken four or five teaspoons of liquid garlic extract (equivalent to 20 to 25 capsules of powder) with no problem."[55]

More can be taken if the garlic is cooked or baked without losing its health benefits.

Grapefruit Seed Extract

Grapefruit seed extract (GSE) is a powerful, broad-spectrum antimicrobial that can be used (always diluted) topically and internally without any side effects. It has received approval from the FDA, USDA (United States Department of Agriculture) and the Pasteur Institute in France, and is used by many health care providers worldwide. It is typically derived from the seed, pulp, and fruit peel of the grapefruit (*Citrus paradisi*) through a pro-

prietary extraction process. I have chosen GSE as one of the mainstays of the specific line of defense because it has so many simple and beneficial applications. The master herbalist Louise Tenny has outlined these qualities in her booklet *Grapefruit Seed Extract*[56], from which I paraphrase the following selections:

- As a broad-spectrum antimicrobial it has demonstrated the ability to fight off a wide variety of bacteria, viruses, fungi and other microbes.
- As a concentrate GSE is a very powerful disinfectant outperforming iodine, clorox bleach, tea tree oil, and colloidal silver. Researchers found it to be ten to one hundred times more effective than chlorine. It was still effective even when diluted to 10 ppm, or 1/100,000 dilution.
- GSE is nontoxic to animals and humans, including pregnant women and children. A person weighing 132 pounds could safely consume 300,000 mg a day!
- GSE poses very little threat to beneficial intestinal bacteria (such as Lactobacillus and Bifidobacterium). (However, Stephen Harrod Buhner states that excessive use of the GSE could disturb the intestinal flora. I always recommend supplementing with probiotics when using any form of antimicrobial.)
- GSE is supported by continuing research done in more than eighty scientific laboratories and forty universities.
- Because GSE is biodegradable it is friendly to the environment.
- GSE rarely causes side effects such as can result from some commercial antibiotics.
- GSE is affordable, widely available, and small amounts will go a long way.

---

[53] Buhner, S. previously cited. (P. 35.)
[54] See: Lau, B., Garlic And You, cited above.
[55] Buhner, S., cited above. (P. 108-9.)

[56] ... (2000).... Woodland Publishing: Pleasant Grove, UT.

Its effect does not diminish over time, and so it requires no expiration date.

- GSE is very compatible with other treatments and products. It can be mixed with vegetable oils (except when used for cooking), alcohol, water, shampoos, lotions and other substances for topical use, and with water, juices and syrups for internal use. It can be mixed into pet foods to treat sick animals. However, it must always be diluted.

Dosages:[57] For human internal use add 3-15 drops in citrus juice 2-3 times a day. Start with the minimal dose and increase if the condition worsens. Douche: 6-12 drops in 1 pint (475 ml) of warm or room temperature water 2 times daily for up to one week. Nasal spray: use 6-12 drops in spray bottle up to 6 times daily. As a Wash place 20-40 drops in 1 pint (475 ml) in room temperature water for infected wounds. As a preventative for Diarrhea or Dysentery use 3 drops per day when traveling. To Purify Water add 3 drops per 8 ounces (237 ml) of water. As a Disinfectant add 30-40 drops per 1 quart (1 liter) of water. Use to clean hands, surgical instruments, rooms, and linens. It is as or more effective than hypochlorite solutions, which can destroy all biological agents mentioned in this book. For use with Bandages add 30-40 drops in 1 quart (1 liter) of distilled water in a spray bottle, and spray on bandages before use. Always use diluted. Citrus juices mask the strong bitter taste of GSE. **Do not use on eyes**.

GSE also comes in capsule form (125 mg is equal to 12-15 drops of the liquid) together with 200 mg of Echinacea Angustifolia Root and 200 mg of Artemesia (by **NutriBiotic®**).

GSE has been found to be effective in fending off secondary infections that often emerge with immune-deficient individuals.

Wild Mountain Oregano

I learned about medicinal grade oregano from Dr. Cass Ingram's book, *The Cure is in The Cupboard*.[58] Since then, I've used it very successfully on myself, my family, and in my practice. "Wild Mountain Oregano", as it is called, differs significantly from the popular kind found in stores for cooking. In fact, this so-called oregano is not oregano at all but is actually marjoram or sweet oregano. Many other forms of oregano found in the market on the West Coast are oregano-like species that come from Mexico. All these herbs dubbed as oregano, and the health products derived from them, do not possess or come near to the healing properties of wild mountain oregano (WMO).

WMO has powerful antimicrobial (in research it inhibited growth of 25 pathogens), anti-inflammatory, antioxidant (scavenges free radicals)[59], anti-venom, mucolytic (liquefies and mobilizes mucous), antitussive (eases cough), and antispasmodic (relieves spasm) properties. This makes it a versatile supportive natural agent against many infectious diseases.

More specifically, in 1995 Greek researchers at the University of Thessoloniki found that a 1-to-4000 dilution of WMO sterilized septic water. "A study published in 1996 in *Medical Science Research* found that oil of oregano destroyed viruses. RNA and DNA viruses, including the type that cause shingles, cold sores and genital herpes, were obliterated when exposed to the oil. Apparently, the oil of oregano shattered the virus' outer coating, essentially disintegrating them. Other studies on bacteria indicate that potent

---

[57] According to Buhner, cited above.

[58] …(2001). …. Knowledge House: Buffalo Grove, IL.

[59] Researchers at the U.S. Department of Agruculture have determined that herbs are higher in antioxidant levels than fruits, vegetables and even spices such as garlic. Shiow Y. Wang, a biochemist at the USDA Beltsville Agricultural Center In Beltsville Maryland, stated in the November issue of the *Journal of Agricultural and Food Chemistry* that the herb "oregano had 3 to 20 times higher antioxidant activity than other herbs studied.„

phenols of oil of oregano are responsible for this cell wall fracturing action. However, the oil is harmless to human cells."[60] In a comparative study involving 40 herbs, Polish researchers found that WMO was the only herb to dramatically stimulate the immune system and the release of interferon. Interferon is the immune systems' antiviral.

A company that manufactures quality WMO products is the **North American Herb & Spice Company**. They produce the brand names known as *Oreganol*, which contains the WMO, *Oregacyn (P73)*, which is a blend of P73 WMO plus antiseptic spice extracts including cumin and sage, and a *SuperStrength Oil of Oregano*. They also produce a crushed-leaf form known as *Oregamax*. These are all food-grade products safe for all ages.

- **Oral dosage:** Minimal amounts of the WMO oil are more effective. Use 1-3 drops of Oreganol placed under the tongue 1-3 times daily for mild conditions, and up to 2 drops hourly of SuperStrength Oil of Oregano* for more severe conditions. Once symptoms clear, taper the dosage down.

- **For wounds:** According to Dr. Ingram: "Oil of oregano supercedes all other over-the-counter antiseptics.... For instance, while iodine, hexachlorophene, and hydrogen peroxide can kill microbes, all have been found in scientific studies to also kill human cells. Furthermore, hydrogen peroxides causes extensive tissue damage and thus interferes with wound healing. Also, scientific studies show how hydrogen peroxide and hexachlorophene are carcinogenic when applied directly to open wounds. Iodine is less toxic to human tissue than hydrogen peroxide, but it is highly toxic if ingested.... In contrast, oil of oregano

destroys germs as well as their spores without damaging human tissue."[61]

- **How to use:** apply in the wound and along the edges 2-6 times daily. Use SuperStrength Oil of Oregano. **Also:** take 3 Oregamax capsules 2-4 times daily.

- **Topical application:** WMO oil can be applied directly on the skin to be absorbed internally. To reduce the intensity of the oil for sensitive-skin types mix 1-5 drops in a fatty medium such as olive oil, sesame oil, cocoa butter, lanolin, coconut oil, or castor oil for deeper penetration. (Non-wound use.)

- **Inhalant:** the oil can be vaporized, nebulized, diffused and inhaled. This helps with lung conditions and is a way to deliver the oil into the system. Also, it can be used in a humidifier to freshen and reduce the microbe load in the air of a house or office space.

Olive Leaf Extract

Olive Leaf Extract (OLE) is derived from the leaf of the olive tree. Scientific research has shown it to have antimicrobial activity to 132 pathogens. This wide antimicrobial activity of OLE has been attributed to the active agents *elenolic acid* and the salt compound *calcium elenolate*.

In addition to these properties, OLE is an antioxidant and an anti-inflammatory. It is very safe to ingest, prophylactically and therapeutically. Furthermore, it won't destroy the friendly flora in the intestines. Nevertheless, I still recommend taking probiotic factors when using natural or synthetic antimicrobials.

In his well-researched book, *Olive Leaf Extract*, Dr. Morton Walker[62] lists 137 infectious diseases for which OLE acts as an antimicrobial agent. "The listing is taken from numerous published medical sources and

---

[60] Ingram (Do), C. Wild Oregano: Germ Killing Spice. March 1999 issue of HSR Health Supplemental Retailer. (P. 74.)

[61] Cited above, p. 136.

[62] ...(1997). .... Kensington Publishing Corp: New York, NY. (P. 64-5.)

from the clinical experiences of currently practicing health professionals who utilize olive leaf extract as part of their armamentarium for patients with internal and external infections...." Of the 137 diseases listed, I have opted to mention only those that have relevance to the topic at hand. They are:

- Anthrax
- Botulism
- California Encephalitis
- Cholera
- Clostridium Perfringens Infection
- Eastern Equine Encephalitis
- Ebola
- Encephalitis
- Hantavirus Pulmonary Syndrome
- Marburg Virus
- Plague
- Rocky Mountain Spotted Fever
- St. Louis Encephalitis
- Smallpox
- Staphylococcal Food Poisoning
- Tuberculosis
- Toxic Shock Syndrome
- Yellow Fever
- Yersenia (Yersinosis)

Dr. Walker quotes James R. Privitera, M.D., of Covina, California on how OLE helps destroy viruses. According to Dr. Privitera, "It interferes with critical amino acid production essential for viruses, and has the ability to contain viral infection and/or spread by inactivating viruses or by preventing virus shedding, budding or assembling at the cell membranes. It directly penetrates infected cells and stops viral replication."

- **Oral Dosages for Maintenance or Prevention:** 1 (500 mg) capsule or tablet 2-3 times daily on empty stomach at least 45 minutes before food or 2 1/2 hours after eating.
- **Therapeutically:** 1-4 capsule(s) or tablet(s) every six hours on empty stomach (as above). Increase the dosage to match the severity of the infection. Also, take into consideration age and health status. Children can take 1/4 to 1/2 of the adult dosage.
- **Pets:** OLE has been used with experimental animals and has proven to

be quite safe. However, no exact dosages have been determined. I would recommend 1/8 to 1/4 the adult dosage per 10 pounds of body weight. Consult with a holistic veterinarian.

ASAP Solution

Since antiquity, silver has been recognized for its capacity to preserve perishable liquids, and to heal the body when water was drunk from a silver vessel. People would place silver objects into wells, store raw milk in silver pails, and, during the plagues in Europe, wealthy families gave their children silver spoons to suck on to protect them from the infestation. Hence, the saying "Born with a silver spoon in his mouth" was indicative of the protective characteristics of silver. Although widely used, no one knew exactly why silver had these protective qualities.

Towards the end of the nineteenth century, scientists discovered that the blood and other vital fluids of the body contained colloidal suspensions of ultra-fine particles. This spurred studies on the colloidal nature of silver, and the discovery that it had broad antimicrobial properties. Using a rather expensive electro-colloidal process, it was manufactured as an antibiotic. Up until 1938 physicians used colloidal silver (of varying formulations) as the antibiotic of the time. Thereafter, the pharmaceutical industry took over with the production of penicillin as the wonder drug of the age, displacing the emphasis on colloidal silver. However, with the rising microbe resistance to antibiotics, interest in colloidal silver has resurfaced.

Considerable amounts of research, and better and cheaper production methods, have given colloidal silver a new standing as an antibiotic. For instance: The March 1978 issue of *Science Digest*, in an article *Our Mightiest Germ Fighter*, reported: "Thanks to eye-opening research, silver is emerging as a wonder of modern medicine. An antibiotic kills perhaps a half-dozen different disease organisms, but silver kills some 650. Resistant strains fail to develop. Moreover, silver is virtually non-toxic." The article ended with a quote by Dr. Harry Margraf, a biochemist and pioneering silver researcher who worked with the late Carl Moyer, M.D., chairman of Washington University's Department of Surgery in the 1970s: "Silver is the best all-around germ fighter we have."[63]

Nevertheless, the production of the many colloidal silver products on the market today is varied and unreliable. No standards have been developed since the FDA grand-fathered it into use with the following 9/13/91 precaution: "These products may continue to be marketed…as long as they are advertised and labeled for the same use as in 1938 and as long as they are manufactured in the original manner." Only one company I know of has exceeded this requirement.

American Biotech Labs has developed the only patented form of colloidal silver, known as *ASAP Solution®* (consisting of 10 parts per million of pure elemental silver), that is showing great promise as a broad spectrum antimicrobial. According to extensive research performed on it, at levels of 5 ppm (parts per million)[64], it has killed every bacterium that independent laboratories have tested against it. It has also shown to be an immune stimulant and anti-inflammatory.

"American Biotech Labs' ASAP Solution® has just passed the US-EPA (Environmental Protection Agency) tests for water treatment and also as a hard surface disinfectant. Tested under worst-case conditions, the ASAP Solution® was able to eradicate 177 of 180 strains of Salmonella choleraesuis in less than five minutes. In the testing, the ASAP Solution® was able to kill 179 or 180 strains of both Staphylococcus aureus and Pseudomonas aeruginosa in less than 15 minutes. One of the most notable results of the testing was that the ASAP Solution® passed all of the EPA tests at a concentration of just 4.4

ppm, a dilution of 56% from the 10 ppm supplement currently being sold worldwide."[65]

After 1 1/2 years of adaptive testing, antibiotic resistant bacteria have not been able to adapt to this solution. According to American Biotech Labs, "(We) believe that the ASAP Solution® product is the only non-toxic product that has been **proven to kill the anthrax spore.**"[66]

On May 19th, 2002, the Clifton Mining Company (a part owner of Biotech Labs) announced that Biotech Labs had completed its first set of testing using ASAP Solution® against **Tuberculosis**. "In the tests which were completed at an independent, FDA approved lab in duplicate, the ASAP achieved a greater than 97% kill rate in just 45 minutes at the 10 ppm level." The article goes on to say: "Because the ASAP Solution has been proven non-toxic and because the TB bacterium attacks the lungs directly, our scientific staff has theorized that direct application of the product to the lungs, by use of a nebulizer, may help cure the problem."[67]

Because of its simplicity and broad antimicrobial activity, it is reportedly being tested by the Department of Defense. Currently, it is pending FDA approval to be labeled as an antibiotic. In the meantime, it is being made available to the public as a *mineral supplement* by **The American Civil Defense Association**.

Unlike colloidal silver, ASAP Solution® does not eventually break out of solution, hence has a long shelf life, and, more importantly, does not with prolonged use cause the skin-graying effect known as *argyria*. It is also very safe for human and animal consumption.

---

[63] Derived from: Altered States e-newsletter, 109th issue, 8/16/02.

[64] Similar to but not like colloidal silver products, which consist of ionic rather than elemental 96% silver suspensions.

[65] Moeller, K. (undated document, received via the Internet on 8/7/02). Why Use the ASAP Solution? American Biotech Labs: Alpine, UT. (P. 3.)

[66] Moeller, K., (received via the Internet on 8/12/02). The ASAP Solution® Difference! American Biotech Labs: Alpine, UT. (P. 2, emphasis mine.)

[67] Clifton Mining Company, (News release: www.cliftonmining.com). ASAP Results Against Number One Human Killer. (Emphasis mine.)

Tests have shown that it would take ingesting the contents of 30 bottles daily of *ASAP* Solution for 30 years before reaching any minimal levels of toxicity that the EPA has established.

It can be used to decontaminate water (more quickly than chlorine), using 8 oz per every 6.25 (requiring 2 minutes) or 12.5 (requiring about 20 minutes) gallons of water.

Dosage: Follow directions on container or as recommended under the Specific Line for a particular agent.

DETOXIFICATION

Detoxification: aims at using substances and therapies that evoke or support certain physiological processes involved in neutralizing and/or eliminating biological, chemical, and nuclear toxins from the body.

Antioxidants

Antioxidants are substances, derived from nutrients or made by the body, that protect against the damaging effects of free radicals. Free radicals are molecules or ions that usually contain oxygen.

According to *The Encyclopedia of Nutrition & Good Health*: "Free radicals possess a single electron; unlike stable molecules with pairs of electrons, these renegades attack innocent bystander molecules of the cell by removing one electron to make up for their own electron deficiency. Once they have been produced, free radicals can multiply via chain reactions, making them even more dangerous to the cell. Free radicals likely to be encountered in the body include superoxide, nitric oxide, hydroxyl radicals, and lipid radicals. Certain activated forms of oxygen, including singlet oxygen, lipid peroxides, and hydrogen peroxide can generate free radicals, though they are not radicals themselves."[68]

Because the body requires oxygen for energy and for immune antimicrobial functions, the production of oxygen-related free radicals is inevitable. To compensate for this side effect of normal metabolic activity, the body produces it own free-radical control substances that either prevent or break the free-radical chain reaction.

Free radicals can also be derived from exposure to toxic industrial and household chemicals, environmental pollution, excessive exposure to the sun's rays, smoke, radiation, and from immune activity during exposure to pathogens and illness.

As was mentioned earlier, during the disease process free-radical activity increases exponentially. Bacteria and viral agents produce free radicals when they release their toxins (exotoxins, and endotoxins) into the body as part of the Herxheimmer reaction, which is further aggravated when antimicrobial or other kinds of drugs are introduced.

To prevent the negative free-radical reaction, the body manufactures enzymes such as catalase, superoxide dismutase (SOD), methione reductase, and glutathione peroxidase. Trace minerals—copper, manganese, zinc, and selenium—contribute to the antioxidant process when they act as cofactors with the enzymes. During illness the use of micronutrients and other substances to support the production and function of these enzymes can be the deciding factor between life and death.

Other substances that contribute to antioxidant production and activity are:

Alpha-Lipoic Acid

Alpha-Lipoic Acid (ALA) is not only a powerful antioxidant but also helps to recycle vitamin E and vitamin C. It stimulates the body's production of glutathione and coenzyme Q_{10}, which are powerful antioxidants. Moreover, ALA can protect both water-and-fat soluble substances, which makes it a full-spectrum antioxidant.

However, oral ingestion of ALA remains for only 90 minutes in the system before it is broken down. For this reason, I have opted for several sustained-release formulas in the

---

[68] Ronzio, R., (1997). ... Facts On File, Inc.: New York, NY. (P. 200.)

market[69], which provide 300 mg per tablet that remain working in the system for 3 hours per dose. While the body produces its own amount of ALA it is not enough for the kinds of conditions being addressed in this book.

When ALA is taken with the herb <u>Milk Thistle</u> they work synergistically to protect liver cells. The liver is a major detoxification organ.

Burdock Root

Burdock Root is a powerful antioxidant that works synergistically with vitamin E. It is often used to cleanse the blood and detoxify the liver, and heal damaged liver cells. It prevents cell mutation, and works superbly with the herb milk thistle. This makes it an excellent candidate to protect the liver, the key organ involved in detoxification.

Melatonin

Melatonin (5-acetyl-5-methoxytryptamine) is the principal hormone of the pineal gland in vertebrates. It is also found in extra-pineal tissues in amphibians, and in smaller amounts in plants. It is typically used with sleep disorders. Research has shown that it has considerable antioxidant and antibacterial effects.

"A study published in *Cell Biology Toxicology* (vol. 16, 2000) showed that Melatonin helped counteract lethal toxins from anthrax exposure."[70] Other studies have shown that melatonin in doses of 10-40 mg nightly can protect and restore normal blood cell production that was disturbed by the toxicity of chemotherapy.[71]

Dosage guidelines: The optimal oral dose of Melatonin has not been established. Typically, for sleep disorders between 1-6 mg are used. However, due to biochemical individualities, it could go up to 20 mg daily. Therapeutic dosages with cancer patients have been as high as 50 mg daily. With exposure to bacterial agents and chemical toxins the maximum therapeutic amount would be suggested. Taper dosage down as the disease subsides.

Use to ensure sound daily sleep because immunity is at its peak during deep fourth-stage sleep (the *delta* band of brainwave measurements). Take with a glass of non-tap water on a relatively empty stomach one hour or so before bedtime. With interrupted sleep take a smaller amount to re-establish sleep.

Caution: Melatonin is not recommended during pregnancy and lactation. It is safe when used orally or injected for short term. It is possibly not safe to use with people under 20 years of age, who most likely produce high levels of Melatonin. Avoid taking during daylight hours. Could be useful for treating thrombocytopenia (reduction of platelets in bleeding disorders). Protects cells from oxidative damage of free radicals.

<u>**Interactions (+ & -):**</u> <u>Benzodiazepines</u> can be phased out with the supervision of a physician or health care provider. Melatonin can reverse the negative effects of <u>Beta Blockers</u> (such as Inderal, Tenormin, but <u>not</u> Coreg) on nocturnal sleep. Melatonin may increase the effects of central nervous system depressants such as alcohol or sedatives (such as benzodiazepines).

Oligomeric Proanthocyanidins

Oligomeric proanthocyanidins (OPCs) are phytochemicals found in a variety of plants. They are more commonly known as *flavonoids*,[72] which are excellent antioxidants. Their value against WMD is augmented by the fact that they are able to cross through the blood-brain barrier, which prevents or slows down the passage of certain biochemicals,

---

[69] Medical Research Institute. Glutotize Controlled Release Alpha Lipoic Acid (Product Reference Guide for Healthcare Professionals). San Bruno, CA.

[70] As reported in Alternative Medicine magazine, issue 45, January 2002. (P. 17.)

[71] See: Segala, M. Ed., previously cited, p. 45.

[72] Research led by Dr. Maurice Iwu, of the London-based Bioresources Development and Conservation Program in West Africa, has found that flavonoid compounds from the *Garcinia Kola* plant might be effective against the Ebola virus. This research is in keeping with the orthomolecular concept that capillary fragility during illness is the cause of scurvy-like symptoms of hemorrhagic diseases. Vitamin C and bioflavonoids are known to strengthen capillaries, especially in the brain.

drugs, and disease causing organisms from the blood into the brain and the spinal cord. This allows them to provide protection to the central nervous system (brain and spinal cord) from free-radical damage. OPCs can help to strengthen and repair connective tissue, and to reduce allergic and inflammatory reactions by decreasing the production of histamine.

Moreover, OPCs have a dual antioxidant benefit that can defend against fat-soluble and water-soluble free-radical activity. Therefore, they can make up for the antioxidant role of vitamin E for lipids and that of vitamin C for water-soluble oxidants.

The green-food supplement (**Magma Plus**) that I recommend in the Preventative Line is rich in OPCs. However, when it is suggested to not use it therapeutically one can substitute the pine-bark extract commercially known as **Pycnogenol** and/or **grape seed extract**, both rich sources of OPCs.

Chelation

The strategy of chelation involves the capture of disease causing toxins (or their dangerous by products) in order to excrete them from the body before they can continue to do harm. For instance, antidotes, absorbents, and chelators can be used. The key idea here involves the process of capturing and taking out.

The word *chelate* is derived from the Greek word for *claw*. Therefore, a chelator is a substance that grabs onto another substance and takes it out of the body. While some chelators may take out a useful element or micronutrient the ones mentioned here are used to take out substances that are poisonous or would be harmful under certain conditions. When taking chelators its is well advised to replace certain nutrients that might be taken out.

IP₆

IP$_6$ (inositol hexaphosphate or phytic acid) was originally introduced as a cancer fighter. It performs many other protective functions in the body. In addition to being a powerful antioxidant, it is one of the best natural iron chelators, which is beneficial with infectious

diseases since the germs need iron to regenerate. This makes it a valuable substance against biological WMD, since, in a way, it mimics the iron-chelating or blocking activity of a number of synthetic antibiotics.[73]

Oral Chelation Formula

This proprietary formula was developed by **Extreme Health**. Many holistic doctors and practitioners have used it successfully to take out toxic metals (arsenic, lead, mercury, cadmium, etc.) from the body. Three (3) capsules of the following (proprietary blend, PB) of ingredients provide a broad spectrum of chelators, antioxidants, and enzymes:

• Activated Attapulgite (Clay)	PB
• Alpha-Lipoic Acid	PB
• Carrageenan (Irish moss)	PB
• Chlorella	PB
• Garlic	PB
• L-Cysteine	PB
• L-Lysine (Hcl)	PB
• L-Methionine	PB
• Sodium Alginate	PB
• EDTA	PB
• Trimethylglycine (TMG)	PB
• Vitamin C (Ascorbic Acid)	300 mg
• Bromelain 2000 (GDU)	25 mg
• Lipase	25 mg
• Catalase	5 mg

Dosage: up to 3 capsules near bedtime with 8-10 oz glass of water. See the specific agent recommendations. This dosage is followed by a (compensatory) formula, Age-Less Formula, taken in the morning with food. Age-Less Formula contains the following proprietary blend (PB) per 3 caplets.

Beet Juice Powder	PB
• Bioflavonoids	PB
• Calcium Citrate	100 mg
• Chondroitin Sulfate	PB
• Chromium (proteinate)	100 mcg
• Cilantro Extract	PB
• Copper (gluconate)	250 mcg
• Ginkgo Biloba Extract	PB
• Grape Seed OPCs	PB
• Green Tea	PB
• Hawthorne Berry Extract	PB
• Hesperidin	PB

---

[73] See: Shamsuddin, M.D., A. (1998). IP6: Nature's Revolutionary Cancer-Fighter. Kensington Publishing, Corp. New York, NY.

- Iodine (as Kelp) — 50 mg
- Inositol — PB
- Artichoke Powder (liver support) — PB
- Lutein — PB
- Lycopene — PB
- Magnesium (oxide) — 50 mg.
- Manganese (gluconate) — 2.5 mg
- Methyl Sulfonyl Methane (MSM) — PB
- Milk Thistle Extract (80%) — PB
- Molybdenum (sodium molybdate) — 100 mcg
- PABA (para-amino-benzoic acid) — PB
- Potassium (Chloride) — 30 mg
- Quercetin — PB
- Rutin — PB
- Selenium (sodium selenate) — 50 mcg
- Vitamin A (beta carotene) — 5,000 IU
- Vitamin B (biotin) — 50 mcg
- Vitamin B (folic acid) — 200 mcg
- Vitamin B1 (thiamine mononitrate) — 12.5 mg
- Vitamin B2 (riboflavin) — 12.5 mg
- Vitamin B3 (niacinamide) — 15 mg
- Vitamin B5 (calcium Pantothenic) — 12.5 mg
- Vitamin B6 (pyridoxine Hcl) — 7.5 mg
- Vitamin B12 (cyanocobalamin) — 25 mcg
- Vitamin D (cholecalciferol) — 100 IU
- Vitamin E (acetate) — 100 IU
- Zinc (sulfate) — 3.75 mg
- Bromelain 2000 GDU — 25 mg
- Lipase — 25 mg
- Catalase — 5 mg

Lung Detoxification

Clear Lungs (Ridge Crest Herbals) is an excellent Chinese formula to clean and tonify the lungs. It contains:
Dong Quai, Hoelen Ophiapogon, Almond Seed, Asparagus, Citrus, *Fritillary*, Gardenia, Morus Root, *Platycodon, Scute, Shizandra,* Licorice Root.

Dosage: 2 capsules 3 times a day with meals.

Oregacyn (North American Herb and Spice Co.) is also an excellent lung formula to dotoxify and balance the lung tissue. It contains a proprietary blend of: Wild Mountain Oregano, Wild Mountain Sage, and Cumin.

Dosage: 1 capsule 1-6 times a day with or without meals.

Homeopathic *Arsenic* 7c

A study has shown *Arsenic* 7c to speed up the elimination of arsenic from poisoned rats;[74] and to protect against mustard gas burns.[75]

Absorbents

Activated charcoal is a highly absorbent (pharmaceutically produced) black-carbon powder that can be used in a variety of therapeutic ways. Historically, the use of charcoal goes back to antiquity. For instance, Dr. David Cooney reports in his book, *Activated Charcoal*,[76] "In the times of Hippocrates (400 B.C.) and Pliny (50 A.D.), wood charcoal was used to treat epilepsy, vertigo, chlorosis, and anthrax.[77]" It can be used as an antidote, a remedy, and a health aid. The following applications make it a valuable method to protect against WMD.

- To absorb ingested toxins, drug overdoses, and poisons (e.g., paralytic shellfish poisons).
- To absorb harmful intestinal bacteria, fungi and viruses.
- To absorb excessive production of stomach and intestinal acid.
- To absorb excessive amounts of bile in the intestines.
- As a poultice to absorb toxins and bacteria from ulcers and wounds.
- As a topical (mixed with bentonite powder and/or chickpea flour) to absorb vesicants (e.g., mustard particles) from the skin (not the eyes).
- As a remedy to reduce diarrhea. Its activity as a powerful astringent with no toxic effects makes it the perfect anti-diarrheal. "Sebedo et al. (1982) studies the effect of activated charcoal (Norit) on diarrhea in 39 children in Indonesia. Group 1 (23 children) received only oral glucose electrolyte

---

[74] Manning, C.; Vanrenen, L. (1988). Bioenergetic Medicines East and West: Acupuncture and Homeopathy. North Atlantic Books, Berkeley, CA. (P. 83.)
[75] Manning, C.: Vanrenen, L. Cited above. (P. 84.)
[76] ...(1995). ...Teach Services, Inc.: Brushton, NY. (P. 5.)
[77] Probably the intestinal form of the disease.

solution (this combats the severe dehydration resulting from diarrhea). Group II (16 children) received the oral glucose solution plus a dose of activated charcoal (166 mg to 750 mg, depending on body weight, 3 times/day). The charcoal lowered the duration of diarrhea from 3.0 days to 2.1 days, a reduction of 30%. It may be that a much larger activated charcoal dose would have had a bigger effect. Unfortunately, only fairly low charcoal doses were employed."[78]

Use the capsule form available in most health food stores and pharmacies. Take 1-4 capsules as needed with 8 ounces (+) water. It can be used to dry up excessive stomach acid or to calm an acidic stomach due to food (e.g., spicy). In this case, take 1-2 capsules right after eating but, since it will absorb much of the HCL, take with 1-2 capsules of a pancreatic enzyme formula (**with no HCL**) to help digest the food. Can be taken on an empty stomach.

- As a remedy to reduce excessive flatulence.
- Taken orally to reduce itching (pruritus), stemming from toxins or pathogens in the gastrointestinal tract.
- To detoxify the blood of chemical and biological toxins. A medical treatment known as *hemoperfusion* draws the blood out of the body and passes it through a special carbon filter, and returns it.

Recommended Dosages: use 100-1000 mg taken orally as suggested in the Preventative Line and for specific WMD. Products are widely available in health-food outlets and in pharmacies. When used after meals, I recommend the commercial product Charco-Zyme (by **Atrium, Inc.**).

Precautions: avoid taking with substances to produce vomiting (emetics such as Syrup of Ipecac) since it might cause the emesis to be drawn into the lungs (pulmonary aspiration). Avoid taking together with prescription medication, since it can absorb them. When taken with dairy products (ice cream, milk, sherbet, etc.) it will not be as effective.

White Oak Bark
White Oak Bark is an herb rich in tannins (8-20%), which exert an astringent and tightening effect on mucosal tissue. It should be used to bind the stool, and discontinued once this occurs.

Dosage: Use 1 tsp of loose herb per cup of tea, or 1-3 capsules can be taken with water 1-3 times daily as needed. Don't use as a bath.

Chickpea Flour
In addition to being a nourishing food, chickpea (garbanzo) flour has tremendous absorbing qualities. Physicians practicing Ayurveda, the ancient and evolving medicinal system from India, have used this flour in poultices to draw toxins out of the body through the skin. Its absorbent qualities make it useful to draw vesicants and other damaging agents off the skin. To increase its ability to absorb, one can add equal amounts of Activated Charcoal to it. This mixture can be prepared in advance and stored in a sealed plastic bag.

Drawing Salves, Poultices, Ointments
These formulas are used to bring boils to a head and/or to extract toxic substances from eruptions. These are also useful for exfoliating the skin and drawing out toxins. They are most effective when used in conjunction with internal use of a natural antimicrobial program or blood purifier such as burdock root tincture (30 drops in water 3 times daily).

Black Ointment
Black Ointment (Dr. Christopher's formula:olive oil, chaparral leaves, comfrey root, red clover blossom, mullein leaves, plantain leaves, chickweed herb, lobelia herb, golden seal root, marshmallow root, poke root, pine tar, and mutton tallow) should be used exter-

[78] Cooney, D., cited above, p. 55.

nally. Apply with a Q-Tip® or spatula to affected area and seal with a bandage, and leave on overnight. Reapply during the morning after cleaning area, and leave on all day if needed.

Bentonite

Bentonite (also known as montmorillonite) is a very fine absorbent clay, somewhat similar in function to activated charcoal. I prefer to use the activated charcoal for poultices and for the extraction of toxins. However, bentonite can be used in conjunction with activated charcoal or alone for intestinal detoxification, and as a topical dry powder to potentially absorb vesicants. Bentonite comes in both liquid and powder forms, and is available in health-food outlets.

Detoxification Through Fasting

Fasting has been used for centuries in every culture to detoxify the liver, kidneys, blood, and gastrointestinal system, and to give the digestive system a rest. Generally, I recommend that people fast two or three times yearly, at the change of seasons, to clear the accumulated toxic load from their bodies. Here the intent is similar, but perhaps more crucial. It would most likely be done as a rehabilitative therapy.

Fasting isn't for everyone. Pregnant and lactating women should **never** fast. The weak, children (except with "mono-fast" mentioned below), and the very sick may use other methods that can yield similar results. Also not everyone should fast alike. Consider the following guidelines based on body types:

- **Catabolic types**, of any size with a thin frame and very little bulk, wiry, skinny, difficulty gaining weight, etc., should not fast for more than 3 days. This type has a fast metabolism and a high need for blood sugar and may tend to have slightly low blood pressure. Fasting can debilitate them. They would do best on a mono-fast of 2 small daily servings of mung beans and brown rice (flavored with a small amount of salt and pepper, with a touch of olive oil) and/or a diluted fruit-juice fast (3 parts juice to 1 part water) drunk between meals. They could have periodic fasts separated by at least 2 months.
- **Anabolic types**, of any size, with a large frame, big boned, gain weight easily, can fast up to 10 days or longer. This type has a slow metabolism and plenty of reserves and would do well with a vegetable juice (carrot, beet, celery, etc.) fast or green drink fast (e.g., with Green Magma or a comparable formula).
- **Metabolic types**, of any size, medium built, sturdy, can gain or lose weight easily, active, can fast 5-7 days on diluted fruit juice or a green drink with a slight amount of a natural sweetener (malto dextrin, etc.) like Magma Plus.

All types can observe the following general guidelines:

- Prepare the body for the fast by eating only raw fruits and vegetables for 2 days before you begin. Catabolic types would do best with homemade vegetable soups. Too many raw vegetables cause excessive flatulence.
- Children could follow the Catabolic Type recommendations. Use 1/2 to 1/4 of any of the recommended dosage/amounts.
- Drink at least 8 eight-ounce glasses of distilled water daily to chelate (take out) the toxins.[79]
- Avoid fasting on water only. It will release toxins too quickly and overwhelm the system.
- Avoid combining fruit and vegetable juices (except organically prepared, enzymatically-intact, powdered forms, and apple juice).
- During and after the fast get some fiber into your system by taking fiber

---

[79] Normally, I don't recommend drinking distilled water because it will take out too much of needed minerals from the body. Distilled water can be improved by adding trace minerals to it. However, pure distilled water has many therapeutic purposes.

tablets or powders. Oat bran is a good source. Avoid wheat. Don't take supplements together with the fiber; wait 2 hours.

- Take a daily probiotic formula that can be mixed in water.
- Use a liquid or powdered daily multi-vitamin with minerals (e.g., All One, Vita Quick). This is especially important for seniors.
- Those with dentures should wear/use them during the fast; otherwise gums could shrink.
- During the fast add 30 drops of Burdock Root non-alcohol based tincture to about 4 ounces of warm or room temperature water and drink 2 times daily with a capsule of garlic or liquid aged garlic (in the drink) each time.
- During the fast, perform mild exercises like walking, Tai Chi, Yoga, light work around the house, etc. Also, get sufficient rest and sleep.
- Take in calming and beautiful impressions (music, visuals, etc.) during the fast to soothe nerves. Perform the Relaxation Response or comparable technique.
- As toxins are released, one may experience some discomfort such as headaches or digestive upset. One may also feel a mild malaise. Usually, these symptoms resolve within a day or so.
- Use fennel-seed and/or ginger tea to calm the digestive system, if needed.
- Take feverfew as capsules or tea for headaches.

Enemas and Colonics

Enemas and colonics help to clear the colon of toxic material. However, before starting a colon-cleansing program it is useful to precede it with a fast or an herbal total gastrointestinal cleansing, including the liver, gall-bladder, and kidneys for about 1-2 weeks. For this purpose, consider using The Ultimate Cleanse (from Nature's Secret) or one of the ReNew Life Formulas, or something similar.

Follow the directions on the container. This will bring down otherwise unreachable toxic material into the colon. Then, finish off with a deep enema or colonic. It is best to have the colonic done by a professionally trained person. They have the know-how and the proper equipment. However, if this is not an option or if you prefer to do it yourself consider the following.

- Different kinds of colonic equipment are available to use in the home. Some of the devices are quite simple.
- Avoid colonics or enemas if you have rectal bleeding.
- Don't use with pregnant women or children under 2 years of age.
- For enema: To 2 quarts of lukewarm distilled water add the fresh-squeezed juice of 3 lemons. If you are sensitive to lemons, use 2 ounces of wheat grass juice or 1 ounce of liquid aged garlic extract (Kyolic). Tap water has toxic chemicals and minerals that can be absorbed through the colon.
- Catnip tea can be used instead of the above formula in order to bring down high fever (over 102° F or 103° F in children over 2). Make 1 quart of the tea and use lukewarm as follows.
- For children use about 1/4 to 1/2 of the above amount.
- Or, use a rubber enema bag and fill with the above solution.
- Lubricate the tip of the insert tube with some vitamin E oil (ok to pierce a soft gel and squeeze out the oil). Use the same oil to lubricate the anal opening. Aloe vera gel can also be used. Those with hemorrhoids might find the aloe to be soothing.
- Position yourself to receive the enema with the head down and pelvis up to provide an incline for the water to enter deeply into the colon.
- If your experience pain during insertion stop the flow from the enema bag and relax; remain in the same position, take a few deep breaths, and continue

If you need to release the liquid, remove the tube, release, then start again.

- After the solution has been inserted you will need to get on your back and roll over and lie on your left side. Then, use your hands to move the liquid through the colon to loosen fecal matter. Start on the lower right side and with gentle pressure move your hand up towards the bottom of the rib cage, then horizontally over to the left, then down on the left side. Do this several times for about 3-4 minutes, holding on to the liquid, then release it.
- Wash and sterilize the insertion tube.
- Perform daily for 3-5 days, and thereafter, as needed.
- Make sure you take daily Probiotic Factors.

Diuretics

Diuretics increase the rate of urination and, in doing so, help to detoxify the kidneys and urinary tract. The following representative formula, produced by **Thompson**, is an excellent diuretic:

Potassium	60 mg.	Parsley Leaf	100 mg
Uva Ursi Extract	33 mg	Short Buchu Leaf	25 mg
Juniper Berry Extract	10 mg		

Sweat Therapy

Sweat therapy is a method by which toxins can be released through the skin. To do this, one can use a sauna or devise a simple sweat tent by placing an electric teapot or steamer under a chair, wrapping a blanket around oneself and draping it down to the bottom of the chair in order to enclose the steam. Start by drinking a cup of ginger tea. Sit in the heated steam until the body starts to sweat profusely. Then take a cool shower. Afterwards, squeeze 1/2 of a lemon into an 8-10 oz glass of room temperature water and drink to replace electrolytes. Initially, this can be performed daily for 4-7 days; thereafter, periodically perform as needed.

PROTECTIVE RESISTANCE

Here we discuss those substances and methods that protect vulnerable cells and their constituents, making them more resistant to invasion.

Cell membrane integrity is vital to prevent the infectious disease process from advancing to a critical stage. Pathogens cause disease only when they adhere to and penetrate cellular membranes. Strong cellular membranes can withstand higher assaults from toxic substances.

Vitamin E

Vitamin E (Alpha-Tocopherol and/or mixed Tocopherols) is an antioxidant that, amongst its many functions in the body, protects cell membranes by inhibiting the oxidation of lipids (fats) and the formation of free radicals. Cell membranes are made from lipids. It also protects other fat-soluble vitamins (D, A) and essential-fatty acids from being damaged by oxidation.

Dosage: 400-1000 IU daily with food.

Echinacea Purpurea

Echinacea Purpurea has shown antibacterial and antiviral activity in scientific research. However, here it is being used for its cell membrane protective qualities (**the Purpurea is superior to the angustifolia and the pallida species**), which is how it may defend against pathogenic invasion. Hyaluronic acid is a substance that helps to maintain cell membrane integrity. A variety of pathogens excrete an enzyme known as hyaluronidase that breaks down hyaluronic acid and thereby weakens the membrane.

In one study "Echinacea extracts helped to raise the tissue resistance against pathogens by stabilizing hyaluronic acid and inactivating hyaluronidase produced by the bacteria."[80]

Dosage: 30 drops of the tincture (alcohol or water base) every 2-3 hours beginning with the onset of symptoms for 2-3 days. Thereafter, use 3 times daily for up to 8 weeks. If

---

[80] Foster, S., (1991). Echinacea: Nature's Immune Enhancer. Healing Arts Press: Rochester, VT. (P. 42.)

needed beyond this time, pause a few days and go the full course again.

REGULATION/BALANCE

These modalities help to monitor and regulate different vital physiological functions to support life and healing activity.

Therapeutic Yoga

The practice of yoga is highly recommended. There is a school of yoga that focuses on gentle therapeutic exercises for people who are ill or in rehab, or for those who prefer the gentle approach instead of the more rigorous methods. Nowadays, there are many locally available sources. One book that is an excellent resource in this regard is *Gentle Yoga* by Lorna Bell, R.R., and Eudora Seyfer.[81] The method they use covers yoga for special needs, the breathing exercises known as *Pranayama*, the use of postures, stress management, nutrition, and philosophical attitudes that one can develop for personal growth and development.

Movement

Movement has a beneficial effect on the circulation, especially on the lymphatic system, which relies on movement as its pump. It increases the delivery of oxygen to the tissues. It also stimulates the production of *growth hormone* to maintain vitality and muscle tone. Exercise is very important, not only for fitness but also because it can help the body to mobilize and excrete toxins. It is also useful for body balancing, since it brings all systems into a state of harmony. We can get exercise when we clean the car, dance, go hiking, swim, and the like. Those who want a more gentle kind of movement might consider Tai Chi. Those who are incapacitated or can't move very well might need mechanical assistance, such as from machines such as the **Oxy-Flow** or **Chi Machines**.

Hot/Cold Applications

Hot/cold therapies are part of a wider spectrum of naturopathic treatments known as *hydrotherapy*. While there are many do-it-yourself books[82] on the subject, it is best to learn from a qualified health practitioner. Hot baths, showers, or steam treatments (e.g., sauna, sweat tent, etc.) increase the body temperature and circulation. When the heat goes slightly above the normal range of 98.6° F, it mimics a slight fever.[83] This stimulates an increase in the white-blood count in addition to the excretion of toxins through the sweat and urine. Immersing oneself in tolerable cold water afterwards (e.g., shower, bath, pool, etc.) causes the cells of the body to contract. Alternating this process several times causes the organs to expand and contract. In most instances, this kind of therapy would be recommended as part of one's rehabilitation.

Contraindications: Acute fever, severe heart complications, seizures, acute bleeding, open wounds, pressure sores, acute skin infections, vascular disease, thermal nerve deficiency, incontinence of bladder/bowel, malignancy or active tuberculosis.

Precautions: check with physician or qualified health care professional if you're pregnant and/or have: loss of sensation, cardiac history, diabetes, obesity, physical disability, impaired balance.

Bodywork

Bodywork is a broad term to represent a number of techniques such as **Chiropractic**, **Massage**, and **Osteopathy**. These methods seek to manipulate the body structurally and/or to stimulate certain nerve and muscle systems to bring the overall system into balance. The main concept is to clear physical blockages to the neural and subtle energy systems. Once these systems are aligned, energy begins to flow properly, and health is restored.

---

[82] See: Dail, (M.D.) C., Thomas C. (Ph.D.), (1995). Hydrotherapy: Simple Treatments For Common Ailments. TEACH Services, Inc.: Brushton, NY. Also: Buchman, (Ph.D.), D. (1994). The Complete Book Of Water Healing. Instant Improvement, Inc.: New York, NY.

[83] Treatments that use heat at higher temperatures are known as *hyperthermia*, which must be given by a physician or qualified practitioner.

...(1987).... Celestial Arts. Berkeley, CA.

Research has shown that bodywork also stimulates the production of *melatonin* (a hormone that helps the body to relax and sleep well) and *growth hormone* (which helps to tone and rejuvenate the body). Melatonin works with the healing potentials during passive recuperative states (the immune system is most active during periods of deep sleep), while growth hormone supports the more active elements of voluntary and involuntary muscle tone.

Subtle Energy Work

As was discussed in the Psychological Line, subtle energy work involves balancing the energy system to promote healing and wellness. Highly trained, sensitive practitioners see themselves as conduits of a higher energy field. Services are provided by: **Network Chiropractors**, **Reiki** practitioners, and **Cranio-Sacral** practitioners, amongst others. This is an excellent line of healing for anyone, and especially for children, pets, the very old, or the disabled.

Dietary

While not fully covered in this book, therapeutic dietary advice is very important for the healing process. One of the better therapeutic dietary approaches comes from the ancient healing science from India known as *Ayurveda*. It recommends foods to individuals based on the concept of body types (*Vata* or catabolic, *Pitta* or metabolic, *kapha* or anabolic)[84], and for use with particular conditions and disease states.

For example the *vata* type has a tendency toward tissue dryness. They should avoid eating too many drying foods (such as beans). Conditions of dry tissue (e.g., dry unproductive cough, excessive thirst) should also compensate with non-*vatagenic* foods. *Pitta* types generate a lot of body heat. They need to compensate with cooling foods, avoiding hot/spicy ones. Inflammatory conditions, as the term implies, are very heating to the body. During inflammatory conditions a person would do better with non-heating foods to avoid aggravating the condition. *Kapha* body types tend to build body tissue quite easily, and as a consequence they tend to be corpulent or heavy. They need to avoid saturated fats, sugars, and foods that can cause one to gain weight. An indication that this quality is aggravated is when the production of mucous is excessive. Conditions characterized by *kapha* need drying and heating foods.

A certain amount of training is required before one can use this approach during the disease process. It is used here as an adjunct during the rehabilitative stage. Nevertheless, whenever appropriate, mention will be made of certain foods to use or avoid for each agent.

An excellent book to learn about *Ayurvedic* foods for healing is Amadea Morningstar's *Ayurvedic Cooking for Westerners.*[85]

Anti-inflammatory

Inflammation manifests at the fifth stage of the disease process with the appearance of overt symptoms. As was previously noted, it can be a double-edged sword in that it is needed to mobilize the immune system, but when it continues activity beyond the borders of necessity it can aggravate the advancing disorder.

When the immune system becomes activated certain bio-chemicals known as cytokines (one of a large group of proteins secreted by various cell types involved in cell-to-cell communication, coordinating antibody and T cell immune interactions, and amplifying immune reactivity) are released that signal the onset of inflammation. Inflammation facilitates the transfer of white blood cells from the blood vessels into the lymphatic fluid between cells. At the same time the inflammatory response isolates the site of immune concern in order to fence off the problem.

To launch the inflammatory response, the body employs several enzymes known as cyclooxygenase 2 (COX-2) and 5 lipooxygenase to convert arachidonic acid, a dietary fatty

---

[84] These are approximate English translations of these Sanskrit terms.

[85] … (1995) … Lotus Press: Twin Lakes, WI.

acid obtained from animal fats, into pro-inflammatory substances. The most active pro-inflammatory ones are: prostaglandin E2 (PGE2), tumor necrosis factor (TNF-á)[86], interleukin-6 (IL-6), interleukin-1 beta (IL-1(B), leukotriene B(4) or LTB(4). Under certain conditions, these substances can over-stimulate acute and chronic states of inflammation, which often exacerbate the disorder.

To curtail the excessive inflammatory response, conventional medicine uses non-steroidal anti-inflammatory drugs (NSAID's)—such as aspirin, Celebrex, Vioxx, and other similar compounds—that specifically inhibit the body's production of these pro-inflammatory substances, especially COX-2. At one time, aspirin was the anti-inflammatory of choice. However, the problem with aspirin is that it also inhibits another important non-inflammatory enzyme known as cyclooxygenase-1 (COX-1). COX-1 is involved with vital body functions such as mucous and acid regulation in the gastrointestinal system, water regulation in the kidneys, and the production of blood-clotting platelets (which has contributed to internal-bleeding disorders). Celebrex and Vioxx were designed to be more specific for COX-2 and avoid inhibition of COX-1. However, these drugs also have significant side effects.

Research into natural substances has found that many plants and oils inhibit the COX-2 pro-inflammatory enzyme without any debilitating side effects.[87] The complex nature of the plant-based approach is what makes it so useful. It provides the system with a healthy, synergistic complexity that supports inner balance as the medium of healing.

Research has implicated chronic inflammation with many degenerative diseases such as cancer, heart disease, lupus, arthritis, and others. In those with inflammatory syndromes, **C-reactive protein** is often sharply elevated in their blood tests.[88] The below-mentioned supplements have been shown to reduce the levels of inflammation and the presence of these indicators in their cytokine-blood-profile tests.

In some conditions, anti-inflammatory agents in general may be contraindicated, and one should refer to the specific condition before embarking on using them in the higher range of the recommended dosages (or at all).

Caution in using these agents should be exercised by those who are on medications or supplemental programs that thin the blood (e.g., Coumadin, anticoagulants, platelet separators, aspirin, ginkgo biloba, etc.). They are also contraindicated for those with bleeding disorders (such as those that present with hemorrhagic fever virus infections).

Anti-inflammatory Enzymes

Enzymes are protein-based substances that speed up and/or evoke all the chemical reactions that take place in every form of organic life. This includes single celled organisms, plants, animals, and human life. Together with the synergistic effect of vitamins and minerals they are involved in every metabolic process that either takes substances apart (catabolic) or brings them together (anabolic).

There are enzymes that facilitate digestion, respiration, the expansion and contraction of the heart, the movement of the muscles, and so on. Enzymes are known to catalyze (speed up) these reactions without being altered by the reaction itself.

Of the millions of enzymes occurring in the body over 3000 have been identified. Each enzyme is uniquely formed from amino acids, the structural units of all protein. The body manufactures a number of these amino acids, which are considered to be non-essential. It also acquires other necessary or essential amino acids from the diet. "As long as our bodies can make enzymes we live. But

---

[86] It is important to note that the body does use tumor necrosis factor-alpha (TNF-á) to acutely fight infections. In such instances it would be wise to pause or discontinue the use of anti-inflammatory agents during the period of active infection.

[87] See. Newmark, T., Schulick, P., previously cited.

---

[88] See Testing in Resources for more information.

our bodies' production of enzymes can be decreased by illness, injury, stress, or aging."[89]

As was discussed, the process of inflammation is controlled by a series of enzymes of which the COX-2 pro-inflammatory enzyme plays a key role.

Proteolytic Enzymes

Proteolytic Enzymes, when taken on an empty stomach, enter the blood stream and have anti-inflammatory effects throughout the body. They include epress, pepsin, trypsin, chymtrypsin, and pancreatin.

To ensure that the different Ph requirements don't obstruct the anti-inflammatory purpose, a variety of enzymes are often formulated with varying Ph requirements so that if one doesn't work the others will as they go through the intestinal tract. These enzymes should be enterically coated so that they can bypass the stomach acid and dissolve in the small intestine.

Wobenzyme®N (Naturally Vitamins) is an excellent product. Three tablets contain: Papain 180 mg, Bromelain 135 mg, Trypsin 72 mg, Chymotrypsin 3 mg, Rutosid (Sophora japonica) 150 mg.

Typical Dosage: take 60 minutes before eating or two hours after meals with water only, up to 3 times daily.

DHA

Of its numerous health benefits, the docosahexaenoic acid (DHA) fraction of fish oil or marine algae has been identified with being able to reduce blood levels of pro-inflammatory cytokines.[90] "Studies on healthy humans and those with rheumatoid disease show that fish oil suppresses these dangerous cytokines by up to 90%."[91] A 1000 mg gel caps of fish oil typically yields about 500 mg of DHA.

Typical Dosage: 1000-2000 mg of DHA daily in divided amounts taken with food.

Interactions: May increase the risk of bleeding when taken with anticoagulant medications (e.g., heparin, warfarin, salicylates = aspirin).

GLA

In scientific research, oils containing Gamma Linolenic Acid (GLA) have demonstrated the propensity to lower inflammatory cytokine activity. Gamma linolenic acid can be converted to compounds that have anti-inflammatory properties.

Typical Dosage: 1000 mg 3 times daily. A supplement of 4000 mg of borage oil yields about 920 mg of GLA.

Interactions: May increase the risk of bleeding when taken with anticoagulant medications (e.g., heparin, warfarin, salicylates = aspirin).

Super GLA/DHA

Super GLA/DHA is a balanced omega-6/omega-3 formula produced by the Life Extension Foundation that provides all the anti-inflammatory benefits mentioned above. Three softgel capsules contain:
Borage seed oil 2000 mg, GLA 460 mg, Marine lipid concentrate 1000 mg, DHA 500 mg.

Barberry

In addition to being one of the most effective herbs for fighting bacterial infections, barberry (*Berberidaceae vulgaris*) contains substances known as berberine and berbamine that produce anti-inflammatory activity. Studies have shown that barberry is an effective COX-2 inhibitor.[92]

Dosage: Here barberry is used as part of an anti-inflammatory formula such as Zyflamend described below.

Cat's Claw

An herb widely used throughout South America, Cat's Claw (*Uncaria tomentosa*) is known for its anti-inflammatory activity, especially with the gastrointestinal system.

Dosage: 300-500 mg 1-3 times a day in capsules or as tea.

Feverfew

Feverfew (*Tanacetum parthenium*) has been traditionally used to quell headaches (espe-

[89] Cichoke, A. (1999), previously cited. (P. 2.)
[90] See: Ley-Jacobs, B. (1999). DHA: The Magnificent Marine Oil. BL Publications: Temecula, CA.
[91] Segala, M., Ed., previously cited, p. 14.

[92] See: Newmark, T. and Schulick, P. previously cited. Also: Balch, P. Prescriptions for Herbal Healing.

cially migraines), lower fever, for stomachache, and for nausea and vomiting. Its effectiveness with these conditions is probably due to its reported ability to inhibit 86-88% of the pro-inflammatory prostaglandin synthesis, especially the formation of COX-2 and lipoxygenase. The active constituent is thought to be 0.2% parthenolide (amounts less than 0.2% might not be effective).[93] Other biochemicals that add to its anti-inflammatory properties are its rich source of *melatonin* and apigenin.

Typical Dosage: Capsules 300-400 mg 3 times a day. Tincture: 15-30 drops in 4 oz of warm water 1-3 times a day. Freeze dried extract 25 mg 1-3 times daily.

Caution: May interfere with anticoagulant medications (e.g., heparin, warfarin, salicylates = aspirin).

Chinese Goldthread

As the name of this herb implies, Chinese Goldthread is found in the mountains of China, and it is notorious for its rich source of berberine, which has antimicrobial and anti-inflammatory properties. "A 1999 article published in the *Journal of Ethnopharmacology* confirmed that berberine found in…Chinese goldthread inhibits the COX-2."[94]

Dosage: Here Chinese goldthread is being used as part of the anti-inflammatory formula Zyflamend described below.

Green Tea

Green tea (*Camellia sinensis, Theaceae*) is made from the young leaves of the plant. Black tea and oolong tea come from the same plant but undergo degrees of fermentation, which reduces the levels of their natural constituents. Green tea is rich in substances known as polyphenols, which have antioxidant, antibiotic, and anti-tumor properties. One of the polyphenols is over 200 times more potent than vitamin E in scavenging free radicals. Research has confirmed that it also contains 51 anti-inflammatory compounds.

Green and black tea also contain a chemical known as *theophylline*, which is pharmaceutically extracted and used for conditions of bronchial constriction such as asthma and bronchitis. Theophylline relaxes the smooth muscles of the lungs and opens the airways.

Dosage: 1 tsp of the leaves (with or without caffeine) added to 8 oz of boiling water to make tea. Do not steep too long as the tea will become bitter. Three cups provide about 240-320 gm of polyphenols.

Caution: for people with hypersensitivity to green tea (with caffeine), those with hypertension (due to caffeine content), cardiovascular complications, nervousness, insomnia, kidney inflammation, gastrointestinal ulcers.

Ginger Root and Essential Oil

Ginger (*Zingiber officinalis*) has been used since ancient times all over the world as a medicinal agent. It is a very complex herb, consisting of up to 477 ingredients. It is used for digestive problems, nausea, inflammation, as an antioxidant, as an anti-parasitic, and as an antibacterial (studies have shown it to enhance the effectiveness of antibiotics as much as 50%).[95] It has been discovered that ginger inhibits the COX-2 enzyme, which explains why it is an effective anti-inflammatory.

Typical Dosages: Fresh ginger up to 8-10 grams (1 gram=1000mg) daily. Fresh cut root can be used to make tea. Drink 1 cup periodically as needed. One or two drops of the food-grade essential oil can be added to: hot water for tea, food or marinade as a condiment, salad dressings, soups, juice. Dried Ginger: 500 mg. 3 times a day. Tincture: (1:5 dilution) 30 drops 3-6 times daily in warm water, tea, juice.

Caution: May increase the absorption of all oral medications. May increase risk for bleeding when taken with anticoagulant

---

[93] See: Natural Medicines Comprehensive Database, cited above. (P. 430.)

Newmark, T., Schulick, P., previously cited, p. 58.

[95] See: Schulick, P. (1994). Ginger: Common Spice & Wonder Drug. Herbal Free Press, Ltd.: Brattleboro, VT.

medications (e.g., heparin, warfarin, salicy-lates = aspirin).

Holy Basil

Indigenous to India, holy basil (*Ocimum sanctum*) has been used as a spiritual plant in holy sites. It has also been used in Ayurvedic clinics to purify the air, since it oxygenates the environment in a manner unusual to other plants. Unlike the culinary spice (*Ocimum basilicum*), holy basil contains substances known as eleanolic and ursolic acids that have significant COX-2 inhibitory effects. "In research conducted at the Dartmouth Medical School, a study confirmed that derivatives of eleanolic acid and ursolic acid possessed potential anti-inflammatory and cancer-preventing activity related to their inhibition of COX-2."[96]

Dosage: Here holy basil is being used as part of the anti-inflammatory formula Zyflamend described below.

Hu zhang

Hu zhang (*Polygonum cuspidatum*, also known as Japanese knotweed) contains one of the richest sources of the substance resveratrol, a powerful suppressor of the COX-2 pro-inflammatory enzyme. In addition to its anti-inflammatory properties, Hu zhang helps to restore glutathione levels and is a powerful antioxidant in its own right, and cancer research has found it to have anti-tumor properties.

Dosage: Here Hu zhang is being used as part of the anti-inflammatory formula Zyflamend described below.

Oil of Oregano

In addition to being a powerful antimicrobial (see Antimicrobials), wild mountain oil of oregano also has anti-inflammatory properties. An article published in *Phytotherapy Research* describes how oregano oil superseded other anti-inflammatory herbs in reversing pain and inflammation, comparable to morphine.[97]

Dosage: The food-grade oil of oregano produced by the North American Herb & Spice Company is, in my opinion, of the highest quality. Can be applied to any region of the skin (for sensitive skin dilute a few drops in 1 tbsp of olive or sesame oil). A few drops can be taken under the tongue periodically as needed (has a strong taste and produces a vigorous sensation). For children, it blends well with milk.

Oil of Wild Lavender

A flower derived from a Mediterranean shrub, lavender (*Lavandula angustifolia*, etc.) has been used for centuries for skin disorders, anxiety, sleeplessness, digestive problems, and infectious diseases. The effectiveness of lavender as an anti-inflammatory for burns was discovered by René-Maurice Gattefossé, who in 1928 founded the science of aromatherapy.

As the story goes, "One day, Gattefossé scalded his hand whilst working in his laboratory and instinctively immersed it in pure lavender oil. The burn healed much quicker than expected, leaving no scars at all, and this remarkable event inspired him to devote all his energies for the rest of his life to the scientific exploration of essential oils and their properties."[98]

Studies now have confirmed that lavender is a COX-2 inhibitor that can work through the skin (transdermally) to block inflammation and protect the burned skin from secondary infections.

Typical Dosage: As an inhalant use the food-grade essential oil of lavender, 5-10 drops per 1 pint of water in a mister or diffuser. A few drops diluted in 1/2-1 ounce of distilled water can be placed into a nebulizer[*] cup to produce a vapor. Topically, it can be diluted in water or used directly on the skin (or from a spray bottle) onto the affected areas.

---

[96] Newmark, T.; Schulick, P., previously cited, p. 64.
[97] Research information provided by the North American Herb and Spice Co.

[98] Tisserand, M.; Jünemann, M., (American edition, 1994). The Magic and Power of Lavender. Lotus Light Publications: Wilmot, WI. (P. 11.)
[*] May require physician's prescription to obtain. Check the laws in your area.

Caution: Essential oils are volatile. It is best to diffuse without heat. Avoid ingesting the oil. Should not be used by pregnant women or nursing mothers. Use only food-grade. Excellent quality can be purchased from the North American Herb & Spice Company.

Rosemary Leaf and Oil

Rosemary (*Rosmarinus officinalis*) grows abundantly in the Mediterranean area. The herb is rich in antioxidants more powerful than vitamins C or E. It has been traditionally used as a spice and for enhancing concentration and memory, and to relieve headaches. It has antibacterial and antifungal properties. Research has shown that the *whole leaf* of rosemary has a (growing) number of constituents that inhibit the pro-inflammatory COX-2 enzyme. This explains why the oil has been traditionally used to relieve aching, rheumatic muscles.

Typical Dosage and Use: 1000-2000 mg of the leaf powdered in capsules or in tea 3 times a day. Tincture (1:1 in 45% alcohol) 30 drops in warm water, tea, or juice 3 times daily. The oil has all the properties of the leaf and is more versatile to use with all age groups. Five or more drops can be added to juice or water. Works well with grapefruit juice. Here rosemary leaf is being used as part of the anti-inflammatory formula Zyflamend described below.

Caution: Avoid during pregnancy or with heavy menstrual flow since it is a uterine stimulant.

Scutellaria

Scutellaria baicalensis (also known as Baikal skullcap, skullcap, Chinese skullcap, Huang Quin, Ogon, scute, and Wogon)[99] has been used in Asian medicine for over 2000 years. It is a versatile herb that is used for: allergies, asthma, pneumonia, anxiety, headache, stress, cardiovascular problems, bacterial and viral infections, and inflammatory conditions. "Baicalin, a Baikal skullcap glycoside consti-uent, has potent anti-inflammatory and anti-tumor properties."[100] The herb has been used to resolve high fevers that most likely result from interleukin-1, a constituent of the pro-inflammatory cascade. Studies have shown that it inhibits the lipoxygenase metabolism from arachidonic acid. "In research from Barcelona University in Spain published in 1999, scientists determined that baicalein (another constiuent) inhibits COX-2."[101]

Dosage: Here scutellaria is being used as part of the anti-inflammatory formula Zyflamend described below.

Caution: Excessive use of this herb may cause liver problems. Avoid if one has diarrhea.

Turmeric

Turmeric (*Curcuma longa*) has a history of use in both Chinese and Ayurvedic medicine to treat a variety of disorders (including inflammation occurring in a number of bodily systems). "Researchers from New York Presbyterian Hospital and the Weill Medical College of Cornell University reported in the 1999 article in *Cancer Research* that curcumin, a major phytochemical in the bright orange root of the turmeric plant, directly inhibited the activity of COX-2."[102]

Dosage: Here turmeric is being used as part of the anti-inflammatory formula Zyflamend described below.

Caution: Not to be used during pregnancy or lactation, with bile duct obstruction, peptic ulcer, hyperacidity, gallstones, bleeding disorders, hypertension, or by those who are hypersensitive to it.

Zyflamend™

Zyflamend is an anti-inflammatory (COX-2 inhibitor) formula developed by **New Chapter**, which contains the following herbs, which were discussed above:

---

[99] Should not be confused with American skullcap (Scutellaria laterifiora).

[100] Natural Medicines Comprehensive Database (3rd Edition, 2000). Therapeutic Research Faculty: Stockton, CA. (P. 94.)

[101] Newmark, T.; Schilick, P., previously cited, pp.79-80. (Parenthesis mine.)

[102] Newmark, T.; Schilick, P., cited above, p. 70.

Rosemary Leaf, 150 mg, Turmeric root 110 mg, Ginger root 100 mg,, Holy Basil 100 mg, Green Tea 100 mg, Hu Zhang 80 mg, Chinese Goldthread 40 mg, Barberry Root 40 mg, Oregano Leaf 40 mg,Scutellaria baicalensis 20 mg.

Interactions: May increase bleeding when taken with anticoagulant drugs (e.g., heparin, warfarin, salicylates = aspirin). May decrease the effectiveness of immunosuppressant drugs (e.g., cyclosporin).

MSM

MSM (methylsulfonylmethane) is an organic-sulfur compound found in plant and animal cells. It plays a vital role in maintaining the integrity of collagen in the connective tissues such as around joints, arteries, and the skin (also nails and hair). MSM also has potent anti-inflammatory properties.

Dosage: 500 mg for every 30 lbs of body weight. When used therapeutically this amount should be doubled. This substance is safe for use with dogs and cats.

Vitamin K

Vitamin K1 (phytonadione) is a factor involved in the clotting of blood. It has also been shown to be an effective anti-inflammatory agent capable of lowering cytokine production.

Dosage:

Age	Mcg
0-6 months	5
6-12 months	10
1-3 years	15
4-6 years	20
7-10 years	30
11-14 years	45
15-18 years (Males/Females)	65/55
19-24 years (Males/Females)	70/60
25+ years (Males/Females)	80/65
25+ years (Pregnant, lactating females)	65
Therapeutic:	**100-500**

Caution: Antagonizes the effectiveness of oral anticoagulants (e.g., warfarin, heparin, salicylates = aspirin).

HOMEOPATHIC REMEDIES

While the Homeopathic Formulary is one of only two forms of medicine officially recognized by the Congress of the United States, many homeopathic practitioners in the U.S. are concerned about how this form of therapy is being ignored.

The President-Elect of the American Institute of Homeopathy, Joyce Frye, DO, MBA expresses her concern about the neglect on using homeopathic medicine to help with the treatment of disease for the bioterrorist threats that we currently face. She writes: "In this time of national threat from terrorists, it is essential to consider every possible means of preparing for and treating the potential consequences of assault in any form. Homeopathic medicine has a two hundred year history of success in the treatment and prophylaxis of thousands of cases of epidemic disease. Additionally, it has uses in the treatment of anxiety and the effects of trauma and shock. Yet, public health officials in our current crisis are overlooking it."[103]

In an article by Wayne B. Jonas, M.D. (entitled *Directions for Research in Complementary Medicine and Bioterrorism*, in the March/April issue of *Alternative Therapies Journal*) he discusses some of the documented successes homeopathy has had with epidemics of infectious diseases in various parts of the world.

"Two examples from that literature include the cholera epidemic in Europe in 1831 and the influenza pandemic of 1918. The mortality rate under conventional treatment was between 40% and 80%. Out of every 5 people who contracted cholera, 2 to 4 died under regular treatment. Dr Quinn, in London, reported the mortality in the 10 homeopathic hospitals in 1831 and 1832 as 9%; Dr Roth, physician to the king of Bavaria, reported that under homeopathic care the mortality was 7%. Admiral Mordoinow of the Imperial Russian Council reported a 10% mortality

---

[103] .... Homeopathy In Crisis Intervention. (P. 1.)

rate under homeopathy."[104] Because of this he feels homeopathy and other forms of alternative therapies should be seriously studied for use against bioterrrorism.

In other areas around the world, such as in Europe and India, homeopathy is used as a viable medical treatment. It is even used during emergency situations. Considering this information I've opted to include homeopathy as part of the supportive lines of defense.

What is Homeopathy?

Homeopathy is a natural system of medicine developed by the German physician Samuel Hahnemann over 200 years ago. It is based on two key principles: the *law of similars*, and *potentization*.

The law of similars means "like cures like", which attributes the power to heal from a disease to the very substance that caused it (or produces similar symptoms). For example, the herb *Belladonna*, if taken in its original form, causes tightness in the throat, difficulty swallowing, vomiting, delirium, and possible coma and death, but, when given in minute amounts, it can relieve conditions that manifest with similar symptoms. The diluted substance is called a *remedy*, and the strength of this remedy depends on how much it has been diluted or *potentized*.

Potentization is the process by which the strength of a remedy is increased through incremental dilutions. In his book, *Homeopathy: Medicine of the New Man*, the renowned homeopath George Vithoulkas describes the staggering extent to which a remedy can be diluted and still remain effective. He writes: "A substance shaken and diluted to a dilution of 1 in 100,000 parts, even to a total of 60 zeros and more, still acts to cure disease, quickly and permanently, and without side effects!"[105] When a substance is diluted to such an extent it becomes impossible to detect its molecular presence by even the most sensitive scientific instruments.

The label of a homeopathic remedy will indicate its strength by a number followed by the letter "C" (to represent centesimal scale) or "X" (to represent the decimal scale). Higher numbers signify a more potent remedy, which may be used with serious diseases. For example, when 1 part of a substance is mixed into 99 parts of a diluting medium (water, alcohol, etc.) and shaken (succussed), and this is repeated 6 times, it will be represented by 6C. A potency of 30 C has been through a similar process 30 times, and so on.

The theory behind potentization, as I understand it, is that the energy configuration of the substance is transferred to the diluting medium (e.g., water, alcohol, etc.) Because of this homeopathy is sometimes referred to as an energy form of healing that reaches the subtle energy field of a living system. The subtle energy field is considered to be the opposite yet complementary template of its physical expression, the body. Therefore, when it receives the cause of the disease it will reverse it into a cure.

Because the substance represents the symptoms of the disease it is important for homeopaths to match the remedy with the symptoms. If the match is a good one, the remedy will more accurately evoke the healing potential of the subtle energy field. Healing is aimed not at the symptoms but to the deeper underlying cause of pathology.

The clinical aspect of homeopathy relies on Hering's "law of cure", developed by one of Hahnemann's pupils, Constantine Hering, which describes the nature of how the disease will be released by the system. According to this law:

- The symptoms should disappear in the reverse order of how they originally appeared;
- Healing progresses from more vital organs to less vital ones;
- Healing progresses from the top of the body downward;
- The disease is released toward the exterior of the body.

[104] .... (P. 30.)

[105] .... (P. 21.)

These stages help one to evaluate if the remedy is working. Various remedies may be used until a complete cure has taken place. The homeopathic repertoire has over 3,000 remedies.

The Practice of Homeopathy In Emergencies

Homeopathy is used for ordinary and serious diseases. It is also used for medical emergency situations. In their book, *Homeopathy 911: What to Do in an Emergency Before Help Arrives*, Eileen Nauman, D.H.M, EMT-B, and Gail Derin-Kellogg, O.M.D., EMT-B, offer instructions on how to utilize homeopathy during an emergency. The following advice is gleaned from this valuable book.

- NEVER use more than the recommended dosage of 6 C. More than this could cause complications (however not life threatening).
- If the person is fully conscious and there are no problems with the airway or breathing hold the open bottle of the remedy close to their nostril so it can be inhaled. If the symptoms do not clear within 10 minutes, then place one drop under the tongue. Applying the remedy on the skin is a better method if there are any doubts about the person's consciousness, airway, and breathing.
- When the injured or sick person is unconscious NEVER put dry pellets or liquids in their mouth. Apply a liquid form of the remedy on the skin to be absorbed into the system.
- Place one drop of the chosen remedy onto the underside of the person's wrist and **gently** rub it in. Or, if not possible to use the wrist, place it behind the ear and **gently** rub it in. Apply it in a circular motion to cover an area about the size of a dime. Do not use more than one drop.
- Do this every 15 minutes until the symptoms stop and/or help arrives. Once the symptoms stop do not continue to give the remedy.

- Homeopathic pellets can be converted into the liquid form, if necessary, by placing 10-20 pellets into a 1 ounce eye dropper bottle filled with brandy.

Homeopathy and Bioterrorism

While the authors of *Homeopathy 911* address typical emergency situations (many of which can be very serious) there are homeopathic practitioners who are offering advice for emergencies from a terrorist event. In this regard, Nancy Eos, M.D., of South Fallsburg, New York, has written a series of three articles entitled *Homeopathy for Major Emergencies*, which have been placed on the Internet. The following advice is gleaned from these articles.

- Homeopathy is not to be used as a substitute for medical treatment. It can be used adjunctively or until help arrives.
- Homeopathy emphasizes a preventative approach.
- For **prophylaxis** they recommend: *Arsenicum* (for viral or bacterial diseases such as anthrax, yellow fever, etc.; *Nux-vomica* (for chemical toxins such as sarin, cyanide, etc.); *Hypericum* (for tetanus); *Baptisia* (for Typhoid or Typhus); *Cuprum* or *Camphor* or *Veratrum-album* (for cholera); *Variolinum* (for smallpox); and *Anthracinum* (for anthrax).

She recommends 12 BASIC REMEDIES that could be useful to deal with the possibility or the occurrence of a bioterrorist event. These are:

Aconite: for fright or terrors, cold, sudden and intense fevers, cough; for bright red hemorrhages, nervousness; first stages of infectious diseases.

Arnica: the "accident remedy"; for injury, head trauma, bruising, as well as muscle aches, surgery, and shock; "It's never too late for arnica".

Arsenicum: for food poisoning; exhaustion that is out of proportion to the illness, or physical and mental restlessness.

Bryonia: for irritability, wanting to cool the body temperature, reduce stimulation and remain isolated; symptoms become worse after any motion and/or become worse after eating.

Carbo-veg: after sudden collapse with limbs cold, bluish, sweat cold, and clammy, for that condition we describe as having "never fully recovered".

Gelsemium: for "butterflies" in stomach; general weakness and trembling; and all viral symptoms.

Hepar-sulph-cal: for any infection especially abscesses, bacteria in the blood, pus, sore throats; very irritable and impatient.

Hypericum: for nerves; sharp pains; seizures; nervous depression; headache; for superficial puncture wounds after Aconite and Arnica.

Ledum: for deep puncture wounds after Aconite and Arnica; deep bruising; dark red hemorrhages; joint pains; itching; wounds cold to the touch.

Nux-vomica: for "too much of anything bad"; feeling overly sensitive; abdominal complaints; working to the point of exhaustion; irritable type of anger associated with stress.

Rhus-tox: itchy, burning rashes; complaints of arthritis; anxious restlessness; stiffness after resting; paralysis; fever with cough and diarrhea.

Sulphur: taken after other remedies, it helps them work; diarrhea; skin eruptions; restless; relapsing symptoms; always burning.

How to Use the 12 Basic Remedies

According to Dr. Eos, "In any situation always give immediately: Aconite or Arnica. Give Carbo-veg or Sulphur if the symptom is total physical collapse. Then try to match a more specific remedy with the following symptoms. One dose of 3 pellets in an emergency is usually enough to feel a little better in a few minutes. If no effect, try another remedy. If we choose a "wrong" remedy for what ails us, it won't help, yet it will not harm us, so keep trying different remedies until improvement is seen."[106]

---

[106] Eos, N., cited above (emphasis mine).

- Abscesses, boils infected lumps: Hepar-sulph-cal, Sulphur, Arnica, Arsenicum
- Abdominal complaints, belly pain: Nux-vomica, Arsenicum, Sulphur, Carbo-veg, Rhus-tox
- Backache: Arnica, Rhus-tox, Nux-vomica, Hypericum, Bryonia
- Bleeding: Arnica. Aconite. Arsenicum, Bryonia, Rhus-tox, Carbo-veg
- Buboes, swollen, inflamed, suppurating lymph nodes: Hepar-sulph-cal, Arsenicum, Arnica
- Chest pain: Bryonia, Aconite, Arsenicum, Sulphur
- Chills, rigor. Aconite, Arsenicum, Carbo-veg
- Cough: Aconite, Bryonia, Arsenicum, Sulphur, Hepar-sulph-cal
- Coma: Carbo-veg, Arnica, Aconite
- Confusion, severe: Gelsemium, Aconite, Arsenicum, Sulphur, Bryonia
- Constipation: Nux~vomica, Sulphur, Bryonia
- Dehydration: Bryonia, Arsenicum
- Diarrhea: Arsenicum, Nux-vomica, Rhus-tox, Sulphur
- Eye problems, conjunctivitis. Ledum, Aconite
- Fever – High: Aconite. Gelsemium, Sulphur, Hepar-sulph-cal
- Fever – Low grade: Arsenicum, Sulphur, Hepar-sulph-cal
- Fever – Intermittent, spiking: Gelsemium, Sulphur, Hepar-sulph-cal
- Gangrene, gas: Carbo-veg, Arsenicum
- Headache Nux-vomica, Gelsemium, Aconite
- Heart irregular: Gelsemium, Aconite, Nux-vomica, Carbo-veg
- Itch: Rhus-tox, Sulphur
- Liver problems, jaundice: Bryonia, Arsenicum, Nux-vomica, Hepar-sulph-cal, Sulphur
- Muscles aching, cramping: Bryonia, Aconite, Gelsemium, Arnica, Nux-vomica, Rhus-tox
- Nausea: Nux-vomica, Carbo-veg, Arsenicum, Bryonia
- Nervousness: Gelsemium, Aconite, Rhus-tox
- Pain – in general: Arnica, Hypericum, Rhus-tox, Bryonia, Arsenicum, Ledum
- Pain – Joints: Bryonia, Sulphur, Rhus-tox, Ledum, Aconite
- Pain – moving eyes: Arnica, Ledum, Hepar-sulph-cal, Arsenicum, Hypericum
- Paralysis – ascending legs to head: Gelsemium, Hypericum
- Paralysis – descending head to legs: Aconite, Hypericum, Arsenicum
- Paralysis – in general: Hypericum
- Pneumonia: Aconite, Bryonia, Arsenicum, Sulphur, Hepar-sulph-cal
- Rash: Rhus-tox, Gelsemium, Sulphur, Ledum, Arsenicum, Hepar-sulph-cal
- Seizures: Hypericum, Sulphur, Nux-vomica, Gelsemium
- Shock: Carbo-veg, Arsenicum, Hepar-sulph-cal, Sulphur, Rhus-tox
- Skin red: Aconite, Rhus-tox
- Sore throat: Aconite, Hepar-sulph-cal, Rhus-tox, Bryonia
- Tired, malaise: Gelsemium, Bryonia, Arsenicum
- Vision double or blurred: Gelsemium, Aconite
- Vomiting: Arsenicum, Nux-vomica, Sulphur, Aconite, Bryonia

Care of the Remedies

Dr. Eos recommends that certain precautions should be followed when using homeopathic remedies. "The remedies, which come in the form of pellets, should be touched only by the person who is taking them.[107] Use the cap to measure the dose. If your supply is limited, a dose may be taken by inhalation, being sure to

---

[107] An exception may occur with an unconscious person. In this case, one could consider the procedure recommended above by Nauman and Derin-Kellogg of applying the remedy onto another person.

not breathe into the vial. Recap the vial quickly. Keep remedies away from strong odors, dampness and direct sunlight so that the energy of the pellets is not lost."[108]

Vaccines and Prophylaxis

From a naturalistic perspective, what comes close to the use of vaccinations or prophylaxis can only be found in the work done by homeopathic practitioners using formulations known as *nosodes* and *sarcodes*. Nosodes are made like any other homeopathic remedy except that the material used to create it comes from the disease agent itself (similar to but not like a vaccine). Sarcodes are made from affected organs, tissue, and secretions. "Historically in infectious outbreaks, a nosode of the disease material and/or genus epidemicus once identified, was given orally for prophylaxis against further cases."[109]

Studies with animals have shown the efficacy of this approach. "In one such study, the incidence of illness in pig herds in Germany, particularly susceptible to infections due to their crowded growing conditions, was compared after one of three treatments—a homeopathic combination remedy chosen for the particular symptoms of infection, prophylactic doses of antibiotic, or full doses of antibiotic. The pigs treated homeopathically fared as well as those given prophylactic antibiotics, although both groups had somewhat more illness than those maintained on full dose of antibiotics."[110]

"Other studies have demonstrated protection from salmonella in chickens equivalent to Cipro using homeopathic **Baptisia 30c**, and partial protection from tularemia in mice using the **Tularemia** nosode. Clearly the animal data warrants prompt further study for human applications as the threat of bioterrorism looms. Initial emphasis should be on those diseases for which vaccination and/or antibiotic therapy is ineffective, not readily available, or associated with unacceptable side effects."[111]

In certain parts of the world where homeopathy is an accepted form of medicine there are reports of the successful use of nosodes. For instance, "Reuters (10/1) reported from the Times of India the recommendation of Dr. B. Gangapadhyay, a former head of the Orissa Medical College of Homeopathy and Research, 'Anthracinum (nosode) works like magic. If a person just takes a dose (of anthracinum) for two days in succession, he would be immune from anthrax for at least three months."[112]

In the *Repertory of Homeopathic Nosodes and Sarcodes* by Berkeley Squire[113] the following nosodes and sarcodes are listed: Anthracinum (Anthrax), Botulinum (Botulism), Brucella melitensis (Brucellosis), Enterococcinum (Enterotoxin), Radium (Radium), Serum of Yersin (Yersinia Pestis), Staphylococcinum (Staph), Tuberculinum (TB).

Naturalistic Therapies

Inhalation Therapy

Inhalation therapy involves rendering a substance into an aerosolized state (such as a fine mist) so that it can be breathed into the lungs and into sinus passages. The size of the droplets depends on how the substance is aerosolized. Very fine particle sizes can more effectively penetrate the mucous membranes in the lungs and be absorbed into the system. Of all the home methods, ultrasonic humidifiers and nebulizers* produce the finest particle size without heating the substance. Heating it may change its molecular structure, an effect I personally disfavor. The humidifier is a good method for modifying the air in a room, etc. The nebulizer can be used to directly inhale, for example, an herbal tincture or an essential

---

[108] .... (P. 2.)
[109] Frye, J. Homeopathy In Crisis Intervention. (P. 5.) Note: using homeopathic remedies for prophylaxis has not been sanctioned by the FDA.
[110] Frye, J. Cited above. (P. 5.)

[111] Frey, J. Cited above. (P. 5.)
[112] Frey, J. Cited above. (P. 6.)
[113] ...(1999). .... Jain Publishers (P) LTD: New Delhi, India.
* May require a prescription by a physician to obtain. Check the state and federal laws.

oil of a desired concentration. Both would work synergistically.

A simple method is to add an essential oil to a handkerchief and place it under the nose to inhale the essence. Or, inhale the essence directly from the bottle.

A perfume or fine spray bottle could also be employed to achieve the same purpose. The advantage of the spray bottle is that the substance will not deteriorate as easily. Certain therapies may require a bottle with a nozzle to be inserted as a nasal spray.

Breathing Exercises

The yogic forms of breathing exercises known as *Pranayama* are the most developed in the world. Anyone having gone through an assault by a WMD will most likely have respiratory issues. These exercises can help to restore and strengthen lung capacity. They are also beneficial to any form of psychological and spiritual practice.

PETS

For many folks, a pet has become family. For them, leaving it behind during a terrorist event, or not knowing what to do to protect it from harm could be a heart-breaking experience. The aim of including pets in this book stems from my love of the natural world and my involvement with a wide variety of animals that gave me happiness, love, and knowledge, especially during my childhood. Although my expertise is with natural forms of healing for human beings, there is considerable crossover of nutrients and therapies between humans and animals. Yet, I'm not an expert in this area, and I have had to rely on others to glean information that could be applicable to the subject at hand.

The information here is derived from a variety of sources. Most of my information was learned from CJ Puotinen's books, especially the *Natural Remedies for Dogs and Cats*.[114] The recommendations made in this book are mainly for dogs and cats, considering that these are the most common type of pets. One would need to consult a veterinarian, or similarly trained professional, to learn what approaches could be used with other kinds of animals.

Essentially, there are very few natural substances mentioned in this book that could not be used for a dog or cat exposed to an agent of mass destruction. For example, they can be given the following supplements: enzymes, vitamins, minerals, amino acids, essential fatty acids, hormones and glandular extracts, and a wide variety of herbal preparations. However, the dosages and method of administration might need to be altered.

A number of the naturalistic therapies could also be used to help them. These include: prevention, detoxification, aromatherapy, flower essences, and homeopathic remedies.

In some instances, the animal could be naturally immune to the disease, and in others it may be the carrier and transmitter of a potent pathogen. This is important to know.

The specific information regarding pets will be provided for each agent under the Supportive Lines of Natural Defense. The following supplement could be used to support the immune response in dogs and cats.

Gary Null's Pet's Health[115]

Four tablets provide:

Vitamin C	300 mg.
Garlic	50 mg
Barberry	25 mg
Cayenne	25 mg
Cinnamon	25 mg
Clove	25 mg
Goldenseal	25 mg
Myrrh	10 mg
Onion	25 mg
Rosemary	25 mg
Usnea	25 mg
Angelica	25 mg
Artemeisia	25 mg
Echinacea	75 mg
Pau D'Arco	50 mg
St. Johnswort	20 mg
Reishi	20 mg
Capryllic Acid	45 mg
Citrus Bead Ext.	100 mg
Lemongrass	30 mg

---

[114] ... (1999).... Keats Publishing: Lincolnwood, IL.

[115] Or comparable product.

Milk Thistle	10 mg
Anise	10 mg
Horseradish	50 mg
Hyssop	50 mg
Astragalus	50 mg
Beta Carotene	2500 IU

In a garlic/liver base

Emergency Formulas

From Poutinen's book I've selected various formulas that I thought could be useful for the types of conditions that are being addressed in this book.

Laxative Formula

This is a gentle laxative formula for dogs and cats for short-term use:

"Combine equal parts powdered psyllium husks and apple pectin. Add 1/4 teaspoon powder per 10 pounds of body weight to enough water, juice, or other liquid to soak it well. As the powder expands, the liquid will thicken. Add to food once or twice per day, and give extra fluids."[116]

Formula for Diarrhea

This is an anti-diarrheal formula for dogs and cats: Dry blackberries in dehydrator or oven until hard, and store in a glass jar away from heat and light.

"When needed, grind the dried blackberries and add the powder to vegetable glycerine, a combination most dogs enjoy, or to small amounts of your pet's favorite food, using 1/4 to 1/2 teaspoon powder per 10 pounds of weight. Alternatively, fill capsules of a size your pet will swallow. Blackberry powder should help stop diarrhea almost immediately. Repeat several hours later if needed."[117]

During Serious Illness and Recovery

"Combine 1/4 cup of slippery elm powder with 2 teaspoons acidophilus powder and 1 teaspoon unrefined sea salt. If available, add the contents of 2 Seacure[118] capsules. Add just enough water to make a slippery syrup that you can feed to your pet by spoon, dropper, or infant nursing bottle. ... To help treat a serious illness or diarrhea, give 1 teaspoon per 10 pounds of body weight every 2 to 3 hours. For a vomiting pet, give 1 teaspoon 5 minutes before feeding."[119]

Alleviate Vomiting and to Increase Absorption of Nutrients or Medications

Prepare in advance and have ready a Ginger Glycerite formula for dogs and cats to alleviate vomiting:

"Loosely fill a pint jar with coarsely chopped fresh ginger root. Fill the jar to the top with vegetable glycerine, which is available in some health food stores. Leave the jar in a warm room for six weeks or longer, shaking it every few days. Glycerine has a sweet taste and viscous consistency that most dogs and many cats find palatable."[120] **Dose:** about 1/2 tsp per 20 pounds of body weight on empty stomach. Can be mixed in favorite food, if necessary. Might be more palatable to finicky cats if mixed with some Valerian Root.

Because of the catalytic effects of ginger, this formula would also assist in the absorption of nutrients and to enhance the effects of medications.

Psychological

To help alleviate the stress dogs and cats may experience during a traumatic event, or when their normal habitat and habit patterns are disrupted, or when they pick up the caretaker's stress levels (which they so often do) consider using *Rescue Remedy* flower essence formula. Other flower essences may be selected based on the specific behavior a pet may exhibit; consult with a qualified practitioner or holistic veterinarian.

Excellent behavioral, environmental, homeopathic, herbal, emergency and first aid advice, including "How to Give Your Pet a Check-Up," can be found in *Dr. Pitcairn's Complete Guide to Natural Health for Dogs & Cats* by Richard H. Pitcairn, D.V.M., Ph..D. and Susan Hubble Pitcairn. Another valuable resource, *Natural Healing for Dogs & Cats* by Diane Stein, covers flower essences, acupressure, homeopathy and more, and offers many important references for further research.

It is best to seek the guidance and expertise of a holistic veterinarian for specific advice for

---

[116] Poutinen, CJ, cited above, p. 157.

[117] Poutinen, CJ, cited above, p. 156.

[118] A nutritional supplement made from deep-sea fish that are predigested by a fermentation process. Considered to be a whole-food supplement, containing: natural amino acids, unsaturated fats, and trace minerals. It is reported to improve immune function, joint flexibility, digestion, allergies, wound healing, stamina, and to assist detoxification.

[119] Poutinen, CJ, cited above, p. 157.

[120] Puotinen, C J, cited above, p 151.

your pet in advance of a problem or crisis. Many "conventional" veterinarians are becoming more open to natural approaches and may be willing to help. Local directories can provide listings of holistic vets; ask your local health food store for referrals, or search online. One excellent website is www.altvetmed.com.

In general, a person maintaining a calm and alert state of mind will be very helpful and comforting to pets. *Rescue Remedy* flower essence can be used by both people and pets. 2 drops of the liquid flower essence can be placed in the animal's water, or, rub the drops between your hands and gently stroke your pet to apply it to their fur.

Do not put the drops directly onto a cat's skin, as they are highly sensitive to the small amount of alcohol that is used to preserve the essence (some dogs may be, also.) It can be mixed into food or treats, or placed in a small spray bottle to mist the air, bedding, or carrier that your pet may be in (use your discretion if your pet is frightened by the sound of a spray bottle.)

Other flower essences address specific behaviors that your animal may exhibit; see Diane Stein's book for recommendations, or websites that work with flower essences for animals. Two good examples are:

- www.anaflora.com,
- and www.petsynergy.com.

The Bach flower essence website has a good page for animals, as well.

Absorbents

The use of Acitvated Charcoal is probably the best absorbent for toxins. Follow directions given for each specific agent.

Essential Oils

Because of their fast metabolism cats are very sensitive to undiluted essential oils. I would avoid using them directly with cats and dogs.

Antimicrobials

Even though grapefruit seed extract is an excellent antimicrobial for pets, it has a bitter taste and may be difficult to mask. The capsule form (by NutriBiotic®) may be opened in food. ASAP Solution® as recommended for each agent may also be used. It is tasteless, and large doses are harmless for people as well as dogs and cats.

Basic Supportive Program

The following program is made within the context of the previously discussed *Five Supportive Lines of Defense*. There are specific characteristics of each agent that will require special attention; these are addressed in the sections describing each agent. While the following suggestions are based on research and my own professional experience, they are essentially steps that I would personally take adjunctively to protect myself against WMD. **Select the suggestions that best meet your needs.**

Psychological Line:

- Perform the <u>Relaxation Response</u> (or a comparable form of meditation or mental relaxation method based on your personal belief system) 1-2 times daily or as needed to quell fears and develop calmness in the midst of perceived danger. During an attack, think of the cue word, thought, or image that would elicit the Relaxation Response. Previous development is an advantage. The following preparatory suggestions might be helpful.
- <u>Hypnotherapy</u> from a qualified practitioner or through autosuggestion.
- <u>Thought Field Therapy</u> from a certified practitioner.
- <u>Subtle Energy Work</u>: Reiki, etc.
- <u>5-HTP</u> (5-hydroxytryptophan) 200-300 mg 1-3 times daily between meals at least 45 minutes before food with room temperature or cool non-protein drink (no caffeinated drinks) to increase the calming neurotransmitter seratonin, as a possible anti-depressive. Adults only.
- <u>GABA</u> (gamma-aminobutyric acid) 500-1000 mg 1-3 times daily between meals at least 30 minutes before food with a room temperature or cool non-protein drink (no caffeine drinks), to help reduce anxiety (worry and nervousness about what might happen). Adults only
- <u>Melatonin</u> 3-18 mg 1/2 to 1 hour before bedtime with water if you have difficulty getting deep sleep. Adults only.

- <u>Homeopathic</u>: such as <u>Aconite</u> (for fear, fright, sudden extreme events). Also: <u>Rescue Remedy</u> Flower essence (liquid or cream).
- <u>**Beautiful Calming Impressions**</u> are food for the soul.
- <u>**Trust**</u> in your Divinely given power to heal.

Social Line:

- **Seek medical help.**
- Inform authorities.
- Consider forming or joining a **Neighborhood Defense Support Group**.
- Consider learning First Aid and Home Caring Skills.
- Preplan an exchange of help with friends and/or relatives.
- Attempt to determine if <u>the agent/disease in question is or is not contagious</u>. If you don't know, consider it contagious and take precautions.
- Consider preparing a simple written plan for action should you or any family member, friends, or neighbors need help. Leave it in a conspicuous place.
- It is always important to have a kit of <u>protective supplies</u> available for caretakers and visitors. Ideally, it should contain: (1) disposable emergency gas masks, 2) disposable medical grade mask capable of filtering biological agents (bacteria, viruses, toxins) 0.01 microns in size, (3) non-allergenic medical gloves, (4) goggles (swimmers' ok), (5) a portable supply of oxygen, (6) plastic bags with ties or seals for hazardous waste items (+ a

marker to identify as "hazardous waste"), 7) instructions (e.g., as outlined on the form "Please Read Before Helping Me/Us).

- ❑ A cellular telephone, to use for emergency calls only.
- ❑ A battery operated or wind-up (preferable) radio.
- ❑ If possible, make sure laboratory tests are done to diagnose and confirm what kind of illness you may have.
- ❑ If possible, take the items of your natural health program with you should you need to be hospitalized, plus written instructions of how to use them. While this may not occur immediately there's a chance that it can be used during the convalescent stage.

Preventative Line:

Use this line of defense to bolster immunity. This is important. By strengthening your immune system with the general program your predisposition level to infectious diseases will decrease.

- ❑ Healthy Dietary.
- ❑ All One (Rice Base, by Nutritech, or comparable formula) 1 1/2 tsp added to the Magma Plus.
- ❑ Mighty Vita-Kids: (liquid multi vitamins and trace minerals, by Tropical Oasis, or comparable formula); follow directions on container.
- ❑ Vita Quick (liquid high potency multi vitamin formula, by Twin Lab, or comparable formula); follow directions on the container.
- ❑ Liquid Multiple-Minerals (Innovative Natural Products, or comparable formula) as a complement to Vita Quick. Follow directions on container.
- ❑ Magma Plus™ (by Green Food, or comparable formula) as directed on the container, 1/2 of the recommended measure 2 times daily.
- ❑ Yummy Greens (chewable, by Solar Green, or comparable formula). Follow directions on the container.

- ❑ Udo's Choice (essential fatty acid blend, by Flora Manufacturing & Distributing Ltd., or comparable formula) 1000 mg 3 times daily with food (see Children under Specific line for dosage recommendations).
- ❑ Digestive Aids: OmegaZyme (full enzyme complex, by Garden of Life, or comparable formula); KidZYME (enzymes and probiotic factors for children, by Renew Life, or comparable formula); Betaine Hydrochloride (HCL, stomach acid by various manufacturers); toasted Fennel Seeds, chew 1 tsp right after meal and swallow them, or drink the tea).
- ❑ Probiotics.
- ❑ Digestive Stimulants: Ginger (in almost any form); Trikatu (Three Spices for Sinus Support, by Planetary Formulas, or comparable product). Follow directions on the container.
- ❑ Laxatives: Aloe-V (by Atrium, Inc., or comparable formula, 1-4 caplets near bed time with water); Magnesium Citrate (100-400 mg near bed time with water); KidLAX (by Renew Life, or comparable product).
- ❑ Those with weak immune systems consider adding to your program 500-1000 mg of Olive Leaf Extract daily.[121]
- ❑ Considering the damaging effect toxins and radiation could have on the cell nucleic acids (DNA, RNA), I would add to my daily preventative or specific or rehabilitative program 60-120 mg of Co-Q-10 (coenzyme-Q-10). This enzyme has been shown to protect the DNA/RNA of cells (especially, in the energy-producing mito-

---

[121] Olive Leaf Extract has a tendency to lower blood pressure. Those with very low blood pressure may use Echinacea (capsule or tincture) or garlic (bulb, capsule, or **Kyolic**) instead.

chondria within the cell), and for cell integrity in general.[122]

- In addition to the preventative program, add mycelized <u>vitamin A</u> (use 1/2 the recommended dose 1 time per day) and mycelized <u>vitamin E</u> (200-400 IU 1-2 times a day) and <u>MSM</u> (methyl sulfonyl methane, 500 mg for every 30 lbs of body weight) are useful for strengthening cellular membranes.

- <u>Alpha Lipoic Acid</u> has shown promise in experimental models to prevent chemical poisoning.[123] Consider taking 300 mg of sustained release 2-3 times daily between meals at least 30 minutes before food with water.

- With suspicious food take 2-6 capsules of <u>Charco-Zyme</u>™ (activated charcoal with enzymes, by Atrium, Inc, or a comparable product), as soon as possible after ingesting, with a glass of water. Prolonged use of absorbents may bind the stools and cause constipation. To help prevent this drink plenty of water.

Environmental Line:

- Disposable <u>Portable Emergency Gas Mask</u> and <u>Medical Grade Masks</u> capable of filtering most (if not all) bacterial agents would be useful to have in various places. Keep one in the car, at work, and on your person. **However**, blister/vesicants can penetrate the material of a mask, unless it is made of vesicant-proof materials (see specific nature of the agent). A small pair of swimmers' goggles might complement the medical mask, considering that some bacterial agents affect the eyes.

- Consider using at home and/or at work an ultrasonic humidifier with <u>Grape-</u> fruit Seed Extract</u> and/or tea tree oil added to the water (10 drops per pint of water). Periodically inhaling the mist might make the lung tissue inhospitable to the virus. Place in the room of the sick, and leave it on all the time.

- Consider using an <u>Ozone and Negative Ion Generator</u> in the room and/or house, office, car. Ozone kills germs, and it will freshen the air.

- Consider the work environment to see where protective measures can be used against aerosol of the agent. For example, the barring of access to air conditioning ducts, etc.

- Consider creating a Bio-Safe area or room.

- It's not likely that an attack would occur in the home, except if a powdered form is delivered through the mail or if one eats contaminated food. Any biological agent can be turned into an aerosol powder and sent through the mail.

- If concerned, wear protective mask and rubber gloves to pick up mail and lightly spray mail and/or packages with <u>GSE</u> or <u>ASAP</u> solution before opening. Suspicious powder should be sprayed and placed in plastic bag and sealed. Call authorities.

- Decontaminate the exposed environment with hypochlorite, GSE, or ASAP solutions.

- Hypochlorite solution is capable of neutralizing virtually all known chemical and biological WMD, after at least 15 minutes of contact time. Then it should be rinsed off with plain water.

- 0.5% Hypochlorite: **Add 64 fluid oz (1/2 gallon) of household bleach (regular, no additives or scent) to 5 gallons of water. Add to spray bottle(s).**

- <u>Grapefruit Seed Extract</u> (as a surface decontaminant) 30-40 drops per quart

---

[122] Life Extension Magazine (Collector's Edition 2002), Mitochondria hold the key to cellular life and death. (P. 109.)
[123] Natural Medicines Comprehensive Database, previously cited, p 41.

or liter of water, or <u>ASAP Solution</u>® inactivates the toxin. Add to spray bottle(s). Allow at least 15-20 minutes of contact time. No need to be concerned if it stays on objects longer since it is not a corrosive.

❑ <u>Dräger Detection</u> equipment is available to detect all chemical agents.

❑ Detector might be connected to high power exhaust system to draw agents out into a neutralizing chamber or safe atmosphere. "Most chemical and biological agents that present an inhalation hazard will break down fairly rapidly when exposed to the sun, diluted with water, or dissipated in high winds."[124]

Specific Line: The Specific Line of defense would be used if you suspect or know that you have been exposed to a WMD. Part of this line could be used preventively. It's important not to overuse this line because the body can entrain to the natural substances (develop resistance to them). **<u>This line is not intended as a substitute for medical care</u>**. It may be used adjunctively or alone if medical care is not available.

Foods

❑ Avoid eating heavy flesh foods. Ingest fresh fruits, vegetables, whole grain foods and products. Soups are excellent. Avoid refined sugars, soft drinks, saturated fats (butter, etc.), high calorie meals, and processed foods. Drink plenty of liquids, especially decaffeinated teas, and water.

❑ A <u>14 Day Emergency Food Supply</u>.

❑ <u>Lung Kichadi</u> would help to detox and strengthen the lungs.

❑ Because <u>iron</u> is found in so many foods take **IP6 (Inositol Hexaphospate)**, 1-2 capsules with meals to take out some of it. Iron

feeds bacteria and supports their toxic activity. If you have iron deficiency anemia consult with a physician in advance about temporarily cutting back on it during a bacterial infection.

❑ <u>Green Tea</u> also helps to chelate iron from foods (and it's less expensive). Drink 1 cup with meals.

Micronutrients

❑ Continue taking nutrients for general support. Stay with the <u>All One</u> and the <u>Magma Plus</u> with 1-2 capsules of <u>IP6</u> or mix in 1/2 cup of <u>Green Tea</u> (to help chelate the small amount of iron).

❑ With biological agents **avoid taking** supplemental iron.

❑ <u>Vitamin C</u> (<u>Super C</u> by **Twin Lab**) 1/4 to 1 tsp in one cup of non-tap (bottled or filtered OK) water to bowel tolerance (slightly loose stools); add a small amount of water to the powder to make a paste, then add the rest and stir. After reaching bowel tolerance cut back until stools normalize. If stools are loose to begin with use <u>SuperAscorbate C</u> (**Twin Lab**) or <u>Ester C</u> capsules 3000-10,000 mg daily.

❑ An intravenous form of vitamin C can be given by a physician.

❑ <u>PantothenicAcid</u> (B$_5$) 500 mg 2 times daily with food (to support the adrenal glands).

❑ <u>Mycelized Vitamin A</u> 10,000-20,000 IU 1-3 times daily (depending on need).

❑ If taking antibiotics make sure you take additional <u>B-Complex</u> (50 mg 1-2 times daily with food, without folic acid), <u>Magnesium</u> (200-300 mg 2-3 times daily with food).

❑ <u>Zinc</u> 50 mg 1-2 times daily (depending on need) with food, to stimulate immune system; excellent for wound and burn healing.

Antimicrobials

❑ <u>ASAP Solution</u>®: follow directions on container, and take every 2-6 hrs (depending on the need). Inhaling the

---

[124] United States Department of State, Bureau of Diplomatic Security. Responding to A Biological or Chemical Threat: A Practical Guide.

mist from a nebulizer might prove beneficial.[*]

- Oil of Oregano 2-3 drops sublingually every 3-6 hours (depending on the need).
- Olive Leaf Extract (225 mg leaf extract + 225 mg powder of leaf = 500 mg) 2 capsules every 3-6 hours (depending on the need).
- GSE + Oil of Oregano, consider inhaling the mist from nebulizer[*] 3 + times daily (depending on the need): add 3 drops of GSE + 2 drops of food-grade lavender essential oil in 1/2 ounce of distilled water, mix well, use eye dropper to add to nebulizer cup, inhale mist on-and-off until it is used up.
- SuperStrength Oil of Oregano rub 2-3 drops on the chest, along the lymphatic areas (especially, the neck, underarms, and groin; **men, avoid getting on testicles**), and along the entire length of the spine every 3-4 hours (depending on the need). For sensitive skin 2-3 drops diluted in 1 tsp of olive oil or castor oil (for deeper penetration).
- Ginger (in any form) taken in conjunction with any natural or synthetic healing agent enhances its effect.

Anti-inflammatory

- Super GLA/DHA (Life Extension Foundation, or comparable product) 3 (1000 mg) soft-gels 2 times daily with food.
- Zyflamend™ (NewChapter, or comparable formula) 1 soft-gel 2 times daily, taken in the middle of a main meal with 8 oz glass of water.

Strengthen Blood Vessels

- Circulegs™ (Solaray) 1-2 capsules 2-3 times a day.
- Reduce Salt Intake.

Antioxidants

- Alpha Lipoic Acid (Sustained Release) 300 mg 1-6 times daily (depending on need) between meals at least 30 minutes before food.

Detoxifiers for Blood and Lymphatic System

- Milk Thistle (to protect liver) non-alcohol tincture, 30 drops + 30 drops of Burdock Root (non-alcohol) tincture into 1/2 cup of Aloe Vera Juice diluted with 1/2 cup of non-tap water, 1-2 times daily 30 + minutes before breakfast, and/or near bedtime.
- Sweat Therapy: 3-5 times weekly.

Probiotics

- Take 1 tsp of acidophilus powder + 1/2 tsp of Inner Strength™ (Ethical Nutrients, or comparable product) in warm water 3-6 times daily between meals. Especially important when taking synthetic or natural antibiotics. Don't take at the same time with antimicrobials.
- KidZyme™ or FloraBear For Kids™ can be given to children. Follow directions on the container.

Oxygen

- An available supply of oxygen could be life saving.

Help Clear Lungs

- Oregacyn (North American Herb and Spice Co.) to relieve congestion use 1-2 capsules 1-6 (depending on need) times per day.
- Clear Lungs (blue label, by Ridge Crest Herbals) 1-2 capsule 1-6 (depending on need) times per day.

For Nausea and Vomiting

- Drink 1-3 cups daily of fresh Ginger Tea. Helps with nausea and to freshen the system after vomiting. Or, add 30 drops of tincture of ginger into 4 oz of warm water and drink 1-3 times a day until symptoms clear. Any form of ginger would be immediately helpful.

---

[*] Nebulizer may require a prescription form a physician to obtain. Check laws in your state or country.

- Soft sweetened ginger candy or pellets can be given to children if the tea is not accepted.
- Drink electrolyte-rich fluids (e.g., squeeze juice of 1/4-1/2 lemon into glass of room temperature water, with a pinch of salt) to replace electrolytes (sodium, potassium, calcium) lost in the vomitus. Also use after sweat therapy.

For Diarrhea

- Drink a natural electrolyte replacement like lemon juice in water with raw unprocessed honey as a sweetener).
- Raw Unprocessed Honey will help to retain water and minerals in the cells due to its osmotic properties. Use 2 tbsp to 1/4 cup 6 times daily for adults. Avoid using with children under 2 years of age.
- White Oak Bark tea plus 3-6 capsules of Activated Charcoal 1000 mg every hour until stools firm up (also helps to clear the organism from the intestines).

For Food Poisoning

- Activated Charcoal Formula: 30 grams of activated charcoal in 4 ounces of water. Drink as soon as possible after ingestion of the toxin. Note: 1 tbsp of the activated charcoal equal about 10 grams. Also, continue to take 250-1000 mg of activated charcoal capsules every 2 hours afterwards for that day.
- If vomiting is occurring, or is to be induced, do not give the activated charcoal formula since the powder can be brought up and create respiratory problems. Wait until it stops.
- Dairy products (especially ice cream) and sherbet interfere with the action of activated charcoal.

Diuretic

- Use Thompson's **Diuretic Formula,** follow directions on container.
- Drink lots of water.

Inhalation Therapy

- The inhalation of the mist of Lavender Essential Oil (food grade) 3-6 times daily could have a beneficial effect on the caustic damage to the respiratory system. If possible, consider using a nebulizer* with 4-5 drops of the oil in 1/2 ounce of water. Use eyedropper to fill the cup and breathe in intermittently until the supply is used up.

Topical Absorbents

- "Talcum powder and/or flour are excellent means of decontamination of liquid agents. Sprinkle the flour (e.g., chickpea or other kind, ideally mixed with activated charcoal, see above) or powder liberally over the affected skin area, wait 30 seconds, and brush off with a rag or gauze pad. (Note: The powder absorbs the agent, so it must be brushed off thoroughly.) If available, protective gloves should be used when carrying out this procedure."[125]

Itching

- Activated Charcoal taken internally has been shown to relieve general conditions of itching.[126] Capsules can be used for this purpose. There's no set dosage. However, 1-3 capsules every 4-6 hours.
- Calamine Lotion used topically.
- Aloe Vera Gel, use topically.

Burns

- Lavender Essential Oil (food grade) may be very effective to relieve burns since vesicants are conventionally treated similarly to thermal burns. Lavender is famous as a natural remedy for burns. It has anti-inflammatory properties, which help with pain. I

---

* May require a physician's prescription to obtain. Check local and federal laws.

[125] United States Department of State, Bureau of Diplomatic Security. Responding to A Biological or Chemical Threat: A Practical Guide.

[126] See: Cooney, D. (1995). Activated Charcoal: Antidote, Remedy, and Health Aid. TEACH Services, Inc.: Brushton, NY. (P. 53.)

would use it periodically as a light topical spray (depending on the need).

❏ <u>ASAP Solution®</u> may be sprayed on blisters; its antimicrobial properties may also help with secondary bacterial infection.

Children

❏ The above recommendations could be given to children over 2 years of age. Consult a physician for children under 2 years old.

❏ **Dosages (not specified above for children):** Children between the ages of **2-5** should take 1/4 of the adult dosage; between **6-12** use 1/2 of the adult dosage; and between **13-17**, 3/4 of the adult dosage.

Pregnant/Lactating Women

❏ Should consult with a physician prior to taking any of the recommended supplements.

Pets

❏ Consider giving 1-4 tablets (depending on size) of **Gary Null's** <u>Pet's Health</u> formula 2 times a day.

❏ For animals use 1 drop of GSE per 2 lbs or 1 kg of body weight. The capsule form could be opened and added to food.

❏ <u>ASAP Solution®</u>: similar to the adult dosages, perhaps using plastic syringe-type dispenser or plastic eyedropper to administer under the tongue.

❏ <u>Homeopathic remedy</u> obtained from a veterinarian might be useful.

❏ Prepare in advance and have ready a <u>Ginger Glycerite</u> formula for dogs and cats to alleviate vomiting. "Loosely fill a pint jar with coarsely chopped fresh ginger root. Fill the jar to the top with vegetable glycerine, which is available in some health food stores. Leave the jar in a warm room for six weeks or longer, shaking it every few days. Glycerine has a sweet taste and viscous consistency that most dogs

and many cats find palatable."[127]
Dose: about 1/2 tsp per 20 pounds of body weight on empty stomach. Can be mixed in favorite food, if necessary. Might be more palatable to finicky cats if mixed with some <u>Valerian Root</u>.

❏ Poutinen's formulas: Recovery, Laxative, Nausea, Diarrhea, Psychology.

Homeopathic

❏ Homeopathic physicians might recommend a specific remedy (see agents) together with other remedies (based on the symptoms; see How to Use the 12 Basic Remedies on page 83).

❏ While taking homeopathic remedies, it's important to avoid 1 hr before and after administration: caffeine of all sorts, vinegar, mentholated products, mint, raw garlic, raw onions, and camphor.

Rehabilitation

❏ Continue with the preventative program.

❏ For lingering lung congestion, consider using the Chinese formula <u>Clear Lungs</u> (blue label) or <u>Oregacyn</u> 1-3 times a day.

❏ Consider having <u>Lung Kichadi</u> 2-3 times a week.

❏ <u>Oral Chelation Formula</u> (by Extreme Health or comparable formula) 3 capsules daily near bedtime, + 3 caplets of <u>Age-Less Formula</u> in the morning with food for adults. Children ages 2-7 use 1/2 of a capsule (can be opened in juice) near bedtime + 1/2 caplet in the morning with food (can be crushed and placed in food). Children ages 2-7 use 1/2 of a capsule (can be opened in juice) near bedtime + 1/2 caplet in the morning with food (can be crushed and placed in food). Children ages 8-13 use 1 capsule near bedtime + 2 caplets of <u>Age-Less Formula</u> in the

---

[127] Puotinen, C J, previously cited, 151.

morning with food. Children ages 13 up can take the adult dose.

- Body Work: <u>Massage</u>, <u>Chiropractic</u>, <u>Osteopathic</u>.
- Energy Work: <u>Network Chiropractic</u>, <u>Reiki</u>, <u>Cranio-Sacral Therapy</u>.
- Detoxification: <u>Liver, Gallbladder, Kidney, Intestinal Cleansing</u> program (Renew Life Products, etc.), <u>Fasting</u>, <u>Colonic</u>.
- Daily exercise, gradually increasing to build up endurance.
- And/or <u>Gentle Yoga</u> or <u>Tai Chi</u> 3 times a week.
- Sweat Therapy.
- Drink plenty of water. Frequent sips throughout the day are best.
- Breathing exercises such as <u>Pranayama</u>.
- Perform a mind-body relaxation method such as the <u>Relaxation Response</u> or comparable one based on your personal belief system.

The Specific Nature of Potential Weapons of Mass Destruction

Bacterial Weapons

Bacteria are microscopic single-cell creatures with full metabolic processes for acquiring and utilizing energy for growth and regeneration. They are much larger than viruses, and, unlike viruses, they can be viewed under a common microscope. Most of the harm caused by bacterial WMD is due to the toxins they contain on their coatings (endotoxins) or that they excrete (exotoxins). All forms of therapy must deal with the effects of these toxins. They must also address how the bacteria seek to avoid being destroyed by the immune system. The typical bacterial infection begins with fairly similar symptoms, and undergoes a period of incubation. As the disease progresses, the symptoms will manifest with the peculiar characteristics of the disease.

ANTHRAX
(*Bacillus anthracis*, a gram positive rod)

B anthracis is a bacterium spread by spores that can cause an infectious disease known as Anthrax. This disease can be fatal if not treated in time (24-48 hours, and, recently, up to 60 hours) with antibiotics. In its natural unadulterated state it is associated with animal contact, mostly farm animals.

Because of the enduring nature of the spores, viable for many years, the disease may also be derived from old animal products such as sheepskins, wool blankets (hence, also known as "wool sorter's disease") and the like.

In spite of its potential severity, anthrax is not a contagious disease.

Mechanism of Disease

Macrophages (large killer cells) engulf the spores. Yet the spores are able to survive and germinate inside the macrophage. Eventually, the bacteria escape from the macrophage and begin reproducing (in the millions) in the lymphatic system, and invade the blood where they release a powerful toxin (anthrax toxin).

The toxin has three components: 1) protective antigen, 2) lethal factor, and 3) edema factor. Edema factor needs protective antigen to enter the cell. Once inside, it releases a chemical that causes the loss of chloride ions and water from the cell, producing edema in the tissue. Lethal factor, in the presence of protective antigen, is an enzyme that breaks apart the biochemical phosphokinase, necessary for cell growth. With the destruction of phosphokinase, cells cannot grow and they die.

There are three forms of the disease: the *skin form* (cutaneous anthrax), the *pulmonary form* (inhalation anthrax), and the *intestinal form*.

With skin anthrax the toxins kill the tissue around it. With gastrointestinal anthrax it destroys the tissue there. However, pulmonary anthrax is not actually a form of pneumonia, but develops in the lymph nodes at the center of the chest (the hilar and mediastinal lymph nodes). In this case, the spores were taken up by the macrophages in the lungs and released in this area where they multiply and poison the blood.

Throughout this entire process enormous amounts of micronutrients are being consumed as the body attempts to fight off the infection.

Symptoms

In the **skin form** spores make contact with broken skin (cuts, scratches, wounds).

- If entry is successful a boil (malignant pustule) will form and eventually develop a black center of dead tissue.
- Level of local edema is considerable.
- After lesions form and dead tissue and crusts fall off, infection may infest the blood stream and cause shock, cyanosis (bluish color of skin and mucous membranes due to poor circulation and insufficient blood oxygen), sweating, shock, and collapse.

The **inhaled form** can readily become serious. However, in the naturally occurring state the incidence of inhalation anthrax is very rare. Initially:
- May produce strong flu-like symptoms
- Pneumonia-like symptoms develop rapidly when not caught in time
- Non-productive cough
- Headache
- Mild chest discomfort
- Following these symptoms one may experience a brief period of improvement
- Then an abrupt onset of respiratory distress with high fever

Further complications include:
- Hemorrhagic meningitis (bleeding and inflammation of membranes that cover the brain and spinal cord)
- Mediastinitis (inflammation of the tissues of the space beneath the breastbone containing the heart, aorta, vena cava, trachea, and other vessels and nerves)

The **intestinal form** of anthrax is contracted from the consumption of contaminated food (most often from the meats of hoofed animals), and it is characterized by an acute inflammation of the intestinal tract. (Although this form is rare it is quite lethal.) There will be initial signs of:
- Nausea
- Loss of appetite
- Vomiting

Fever Followed by:
- Abdominal pain
- Vomiting of blood
- Severe diarrhea

Agent Characteristics as a Weapon
Estimated Level of Attraction
Low 1-2-3-4-5 High

- Availability of information about the agent. **5**
- Ease of performing research, and manipulating agent. **5**
- Ease of manufacture with minimal danger. **3-4**
- Availability of the ingredients. **4-5**
- Low cost. **5**
- Easy to store/house. **5**
- Durability of agent. **5**
- Difficulty for being detected. **5**
- Has a quick rate of action /incubation time. **5**
- Ease of transport. **5**
- Ease of delivery by various methods. **5**
- Ability to inflict widespread harm/death. **5**
- Treatable. **4-5**

Assessment

What makes anthrax attractive is its ease of manufacture (not any more difficult than fermenting cheese) and its durability. Its incubation period is short, its capacity to disable and harm is severe, and the spores last a long time. "Small to large quantities can be made at all levels of production ranging from basement petri culture dishes to 5,000-gallon fermenter reactors."[128] However, producing a weapons-grade product is more complicated.

The difficulty lies in the spore's tendency to clump and, therefore, a highly technical method needs to be employed to render them airborne in a particulate state of 1 to 5 microns. Clumping is the result of electrical charges in the spores. To eliminate clumping a technical process is used to render the spores electro-magnetically neutral. This would most likely be the work of sophisticated military and state-run laboratories.

"With weapons grade spores, delivery is as simple as spraying an aerosol can into an indoor HVAC air conditioning system or as

---

[128] From paper presented by Terrence K. Cloonan, Preparedness Specialist/Occupational Hygienist, Scott Health and Safety, Scott Technoligies, Inc., Monroe, NC.

complicated as a bulk aerial spray attack over a metropolis."[129]

Because meteorological conditions such as rain and sunlight can destroy the spores, an aerosol attack would need to take place in a relatively dark and dry environment, or indoors.

To cause infection the dose would need to be quite high (estimated to be greater than 3,000-10,000 spores at one time). One gram of anthrax can contain approximately 1 billion spores! "Non immunized workers in animal-hair mills have been shown to inhale 150-700 infected particles per hour of smaller than 5 microns, but are rarely affected."[130]

Considering these factors and the incidents that have already taken place, I would place it in the **4-5** range of attraction and possible recurrence.

Detection and Diagnosis

Diagnostic testing: With anthrax early diagnosis of infection is essential because the incubation period has ranged between 1-60 days (considering that immune strength was not evaluated). Tests that would be used diagnostically are: blood cultures; chest X-ray; serologic (blood serum) test for anthrax; spinal tap for culture and analysis.

The Mayo Clinic in Minnesota has recently developed a confirming PCR (Polymerase Chain Reaction) test for anthrax, which could deliver results within 1 hour from receipt of a sample. This test is being made available to any licensed clinical laboratory at no charge.

Detection in the field: Detection of anthrax in its natural form is often the ongoing work of state and national health agencies performing epidemiological investigations and environmental sampling, using feedback statistics from local health-care providers.

What makes anthrax difficult to detect by the senses is that it is colorless, odorless, and tasteless.

The biotech lab, Tetracore, Inc., has produced the BTA™ Test Strip for biological agents (to be used by first responders). It is a rapid (1-15 minutes) hand-held on-site screening test for anthrax that recognizes the bacterial and spore forms. However, the results of this test still need to be confirmed in a laboratory.

Conventional Method of Care and Treatment

Emergency pre-hospital care would depend on the identification of the condition. First responders would ideally have protective equipment, which consists of a respirator, head and face protection, impervious boots and gloves, and body protective gear. They would:

Perform airway, breathing, and cardiovascular (ABC) checks on site and/or in the ambulance en route to the site of treatment.

Provide adequate ventilation with high flow oxygen with a non-rebreather mask. Such ventilation increases the chances for survival for it reduces the potential for shock.

More serious respiratory conditions (apnea, no breathing) would require a surgical incision into the windpipe (trachea) and insertion of a plastic tube (orotracheal intubation) to prevent suffocation, or the use of a bag-valve air delivery mask.

Exposure to almost any biological agent can cause dehydration and septic shock. To help prevent this, intravenous solution would be administered to all non-ambulatory patients.

Medical care: In general, isolation of the patient would occur until the diagnosis of the disease has been confirmed; with anthrax isolation is not required.

Non-resistant strains of anthrax can be treated with traditional antibiotics. The skin form is more amenable to such treatment, and if caught in time will not become serious. *Doxycycline* and *Ciprofloxacin* (Cipro) are

---

[129]Terrance K. Cloonan, cited above.
[130]Campbell, S. (M.D). Anthrax in a Biowar Environment.

currently the antibiotics of choice for inhalation cases. These may be used for prophylaxis, but there may be side effects in addition to the development of bacterial resistance if used too often.

Vaccination: There is currently a vaccine for anthrax, but it is only used with military personnel and those who are at risk such as laboratory personnel, veterinarians, etc. The FDA is considering its use with civilian populations. Other forms of the vaccine are also in the works; however, it will take a year or so before they may become available.

Supportive Lines of Natural Defense

Use the **Basic Supportive Program** (found on page 89) for your plan of action. Also, consider the following important points about Anthrax that may be useful:

Specific Line:
- ❑ Melatonin has shown activity against toxins produced by anthrax.

- ❑ Cutaneous anthrax: The powdered (aerosol) spores can cause inhalation anthrax; spores that land on the skin can cause cutaneous anthrax. If you have its symptoms seriously consider these suggestions as soon as possible: **On the boil:** Use Wild Mountain Super-Strength Oil of Oregano as follows.
- ❑ Apply directly with a dropper in the wound and along the edges 2-6 times daily.
- ❑ Apply a topical poultice, (leave on overnight) to draw out toxins, containing 1 part Activated Charcoal mixed with 1 part crushed Flaxseeds and some water to make a paste (placing flaxseeds in blender with some water is best). Make a supply of the flaxseed mix to be added to the activated charcoal as needs arise. Can be refrigerated in a plastic container and brought to room temperature for use.
- ❑ **Also:** take 3 Oregamax capsules 2-4 times daily.
- ❑ Wild Mountain Oil of Oregano (Super Strength): rub 2-3 drops along the lymphatic areas—especially the groin, neck, and underarms—and along the entire length of the spine every 3-4 hours. Important!
- ❑ **Seek Medical Attention.**

BRUCELLOSIS
(Brucella species are classified as gram-negative rods and are named according to the animals they infect: melitensis [goats] abortus [cows] suis [pigs], and canis [dogs].)

Brucellosis (also known as undulant fever, Malta fever, Bang's disease) is an acute infection caused by *Brucella* bacteria. It is transmitted through contact with the secretions and/or excretions from infected animals such as swine, goats, cattle, deer, elk, dogs, and several other animals. The typical routes of human infection occur:
- Through inhalation of contaminated particles, a potential hazard for those working with the slaughter of animals, and laboratory personnel;
- When the bacteria enter the body through broken skin;
- By eating or drinking contaminated non-pasteurized milk products, representing the most common source of infection.

However, person-to-person transmission is rare. Nevertheless, mothers may transmit the organism to their infants through breastfeeding. Sexual transmission is also possible. Tissue transplantation is another (although unusual) source. While dogs may acquire the disease it is not likely that it will be passed on to humans unless one has contact with the blood, semen, or placenta of the dog. People with weak immune systems need to avoid handling sick animals.

Brucellosis may come on as an acute (short) or chronic (long term) disease. Although the illness may be prolonged the disease is rarely fatal.

Mechanism of Disease

Once organisms enter the body, they localize in the lymph nodes and spread to the liver, spleen, and bone marrow. Macrophages (large immune killer cells) kill many of the bacteria, but some survive inside the macrophage where they are protected from antibodies produced by the immune system. Because of this, the organisms are extremely difficult to eradicate even with antibiotic therapy. The condition leads to granular formations on the skin that may advance to abscesses and tissue damage. The complete mechanism of the disease is not completely known.

The nutrient toll may become chronic.

Symptoms

The appearance of symptoms can range from 5 days to several months. Symptoms may vary considerably during the early stages, and may begin suddenly with:

- Chills
- Fever
- Severe headache
- Malaise
- Possible diarrhea

The disease is characterized by two stages: acute, and chronic. The acute phase produces:

- Fevers (reaching 104°-105° F. during the evening, which gradually diminishes to normal or near normal in the morning; this "undulant" pattern is not common, and the fever is considered insignificant)
- Chills
- Profuse sweating (after fever goes down)
- Fatigue
- Headache
- Anorexia
- Myalgia (muscle pain)
- Backache
- Swollen lymph nodes
- Enlargement of liver and spleen
- Weight loss
- Formation of abscesses and granuloma (inflamed tumor-like masses under the skin)
- Depression and emotional instability
- Insomnia

In the chronic form, manifesting approximately one year from onset, it progresses with:

- Recurrent depression
- Insomnia

- Chronic-fatigue-like syndrome
- Arthritis
- Sexual impotence
- Enlargement of lymph nodes
- Abscesses may form in testes, ovaries, kidneys, and brain (meningitis and encephalitis), which may lead to hearing and visual impairment, paralysis on one side of the body, and lack of muscle coordination
- Endocarditis (inflammation of valves and/or membrane lining of the heart) is a possible yet rare occurrence.

Agent Characteristics as a Weapon
Estimated Level of Attraction
Low 1-2-3-4-5 High

- Availability of information on the agent. **3-4**
- Ease of performing research, and manipulating agent. **5**
- Ease of manufacture with minimal danger. **2**
- Availability of the ingredients. **5**
- Low cost. **5**
- Easy to store/house. **5**
- Durability of agent. **3-4**
- Difficulty for being detected. **5**
- Has a quick rate of action/incubation time. **3**
- Ease of transport. **5**
- Ease of delivery by various methods. **4**
- Ability to inflict widespread harm/death. **2-3**
- Treatable. **5**

Assessment

Brucella organisms have been developed and considered for biowarfare for quite some time. They can be easily freeze-dried (lyophilized) and turned into an aerosol powder. They can be easily housed and stored.

While not usually fatal it can mimic natural disease. Untreated cases can be ill for months or years. Chronic cases develop a chronic-fatigue-like syndrome. In large numbers this can have a draining effect on healthcare systems, and also on the economy.

The dissemination of Brucellosis would be characterized as a surreptitious attack to incapacitate a portion of the population. It would lack the news worthy drama terrorists so enjoy to carry out their aims. Therefore, I would assess the likelihood of occurrence in the **3** range of possibility.

Detection

Diagnostic testing: may involve blood tests for antibody analysis, and tests on a sample of spinal fluid to be cultured in the laboratory. Agglutination titers (red cell clumping) are one indicator in 90% of cases within three weeks of onset of the disease, but can be misleading with those vaccinated against tularemia, Yersinia, or cholera. Biopsies of infected tissue provide the most convincing basis for diagnoses. Culturing is most accurate during the acute phase.

Detection in the field: Clinical suspicion with people who have been or may be exposed to infected animals and/or their products. There is currently no form of field detection in place.

Conventional Methods of Treatment

Emergency pre-hospital care would depend on the identification of the condition. First responders would ideally have protective equipment, which consists of a respirator, head and face protection, impervious boots and gloves, and body protective gear. They would:

Perform airway, breathing, and cardiovascular (ABC) checks would on site and/or in the ambulance en route to the site of treatment.

Provide adequate ventilation with high flow oxygen with a non-rebreather mask. Such ventilation increases the chances for survival for it reduces the potential for shock.

More serious respiratory conditions (apnea, no breathing) would require a surgical incision into the windpipe (trachea) and inserting a plastic tube (orotracheal intubation) to prevent suffocation, or the use of a bag-valve air delivery mask.

Exposure to almost any biological agent can cause dehydration and septic shock. To help prevent this, intravenous solution would be administered to all non-ambulatory patients.

Hospital/Medical care involves: bed rest, and treatment with oral *tetracycline* (at least 3 weeks), with *streptomycin* (2 weeks). *Doxycycline* is also effective as part of this combination. Because tetracycline may cause tooth damage in children under 8 years of age other antibiotics are used. Relapses are more common when a single antibiotic is used. Severe cases may require intravenous treatment with *corticosteroids* (3 days), followed by the oral form. *Codeine* may be used to relieve muscle pain.

Temperature (oral or rectal) needs to be monitored periodically. Milk shakes and other supplemental foods may need to be given to counteract weight loss. To ensure proper rest sedatives may be in order.

Supportive Lines of Natural Defense

Use the **Basic Supportive Program** (found on page 89) for your plan of action. Also, consider the following important points about Brucellosis that may be useful:

With brucellosis one might need to deal with the possible delayed onset of symptoms. This may be confusing in trying to figure out how and when the disease may have been contracted. Important as this information may be, it is best to get on with the care that is needed and not dwell on this issue.

Preventative:

❑ By avoiding and eliminating animal and food sources of infection; vaccinating healthy animals; wearing goggles, gloves, and covering broken-skin areas (especially those who deal with animal products on a daily basis such as meat packers, butchers, etc.) Cook meats thoroughly and drink pasteurized milk.

❑ To prevent infection through drinking non-pasteurized milk consider heating it and/or adding 5-10 drops of 35% Food Grade Hydrogen Peroxide (needs caution when undiluted: avoid **undiluted** contact with skin and plastic surfaces) per gallon of milk, OR add ASAP Solution (this would be expensive)

❑ To prevent infection with potentially contaminated foods consider using: Activated Charcoal 200-300 mg capsules 1-4 at a time plus 1-2 tablets/capsules of a Pancreatic Enzyme Complex (with Betaine HCL) with meals.

❑ Homeopathic Remedies: Homeopathic physicians might recommend using the remedy Arsenicum to help prevent bacterial and viral diseases. Also, they might recommend the nosode of *Brucella* with animals and humans alike. (See How to Use the 12 Basic Remedies for symptoms on page 83.)

- ❑ Milk Thistle (to protect liver) non-alcohol tincture, 30 drops + 30 drops of Burdock Root (non-alcohol) tincture into 1/2 cup of Aloe Vera Juice diluted with 1/2 cup of non-tap water, 1 time daily near bedtime and 30 + minutes before breakfast.

Rehabilitation:
- ❑ Sweat Therapy: 3-5 times weekly.
- ❑ Dogs and cats are vulnerable to this disease.
- ❑ Enriched protein shakes (available at your health food store) to help prevent excessive weight loss, a condition possible with this disease.

CHOLERA
(*Vibrio cholera,* a gram-negative rod)

Cholera is a diarrheal, exclusively human disease caused by the bacterium *Vibrio cholera.* Transmission occurs through the feces of infected people. Infected humans who are either in the incubation period or are convalescing, while not manifesting obvious symptoms are capable of transmitting the bacteria. It is acquired by consuming water or food that has been contaminated by the organism. Animal sources are: contaminated, undercooked, marine shellfish (mainly shrimp, oysters). Factors that predispose areas to epidemics are poor sanitation, malnutrition, overcrowding, and inadequate health care.

Mechanism of Disease

V. cholera is quite vulnerable to stomach acid, one of the first lines of defense. In order to survive the acid, at least one billion organisms need to be ingested so that 10-500 of them might be able to pass into the small intestine and cause an infection. Those with abnormally low levels of stomach acid, or those who use antacids (Tums, Peptobismol, etc.) on a regular basis, or those who have had the stomach (or portion of) surgically removed are more susceptible.

Once the organisms attach to the lining of the small intestine, they release a toxin called choleragen. This triggers a series of biochemical reactions that stimulate the release of *adenylate cyclase* (cAMP). The overproduction of cAMP then stimulates the secretion of chloride ions and water from the cells, which is the cause of massive non-inflammatory watery diarrhea. The excessive loss of fluid causes dehydration, loss of electrolytes, and may cause death.

Massive amounts of nutrients (especially electrolytes) are lost because of the diarrhea.

It is important to note that the presence of the toxin alone (in the absence of the bacteria) is capable of producing the disease.

Symptoms

After an incubation period of 12-72 hours victims experience:
- Headaches (possibly very painful)
- Little or no fever
- Abdominal bloating
- No abdominal pain
- Profuse, watery diarrhea (from 5-10 liters of water per day) that looks like rice water (colorless with small flecks of mucous).
- Malaise
- Possible vomiting (increasing loss of fluids and electrolytes)

The results of the massive diarrhea can have the following effects:
- The loss of fluids and mineral electrolytes (sodium, potassium, magnesium) can lead to heart and kidney failure
- Acidosis (low blood Ph) and hypokalemia (loss of potassium in the blood) can also occur as fluid loss increases
- 50% of untreated cases can result in death.
- Children are particularly vulnerable.

Agent Characteristics as a Weapon
Estimated Level of Attraction
Low 1-2-3-4-5 High

- Availability of information about the agent. **5**
- Ease of performing research, and manipulating agent. **5**
- Ease of manufacture with minimal danger. **5**
- Availability of the ingredients. **5**
- Low cost. **5**
- Easy to store/house. **5**
- Durability of agent. **3**
- Difficulty for being detected. **3**
- Has a quick rate of action/incubation time. **5**
- Ease of transport. **5**
- Ease of delivery by various methods. **3**
- Ability to inflict widespread harm or death. **3**
- Treatable. **2**

Assessment

The toxin released by *Vibrio* organisms can reproduce the symptoms of cholera even in the absence of the bacteria. Therefore, it can be produced as a poisoning agent. The aerosolized form, to be directly inhaled, would not be a likely form of transmission. As a WMD cholera would most likely be used to contaminate water and/or food supplies. While the organism is susceptible to heat, drying, chlorinated water, pure water, ozone, and ultraviolet light, it can live for up to six weeks in untreated water in which there is organic matter such as sewage. It can also withstand freezing for up to 4 days. Therefore, ice cubes can become a problem.

Rural areas not having chlorinated water supplies (such as well water) could be targets. This would require special efforts with a more dispersed population.

Considering the delicacy of the organism, the high number required to cause the disease, and the ability to treat it in a modern society I would estimate it to be within the **2-3** range of possibility in non-third world populations.

Detection

Diagnostic testing: Depending on the situation, clinical judgment is often exercised without the use of laboratory tests. However, diagnosis involves the culture of a sample of the diarrhea stool to rule out other possible causes of watery diarrhea—*E. coli*, viruses, food poisoning from the preformed toxins of *Clostridium perfringens, Bacillus cereus,* or *Staphylococcus aureas.*

Field detection: Water and foods can be tested.

Conventional Methods of Care, Prevention, & Treatment

Emergency prehospital care would depend on the identification of the condition. In this case, gloves, eye protection or face shield, mask, and gown are needed. Airway, breathing, and cardiovascular (ABC) checks would be made on site and/or in the ambulance en route to the site of treatment.

Because exposure to cholera causes severe dehydration and septic shock, intravenous solution would be administered to all non-ambulatory patients. Without this initial treatment, a 50% death rate may result from severe dehydration, loss of blood volume and shock (hypovolemic shock).

Medical care: Treatment aims at preventing and restoring the loss of fluids and electrolytes with IV fluid replacement. Use of the World Health Organization or rehydration solution drink (containing: water, sodium chloride, potassium chloride, sodium bicarbonate, and glucose) is successful with adults and some children.

Of secondary importance is the use of antibiotics: *tetracycline* or *doxycycline*. However, resistant strains of the bacteria may require treatment with *ciprofloxacin* (Cipro) or erythromycin. Children should be treated with tetracycline for 3 days, *erythromycin* or *trimethoprim-sulfamethoxazole*, all for three days duration. The risk of staining children's teeth with tetracycline is not considered to be a problem due to the short course of therapy.

Vaccination: A cholera vaccine is available for travelers to areas susceptible to the disease, but it is of limited efficacy.

Prevention: Decontamination of water and food supplies. Drinking boiled water or water decontaminated with iodine or commercially bottled water. Eating only cooked foods.

Supportive Lines of Natural Defense

Use the **Basic Supportive Program** (found on page 89) for your plan of action. Also, consider the following important points about Cholera that may be useful:

Loss of electrolytes can produce mental sluggishness and feelings of withdrawal. It may difficult to hold down solid food and oral supplements.

Psychological/Social Lines:
- ❑ Avoid harsh, fast, loud music and other similar impressions, since these stimulate that part of the nervous system that is related to the fight-or-flight response, and could further aggravate the stomach and intestines.
- ❑ Remember, this disease is not contagious from person-to-person.

Preventative Line:
- ❑ Supplemental HCL (hydrochloric acid), an important first line of defense against ingested pathogens, may be necessary. A combination of Pancreatic Enzymes with Betaine HCL (hydrochloric acid), 1-2 tablets/capsules, and Activated Charcoal (powder in 200-300 mg capsules), 1-3 at a time, can be taken together at the beginning of meals. For children use KidZYME (Renew Life).
- ❑ Homeopathic physicians might use Veratrum-album to help prevent this condition.

Environmental Line:
- ❑ To protect water (especially well water) use a home water purification system that treats water with ozone, ultraviolet light, and passes it through a carbon filter (Ecoquest).
- ❑ Add ASAP Solution to all filtered water to ensure safety and not disturb the taste.
- ❑ Water may be purified with Grapefruit Seed Extract (GSE) 3 drops per 8 ounces or 237 ml of water or ASAP Solution®. Drink this water as a preventative when traveling through or staying in suspect areas. **When using GSE always dilute it.**
- ❑ As a general preventative add 3 drops of GSE in juice and drink 1-2 times daily.

- ❑ Use 20 drops of GSE per pint (475 ml) of water and place in spray bottle to wash fruits and vegetables. **Do not use on eyes.**
- ❑ As a general disinfectant to clean hands and objects use 30-40 drops of GSE per 1 quart (1 liter) of water.

Specific Line:
- ❑ Potassium rich soups (e.g, potato) are excellent.
- ❑ Drink a natural electrolyte replacement like lemon juice in water with raw unprocessed honey as a sweetener.
- ❑ Raw Unprocessed Honey will help to retain water and minerals in the cells due to its osmotic properties. Use 2 tbsp to 1/4 cup 6 times daily for adults. Avoid using with children under 2 years of age.
- ❑ Ginger tea for nausea, and to refresh the system after vomiting.
- ❑ White Oak Bark tea plus 3-6 capsules of Activated Charcoal 1000 mg every hour until stools firm up (also helps to clear the organism from the intestines).
- ❑ Stronger Activated Charcoal Formula: Add 3 tbsp (30 grams) to 4 ounces of water, and drink. Continue to take 25-1000 mg of Activated Charcoal Capsules every 2 hrs afterwards for that day.
- ❑ Continue with the All-One plus the Green Magma (or comparable formulas), and the Udo's Choice supplements, as soon as it is possible to ingest foods.
- ❑ **Very important** to take 1 tsp of Acidophilus Powder + 1/2 tsp of Inner Strength (Ethical Nutrients or comparable product) in water 3-6 times daily. Do not take together (at the same time) with antimicrobials.
- ❑ KidZyme™ or FloraBear For Kids™ can be given to children. Follow directions on container.

Rehabilitation:
- ❑ **Gentle detoxification:** Four weeks after one's system has normalized, consider drinking 1/2 cup of Aloe Vera Juice diluted with 1/2 cup of non-tap (non-chlorinated) water to which is added 30 drops of non-alcohol based Burdock Root tincture, 1 time daily around bedtime, for 4-8 weeks. Adding 1 tbsp of frozen apple juice concentrate improves the taste.
- ❑ Avoid fasting and sweat therapy for 1-2 months

GLANDERS
(Burkholderia mallei, Previously known as Pseudomonas, a gram-negative rod)

Glanders is a highly infectious disease caused by the bacterium *Burkholderia mallei*. The disease is also known as *Malleomyces mallei*, Farcy, Malleus. It is primarily contracted by horses, mules, and donkeys, which are the naturally occurring sources of transmission. Glanders can also be acquired by goats, dogs, and cats. Unlike other *Burkholderia* species, this organism cannot survive in soil, water, or plants.

Infection occurs from:
- Ingestion of contaminated food,
- Bodily discharges, or
- Inhalation of aerosol droplets.

Human-to-human transmission is possible. While very few organisms (only 1) are required to cause infection no naturally acquired cases have occurred in the U.S. since 1945. Yet the disease sporadically appears in Asia, Africa, the Middle East, and South America.

Those with compromised immune systems—premature infants, the elderly, those with debilitating diseases, burns, or wounds—are particularly vulnerable to infection, which can sometimes prove fatal.

Mechanism of Disease

The nature of how the organism causes disease is unclear. However, it excretes toxins (exotoxins) and possesses a toxin on its surface (endotoxin) that contributes to the disease process. Generally, after infection the organism penetrates the mucous membranes at the point of entry in order to enter the lymphatic system. Through the lymphatic pathways it can infect other parts of the body. Eventually, the organism lodges in the lungs where it forms lesions full of thick, sticky pus. The disease may begin in the following four ways:

- Acute localized pus-forming skin infection.
- Acute pulmonary infection with mucopurulent discharge.
- Septicemic (bacterial infestation of the blood) illness, which can prove fatal within 7-10 days.
- Chronic pus-forming cutaneous (skin) infection.

Many valuable nutrients are lost as the disease progresses.

Symptoms

The incubation period ranges from 1-14 days[131] after exposure. Onset of the disease may be quicker with diabetics and immune compromised individuals. The symptoms depend on how the infection was acquired. Generally it presents with:

- Pain and swelling occur at the point of infection (lips, eyes, hand, chest, etc.)
- Several days later (3-4), development of skin abscesses, pustules on skin, nose, and mouth.
- Joint inflammation
- Malaise, fever
- Finally, septicemia (usually fatal)

Inhalation of the bacteria would be in keeping with the most likely form of exposure from a terrorist attack. Inhalation exposure produces:

- Fever, chills
- Rigor (violent shivering)
- Sweats
- Malaise
- Muscle pain
- Headache
- Photophobia (sensitivity to light)
- Lacrimation (tears)

---

[131] Other reports vary from this range by indicating 10-14 days. I have opted to possibly err with caution.

- Diarrhea
- Chest pain (pleuritic)
- Swelling of lymph glands on the neck
- Enlargement of the spleen
- Generalized pimple-like formations and pus-filled eruptions.
- The septicemic form begins once the bacteria invade the blood stream, which is often fatal.

Agent Characteristics as a Weapon
Estimated Level of Attraction
Low 1-2-3-4-5 High

- Availability of information about the agent. **3**
- Ease of performing research, and manipulating agent. **3**
- Ease of manufacture with minimal danger. **1-2**
- Availability of the ingredients. **5**
- Low cost. **4**
- Easy to store/house. **4-5**
- Durability of agent. **5**
- Difficulty for being detected. **5**
- Has a quick rate of action/incubation time. **4**
- Ease of transport. **5**
- Ease of delivery by various methods. **5**
- Ability to inflict widespread harm or death. **4**
- Treatable. **5**

Assessment

B. mallei has been considered by the CDC as a possible agent of bioterrorism. Very few organisms are required to cause disease. It can be aerosolized through freeze-drying techniques (lyophilization). It can be aimed at animal stocks. There's no current vaccine or reliable treatment. It can have a mortality rate of over 50% despite antibiotic treatments. However, handling of the bacterial cultures poses high risks of incidental infection to those who are cultivating it as a weapon. Considering these variables I would estimate its potential use within the **3-4** range of probability.

Detection and Diagnosis

Pre-diagnostic testing may involve clinical consideration of at-risk people such as veterinarians, horse and donkey caretakers, those involved with the slaughter of animals, and laboratory personnel. Because of the rareness of incidents in the U.S., rapid epidemiological

and laboratory protocols remain a challenge for timely detection. Currently no national or state surveillance exists.

Diagnostic testing: Using infected areas to isolate samples in order to determine the antibiotic susceptibility is crucial. Blood cultures are usually negative until the patient is close to death.

Field detection is not currently available.

Conventional Methods of
Care and Treatment

Emergency pre-hospital care would depend on the identification of the condition. First responders would ideally have protective equipment, which consists of a respirator, head and face protection, impervious boots and gloves, and body protective gear. They would:

Perform airway, breathing, and cardiovascular (ABC) checks on site and/or in the ambulance en route to the site of treatment.

Provide adequate ventilation with high flow oxygen with a non-rebreather mask. Such ventilation increases the chances for survival for it reduces the potential for shock.

More serious respiratory conditions (apnea, no breathing) would require a surgical incision into the windpipe (trachea) and insertion of a plastic tube (orotracheal intubation) to prevent suffocation, or the use of a bag-valve air delivery mask.

Exposure to almost any biological agent can cause dehydration and septic shock. To help prevent this, intravenous solution would be administered to all non-ambulatory patients.

Medical care: the standard precautions for healthcare workers are required. Isolation is not mandatory. However, caution needs to be exercised with the handling of infected secretions. Decontamination is effective with 0.5% hypochlorite solution.

Few antibiotics have been evaluated with humans. However, *Sulfadiazine* may be effective in some cases. *Ciprofloxacin, doxycycline*, and *rifampin* have shown effectiveness with in vitro (petri dish) studies.

Vaccination: there is no current human or veterinary vaccine.

Supportive Lines of Natural Defense

Use the **Basic Supportive Program** (found on page 89) for your plan of action. Also, consider the following important points about Glanders that may be useful:

- ❑ Those with **photosensitivity** should **avoid** taking **St. John's Wort**. This disease may present photophobia as a symptom.
- ❑ Remember, this is a highly infectious disease. Wear a mask and take precautions when interacting with other people.
- ❑ Homeopathic physicians might recommend the nosode of glanders together with other remedies based on the symptoms (see How to Use the 12 Basic Remedies on page 83.)
- ❑ Dogs and cats are vulnerable to this disease.

MELIOIDOSIS
(*Burkholderia pseudomallei,* a gram-negative rod)

Melioidosis, also called Whitmore's disease, is an infectious disease occurring in humans and animals caused by the bacterium *Burkholderia pseudomallei* (formally known as *Pseudomonas pseudomallei*). It is ordinarily found in the soil and in stagnant water, and it is transmitted when it comes in contact with skin abrasions, burns, or wounds; may also occur from the ingestion or inhalation of the organisms. Person-to-person transmission is rare. (There have been cases of sexual transmission.)

While reports indicate that it can present in many parts of the world, it is especially prevalent in Southeast Asia. The disease tends to have variable and inconsistent clinical effects, and has been dubbed the "Great Imitator" because of this.

Mechanism of Disease

Knowledge of how it causes disease is lacking. Several lines of study as well as clinical evidence indicate that *B. pseudomallei* is a pathogen capable of adapting to more than one condition, resisting the immune system, and surviving inside the cell. However, it is known to excrete a powerful toxin.

Melioidosis may remain latent for years, and months of treatment with antibiotics may not necessarily eradicate the disease. The disease can come on as:

- An acute localized infection
- A pulmonary infection
- An acute blood infection (septicemia)
- A chronic (long term) infection.

Chronic nutripenia may develop during the course of the disease. Those who survive acquire permanent immunity.

Symptoms

The disease has an inconsistent incubation period, and it may produce a mild or a fulminant condition. The **acute localized infection** is characterized by the following developments:

- A local nodule with ulceration forms
- If infection spreads to nearby lymph nodes fever and muscle aches may develop
- If unattended to, the infection can spread to the blood stream and become septic

The **pulmonary infection** can resemble bronchitis or pneumonia with:

- Cough (dry or wet)
- Chest pain
- High fever (possibly)
- Headache (possibly)
- Loss of appetite (possibly)
- Muscle soreness (possibly)

- There can be abscesses in the lungs
- As the disease progresses (even months later) abscesses on the skin can occur

The **acute blood infection** usually afflicts people with chronic illness (e.g., diabetics). Typical symptoms include:

- Respiratory distress
- Headache
- Fever
- Diarrhea
- Pus-filled lesions on the skin
- Abscesses all over the body
- Muscle soreness
- Disorientation
- Pimples on upper body
- Can be fatal within 24-48 hours

Chronic melioidosis presents:

- Multiple pus-filled abscesses on the viscera (organs in the chest or abdominal cavity), lymph nodes, spleen, brain, liver, lungs, skin, and muscles
- Bones and joints can become inflamed (osteomyelitis)

Agent Characteristics as a Weapon
Estimated Level of Attraction
Low 1-2-3-4-5 High

- Availability of information about the agent: **2**
- Ease of performing research, and manipulating agent: **2**
- Ease of manufacture with minimal danger: **3**
- Availability of the ingredients: **5**
- Low cost: **4**
- Easy to store/house: **4**
- Durability of agent: **5**
- Difficulty for being detected: **5**
- Has a quick rate of action/incubation time: **1**
- Ease of transport: **5**
- Ease of delivery by various methods: **4**
- Ability to inflict widespread harm/death: **3-4**
- Treatable: **4-5**

Assessment

Varieties of *Burkholderia* bacteria have been used as biowarfare agents as early as World War I. However, those were the days when the destruction of mules, horses and donkeys had a military advantage.

This organism would most likely be developed as an aerosolized weapon. Inhalation melioidosis could lead to any of the above symptoms. However, its prolonged incubation period would make it less attractive than, say, anthrax. Yet the lack of a vaccine and its high mortality rate (prior to antibiotics 95% of cases died; with treatment 50% of septicemic cases and 20% of localized forms of the disease perish, producing a 40% overall rate of death) may make it more attractive as a bioweapon.

In spite of its lethality, it appears to have too many inconsistencies, and therefore would have a lower level of attraction, perhaps in the **1-3** range. Nevertheless, it cannot be discounted.

Detection

Diagnosis: Melioidosis (the "Great Imitator") can be difficult to diagnose. It may be confused with many other types of infections presenting similar symptoms. For example, the pulmonary infection may appear as tuberculosis until tests confirm otherwise. This can cause critical delays in diagnosis, since its severest form can be fatal with a few days. Diagnosis is made from culture of blood or sputum samples.

Field Detection: No field detection is available at this time.

Conventional Methods of
Care and Treatment

Emergency pre-hospital care would depend on the identification of the condition. First responders would ideally have protective equipment, which consists of a respirator, head and face protection, impervious boots and gloves, and body protective gear. They would:

Perform airway, breathing, and cardiovascular (ABC) checks on site and/or in the ambulance en route to the site of treatment.

Provide adequate ventilation with high flow oxygen with a non-rebreather mask. Such ventilation increases the chances for survival for it reduces the potential for shock.

More serious respiratory conditions (apnea, no breathing) would require a surgical incision into the windpipe (trachea) and insertion of a plastic tube (orotracheal intubation) to prevent suffocation, or the use of a bag-valve air delivery mask.

Exposure to almost any biological agent can cause dehydration and septic shock. To help prevent this, intravenous solution would be administered to all non-ambulatory patients.

Medical care: Thorough cleansing of the affected skin can help reduce the risk of disease after exposure.

The drug treatment of choice for the seriously ill patient is *ceftazidime*, administered for several weeks, and *piperacillin*. Other drugs that have been used successfully in less serious cases include *tetracycline*, *chloramphenicol*, and *trimethoprim-sulfamethoxazole*. X-ray is used to diagnose and monitor lung complications.

Vaccination: None at this time. There's no information on the use of antibiotic prophylaxis as a preventative measure.

Supportive Lines of Natural Defense

Use the **Basic Supportive Program** (found on page 89) for your plan of action. Also, consider the following important points about Melioidosis that may be useful:

- Essentially, this disease is not contagious. Person-to-person transmission is rare.
- Apply antibacterial topical ointments (such as elemental silver salves), to skin abrasions, wounds, cuts, and burns, cover with bandage, etc., if needed, to avoid entry of this organism.
- Homeopathic physicians recommend the *nosode* of melioidosis or Farcy together with other remedies based on the symptoms (see How to Use the 12 Basic Remedies on page 82).

MULTIDRUG-RESISTANT TUBERCULOSIS
(*Mycobacterium tuberculosis*, an aerobic acid-fast rod)

Tuberculosis (TB) is an infectious disease (caused by the *Mycobacterium tuberculosis*) that typically affects the lungs. Worldwide it is the cause of more deaths than any other microbial agent. In 1993 the World Health Organization declared TB a global health emergency, the only time it has made such a claim for any disease. It has been estimated that 3 million people annually die of the disease while 8 million new cases occur worldwide. The socio-economically disadvantaged, the malnourished, and the immune-deficient (such as those with AIDS) are particularly susceptible. As the name implies, multidrug-resistant tuberculosis (MDR TB) is a form of tuberculosis that has developed resistance to two or more of the drugs used to treat it.

Mechanism of Disease

Humans are the sole natural reservoir of *M tuberculosis*. Therefore, animals are not implicated in the disease. (However, another strain, *Mycobacterium bovis*, found in unpasteurized cow's milk, also causes a mild TB in humans.) *M tuberculosis* is generally transmitted from person-to-person by inhaled infected droplets, dry aerosols, or by ingestion of contaminated food. Roughly 5% of infected people develop TB within a year; the remainder can develop a latent infection. While it usually affects the lungs, multiple organ systems may be involved (such as the liver, spleen, bone marrow, and lymph nodes).

After exposure, the immune system usually controls the organism by killing it. However, the bacterium has a way of protecting itself from being destroyed. The organism does not produce toxins (endotoxin or exotoxin) as many other bacteria do in order to disrupt immune and cellular function. Instead, once engulfed by a phagocyte (a cell that is able to surround, engulf, and digest microorganisms and foreign material), it survives and regenerates within it. It does this inside the space (phagosome or membranous pocket), of the phagocyte that is used to digest microorganisms with the aid of a biochemical called lysosome. *M tuberculosis* survives by producing a protein (exported repetitive protein) that prevents lysosome from fusing with it.

Eventually, the immune cells containing the bacteria go on to form tiny nodules (tubercles) to trap the bacteria. However, the bacillus may lie dormant within the tubercle for years. In the future, these nodules can erode and release the bacteria into other parts of the body via the blood stream, and reactivate the disease.

Factors that increase the probability that TB will reactivate are uncontrolled diabetes, Hodgkin's disease, leukemia, silicosis (a chronic fibrous lung condition due to the prolonged inhalation of silicon dust), AIDS, nutrient and drug related immune-deficiency.

Those infected with strains that are sensitive to antimicrobial drugs have an excellent prognosis. With MDR TB the mortality rate may skyrocket to 50%.

Throughout the disease chronic nutripenia is likely to develop.

Symptoms

The incubation period may take 4-8 weeks. TB usually does not present with specific symptoms, which may manifest (asymptomatically) as:

- Fatigue
- Weakness
- Loss of appetite
- Weight loss
- Night sweats
- Low-grade fever

With reactivated TB one may find:

- Persistent cough
- Mucopurulent sputum (discharge containing pus and mucus)
- Occasional coughing up of blood
- Chest pains

Agent Characteristics as a Weapon
Estimated Level of Attraction
Low 1-2-3-4-5 High

- Availability of information about the agent: **5**
- Ease of performing research, and manipulating agent: **5**
- Ease of manufacture with minimal danger: **3**
- Availability of the ingredients: **5**
- Low cost: **5**
- Easy to store/house: **5**
- Durability of agent: **5**
- Difficulty for being detected: **4**
- Has a quick rate of action/incubation time: **2**
- Ease of transport: **5**
- Ease of delivery by various methods: **5**
- Ability to inflict widespread harm or death: **5**
- Treatable: **4**

Assessment

M tuberculosis is very resistant to dehydration, and can survive in dried expectorated sputum, rendering it a candidate for transmission by a simple powdered aerosol (instead of the more sophisticated use of lyophilization). Because of the worldwide existence of the problem, the drug-resistant infectious material could be easy to come by. The acute and chronic nature of the disease is gradual, and not dramatic.

Therefore, the newsworthiness so essential for terror politics would be diminished. However, the intentional sustained release of contaminants into the environment can have an accumulative toll on affected populations, slowly adding to the existing burden, and overwhelming valuable resources. It would be difficult to determine the source of transmission. One infected asymptomatic person could quite easily infect another 20-30 people. Considering these outstanding factors, I see MDR TB as being in the **4-5** range of attractiveness.

Detection and Diagnosis

Diagnostic Tests: The diagnostic procedures involve physical examination, chest X-ray, tuberculin skin test, sputum smears and cultures to detect the presence of tubercle bacilli. The diagnosis needs to be precise since there are other diseases that mimic TB such as: lung cancer, lung abscess, and other bronchial disorders. Testing to determine resistance of a particular strain has usually taken weeks to complete.

Field Detection: Environmental detection of the disease is primarily epidemiological in nature, based on incidence and location.

Conventional Methods of Care and Treatment

Prehospital emergency care: Most cases of MDR TB would most likely not require first responder emergency services. However, in a biowar scenario where the disease has become rampant, emergency services might very well be required. It is important for first responders to know that one has this disease, for it is contagious.

Emergency care would depend on the identification of the condition. First responders would ideally have protective equipment. Airway, breathing, and cardiovascular (ABC) checks would be made on site and/or in the ambulance en route to the site of treatment.

Given the propensity of respiratory complications from an aerosol attack, priority would be given to maintaining airway and providing adequate ventilation. Such ventilation increases the chances for survival for it reduces the potential for shock.

Because exposure to almost any biological agent can cause dehydration and septic shock, intravenous solution would be administered to all non-ambulatory patients.

Medical Care: Patients need to be isolated in quiet, well-ventilated quarters until sputum tests indicate absence of the bacteria. To prevent spread of the disease, patients need to cough and sneeze into tissue, discard tissue and all secretions properly into a plastic bag. Collection bag needs to be disposed of properly to avoid further contamination.

Patients also need to wear a mask when interacting with other people or when outside of the room. Caretakers and visitors need to wear masks. Those who interact with patients should have tuberculin tests done.

It's important to stress the need for plenty of rest, and for healthy nutrition. Those with poor appetite need to eat frequent small meals.

Monitor for side effects of medications (optic neuritis, peripheral neuritis, hepatitis). Observe for complications such as coughing up blood.

Those with MDR TB require multiple-drug therapy during the possible 6-9 month (or longer) period of treatment. *Isoniazid* (INH), a bactericidal drug, is the treatment of choice, in conjunction with *rifampin*, and *pyrazinamide*. (INH and *rifampin* are given for 6 months, but *pyrazinamide* is stopped after 2 months.)

"In patients who are immunocompromised (eg, AIDS patients), who have disseminated disease, or who are likely to have INH-resistant organisms, a fourth drug, *ethambutol*, is added and all four drugs are given for 9-12 months."[132] (One recent development in TB treatment is the FDA approval of *Rifater*, a drug that combines the aforementioned drugs into one pill. Another is *Priftin*, which can be taken less often with other drugs in the final weeks of treatment.)

Even though the drug therapy may clear the sputum of the organism, metabolically inactive organisms still remain in the system and the infection may resurface in the future.

Those who are discharged from hospital treatment must maintain cautions to prevent spread of the disease, and they need to sustain discipline in taking required medications. This has been a problem.

To counter it, a supervised method known as "directly observed therapy" (DOT) has been very effective. DOT is a system of treatment in which the patient is administered medication by a nurse or health worker and is observed taking the medication. Periodic checkups are required.

---

[132] Levinson, W.; Jawetz, E. (2000). Medical Microbiology & Immunology: Examination & Board Review. Lange Medical Books/McGraw-Hill: New York, NY. (P. 138.)

Supportive Lines of Natural Defense

Use the **Basic Supportive Program** (found on page 89) for your plan of action. Also, consider the following important points about Multidrug-Resistant TB that may be useful:

Psychological and social considerations: MDR TB is often a prolonged illness. It has the propensity to be taxing to the mind-body relationship, and, as a consequence can lead to depression and a sense of indifference. This is a disease with strong social implications that need to be addressed during the healing process. However, much of the statistics on this disease have not taken into consideration the nutrient base. So with a synergistic approach there is much hope. Be calm. Stay focused.

Social Line:

- Remember, this a slow-developing contagious disease. It is spread through the air. Those who are vulnerable are people with whom the infected person has frequent contact.
- To avoid spreading the disease, always cover your mouth with tissue when coughing, sneezing, or laughing.
- Discard tissue in a paper bag and, if possible, spray each tissue with GSE decontaminant. (The bacteria can survive in a dry state.)
- Do not go to work or school if sick. Medical tests are the only way to determine if you are not. If you must have contact with other people, wear a mask scented with a few drops of food-grade lavender essential oil.
- Sleep in a bedroom away from other members of the household.
- Lavender: periodic inhalation of the food-grade essential oil from diffuser, ultrasonic humidifier (10 drops per pint of water) might be helpful. The essential oil can also be dabbed onto a handkerchief and inhaled periodically.

Environmental:

- Inhaling the cool mist of ASAP Solution® from a nebulizer* might be helpful.
- Use Grapefruit Seed Extract (GSE) solution (30-40 drops per quart or 1 liter of water) or ASAP Solution® in a spray bottle to use as a decontaminant for areas that you feel could collect bacteria.
- Get the air to move! If possible, use a fan to vent air from room (apartment etc.), and another one to draw in fresh air. Airflow is important with this disease. If using an air conditioner, spray the filters with GSE decontaminant and scent them with food-grade lavender essential oil. Do this periodically.
- A positive or negative pressure room can be devised using HEPA (or similar) filtering system.
- Consider using an Ozone and Negative Ion Generator in the room and/or house. Ozone kills germs, and it will freshen the air.

Specific/Rehabilitation Lines:

- Lung Kichadi: Ayurvedic stew to support lungs
- Homeopathic physician might recommend the nosode of Tuberculinum. Best to work with a homeopathic physician.
- Periodic Sweat Therapy would be useful.

Pets:

- Humans are the sole reservoir of this disease.

---

* May require prescription from a physician. Check the local and federal laws.

PLAGUE

(Yersinia pestis, a gram-negative rod)

The plague, also known as the Black Death, is a severe infectious disease caused by the bacterium *Yersinia pestis*. During the Middle Ages its infestation killed massive numbers of people. It is usually transmitted by fleas from infected animals, particularly wild rodents, such as rats, mice, squirrels, and prairie dogs to humans and to household pets (especially cats). When the wild animal sources of sustenance become scarce, the hungry fleas will opt for humans and pets.

This disease has also surfaced during modern times. For instance, it occurred endemically in India during the 1990s in the region of Mumbai (Bombay). It also occurs periodically on a smaller scale in the United States. A recent article in the Scientific American reports that: "In 1999 microbiologists identified plague in flea-infested squirrels, chipmunks and other wild rodents in 22 counties surrounding Sacramento, California. In 2000 state health officials began issuing regular warnings about plague-prone areas there." (Vol. 285, No. 3, p. 93.)

Mechanism of Disease

There are a number of factors that contribute to how this germ survives and causes harm. *Y. pestis* has an antigen on its surface called F-1, which enables it to resist being destroyed after being engulfed by a phagocyte. Once inside, it continues to reproduce and migrate to the lymph nodes, usually those in the groin (inguinal nodes), and release other harmful substances. The nodes become inflamed and swell to form the hot painful *bubo*. From there, they invade the bloodstream (septicemia) and proceed to infect other organs throughout the body.

The toxins on its surface (endotoxin) cause intravascular coagulation and subcutaneous hemorrhages, probably the mechanism causing a darkening of the tissue, which may have been the origin of the term "black death."

It can occur as one of four forms: bubonic, pneumonic, septicemic, or pestis minor. In a biowar scenario the bubonic form could be transmitted via infected fleas; the aerosolized pneumonic form would seem more likely to be used.

Severe forms of nutripenia are one of the aggravating side effects of this disease.

Symptoms

Bubonic plague symptoms usually appear 2 to 5 days after exposure to the bacterium, but can appear any time from a few hours to 12 days later.

- Symptoms start suddenly with chills and a fever of up to 106 degrees F.
- The heartbeat becomes rapid and weak and the blood pressure may drop.
- Swollen lymph nodes (buboes) appear with or shortly before the fever. Typically, the nodes are extremely tender to the touch, firm, and surrounded by swollen tissue. The overlying skin is smooth and red but not warm.
- The person is likely to become restless, delirious, confused and uncoordinated.
- The liver and spleen may swell substantially and can easily be felt during examination by a doctor.
- Lymph nodes may fill with pus and drain during the second week.
- More than 60 percent of untreated people die. Most deaths occur between the third and fifth day.

Pneumonic plague can be acquired either from inhalation of an aerosol or from septic blood clots that reach the lungs. The incubation period is 2-3 days. The onset is acute and fulminant with:

- Malaise
- High fever which may suddenly plunge
- Chills
- Headache
- Muscle pain
- Cough with production of bloody sputum

114

- Toxemia (toxins in blood)

The pneumonia progresses rapidly resulting in:

- Shortness of breath
- Loud, harsh breathing
- Respiratory failure
- Circulatory collapse
- Potential bleeding

Septicemic plague occurs when the infection of the bubonic form spreads into the blood. It may cause death even before other symptoms of bubonic or pneumonic plague appear. This may produce the following symptoms:

- Acute fever
- No lymphatic damage or swellings
- Rapid progression to septic shock and fatality.

"Pestis minor is a mild form of plague that usually occurs only in a geographic area where the disease is prevalent (endemic). Its symptoms—swollen lymph nodes, fever, headache, and exhaustion—subside within a week."[133]

Those with pneumonic plague must be isolated, and anyone who may have had contact needs to be examined and tested.

Agent Characteristics as a Weapon
Estimated Level of Attraction
Low 1-2-3-4-5 High

- Availability of information on the agent. **3-4**
- Ease of performing research, and manipulating agent. **3-4**
- Ease of manufacture with minimal danger. **2-3**
- Availability of the ingredients. **4-5**
- Low cost. **3-4**
- Easy to store/house. **4**
- Durability of agent. **5**
- Difficulty for being detected. **5**
- Has a quick rate of action/incubation time. **5**
- Ease of transport. **5**
- Ease of delivery by various methods. **3-4**
- Ability to inflict widespread harm or death. **5**
- Treatable. **3-4**

Assessment

Even though the nature of the disease is not completely known, it doesn't take much technological knowledge to employ plague-infested materials as a bioweapon. It is documented to have occurred during the 14th century when dead bodies foul with plague were hurled over the walls of enemy cities. During World War II infected fleas were used against populations killing hundreds and perhaps thousands of people.[134]

Pneumonic plague is the only form that can be transmitted from person-to-person without the inoculation by an insect. Therefore, the aerosolized form (possibly freeze-dried) would be the most likely used by terrorists. This technology is readily available in the commercial sector, which is used to produce such products as freeze-dried coffee. A number of countries have already produced tons of *Y. pestis* in the powdered form.

The powdered form can be easily housed and stored in sealed containers once the lyophilization (freeze-drying) process has been successfully completed. In this form it can be delivered as any other powdered agent to be carried in the wind or in envelopes (like anthrax). It could be spread on clothing in stores. It doesn't seem like it would be used in warheads, although this is possible.

The aerosolized form, however, is not without its risks, for great care must be taken by laboratory workers to protect themselves from the aerosols that might transmit the infection. While a *Y. pestis* vaccine has been produced in the United States against the natural occurrence, and has been extensively used, its utility against an aerosol challenge is unknown.

Considering all these factors I would assess the use of *Y. pestis* as a biowarfare agent to be within the **4-5** range of possibility.

---

[133] Berkow, R., Editor-In-Chief, (1997). The Merck Manual of Medical Information (Home Edition). Simon & Schuster Inc.. New York, NY.

[134] See: Miller, J; Engelberg, S.; Broad, W., previously cited, pp. 37-38.

Detection

Diagnostic tests: Those who show evidence of the plague must (with the more severe forms) be treated within 24 hours. Because of the short incubation period of the disease, treatment must begin early. This does not allow for extensive confirmatory testing to rule out other pathogens. However, diagnostic tests are becoming more sophisticated with extremely shorter turn-around times. Currently, smear and culture of samples from blood or pus or sputum is the best diagnostic procedure.

Field detection of *Y. pestis* is still in its infancy stage, relying on reports of incidence in non-endemic areas. The **Bio Threat Alert™ (BTA) Test Strip**, produced by Tetracore, Inc., for plague is available for use by first responders.

Conventional Methods of Care and Treatment

Emergency pre-hospital care would depend on the identification of the condition. First responders would ideally have protective equipment, which consists of a respirator, head and face protection, impervious boots and gloves, and body protective gear. They would:

Perform airway, breathing, and cardiovascular (ABC) checks on site and/or in the ambulance en route to the site of treatment.

Provide adequate ventilation with high flow oxygen with a non-rebreather mask. Such ventilation increases the chances for survival for it reduces the potential for shock.

More serious respiratory conditions (apnea, no breathing) would require a surgical incision into the windpipe (trachea) and inserting a plastic tube (orotracheal intubation) to prevent suffocation, or the use of a bag-valve air delivery mask.

Exposure to almost any biological agent can cause dehydration and septic shock. To help prevent this, intravenous solution would be administered to all non-ambulatory patients.

Medical Care: Caretakers should wear protective gear. Prompt treatment reduces the incidence of death to less than 5 percent. Isolation of patients is necessary.

Septic shock and pneumonia are the main life-threatening events.

There is no significant antibiotic resistance. The treatment may involve: *streptomycin, tetracycline, gentamicin, doxycycline, ciprofloxacin*, or *chloramphenocol*. (**Avoid** taking **calcium** and **magnesium** supplements at the same time. They may impair absorption of the drug).

Supportive Lines of Natural Defense

Use the **Basic Supportive Program** (found on page 89) for your plan of action. Also, consider the following important points about Plague that may be useful:

Connotations of the plague may evoke a sense of doom and fear. While this disease progresses very quickly, those who receive treatment have a very good chance for survival. Natural therapies may very well provide that extra help to keep one alive.

Social Line:

- ❑ Remember, this disease can be very risky for caretakers who come in contact with the patient.

Preventative Line:

- ❑ In the research process I've encountered valid scientific research, and I have also found compelling anecdotal accounts. The following account from the book by Maggie Tisserand and Monika Junemann, *The Magic Power of Lavender,* caught my eye: "From the history of the Middle Ages, we learn that people handling lavender never fell victim to the bubonic plague."[135] Also, many of the towns using plant-based essential oils (including lavender) for the production of perfumes were immune to the plague. While it many raise many eyebrows, I felt that this was a powerful statement that should not be ignored.

Environmental Line:

- ❑ Essential Oil of Wild Lavender inhaled using a diffuser or in an ultrasonic humidifier (5 drops per pint of water) might have a protective effect.

---

[135] ... (1994, English translation from the 1989 German edition by Matthias Dehne). Lotus Light Publications: Wilmot, WI.

□ All contaminated clothing, linens, and the like, must be sprayed with decontaminant, placed in plastic bags and tied, and burned later.

Specific Line:
□ Homeopathic physicians might recommend the <u>Serum of Yersin</u>. Then use other remedies for individual symptoms (see How to Use the 12 Basic Remedies on page 83.)

□ Dogs and cats could become a transmitting source. If there are reports of the plague in your area, you may consider placing a sachet scented with lavender around the collar.

Q FEVER
(*Coxiella burnetii*)

Q Fever is an acute systemic disease caused by the organism *Coxiella burnetii*, (a rickettsial organism—resembling gram-negative rods—that shares characteristics of both bacteria and viruses), which thrives primarily in domestic animals like cattle, sheep, goats and cats, and wild animals and ticks. Transmission of the disease typically occurs through contact with contaminated materials that have been subject to an infected animal's feces, blood, placenta, etc., or after inhaling contaminated dust or droplets, or from the ingestion of contaminated food or raw (nonpasteurized) milk. It is not often a fatal disease but can cause serious incapacitation.

Q Fever occurs throughout the world. People who are inevitably exposed to domestic animals (farm workers, veterinarians, etc.) may not be able to prevent this infection. They must take preventative measures, which from a conventional perspective may be the avoidance of unpasteurized dairy products, and the use of antibiotics.

Mechanism of Disease

Unlike other rickettsial diseases (such as Rocky Mountain spotted fever, and scrub typhus), Q fever is transmitted by aerosol of contaminated materials inhaled into the lungs.

Rickettsiae are intracellular parasites that need to derive their energy from the host's cells in order to replicate (like viruses). *C. burnetii* causes inflammation of the inner lining of the blood vessel wall. This increases the transfer of fluids from the small blood vessels into the space surrounding the tissue causing edema and hemorrhage.

There is evidence that it presents a harmful toxin on its surface, and that it may be capable of surviving inside phagocytes. However, the precise mechanism of disease is unclear.

As with other bacterial infections, the consumption of nutrients escalates dramatically.

Symptoms

The initial form occurs as Q fever (early), which may last for about several days to 2 weeks; a chronic relapsing form also exists as Q fever (late), which may last for about 6 months to a lifetime. The incubation period may take from 9-28 days before symptoms appear with a sudden manifestation of:
- High fever
- Chills
- Severe headache
- Cough
- Nausea
- Vomiting
- Extreme weakness
- Muscle aches
- Slow heartbeat (bradycardia)
- Chest pain
- Pneumonitis (inflammation of the lung) without any rash formations

Complications, which could be life endangering can include:
- Endocarditis (inflammation of the valves or lining membrane of the heart)

- Myocarditis (inflammation of the heart muscle)
- Chronic hepatitis (inflammation of liver cells)
- Encephalitis (inflammation of the brain)
- Osteomyelitis (infection of bone)
- Pneumonia

Agent Characteristics as a Weapon
Estimated Level of Attraction
Low 1-2-3-4-5 High

- Availability of information about the agent. **3**
- Ease of performing research, and manipulating agent. **3**
- Ease of manufacture with minimal danger. **4**
- Availability of the ingredients. **5**
- Low cost. **5**
- Easy to store/house. **5**
- Durability of agent. **5**
- Difficulty for being detected. **3**
- Has a quick rate of action/incubation time. **4**
- Ease of transport. **5**
- Ease of delivery by various methods. **5**
- Ability to inflict widespread harm or death. **1**
- Treatable. **1**

Assessment

As a bioweapon it can mimic a naturally occurring form of disease such as the flu. One organism is capable of causing disease. However: "Vaccination with a single dose of a killed suspension of *C. burnetii* provides complete protection against naturally occurring Q fever and greater than 90% protection against experimental aerosol exposure in human volunteers. Protection lasts for at least 5 years."[136] Yet recovery can usually occur without treatment.

Because of these factors I would estimate Q fever to be within the **1-2** range of attraction. However, if used as part of an overall plan that involves widespread incapacitation of citizens, followed by other bioweapons, Q fever could very well become a complicating factor.

---

[136] Pike, J., Ed., (9/15/99): Special Weapons Primer. Federation of American Scientists. (P. 9.) Derived from the Internet.

Detection

Diagnostic tests: Physical examination may appear as hepatitis (with an enlarged liver with elevated enzymes) or pneumonia (with abnormal lung sounds). Chest X-ray, abdominal X-ray, abdominal CT scan, or other testing may be recommended. Diagnosis is verified through serologic tests during the acute and convalescent stages.

Field detection: No field detection devices are available at this time.

Conventional Methods of
Care and Treatment

Prehospital emergency care would depend on the identification of the condition. First responders would ideally have full protective equipment.

Because of the ease with which *C. burnetii* infects, decontamination needs to be thorough. All clothing should be removed and the exposed areas washed with soap and water. Decontamination of the area of bacterial release also needs to be done with hypochlorite solution. They would also:

Perform airway, breathing, and cardiovascular (ABC) checks on site and/or in the ambulance en route to the site of treatment.

Provide adequate ventilation with high flow oxygen with a non-rebreather mask. Such ventilation increases the chances for survival for it reduces the potential for shock.

More serious respiratory conditions (apnea, no breathing) would require a surgical incision into the windpipe (trachea) and insertion of a plastic tube (orotracheal intubation) to prevent suffocation, or the use of a bag-valve air delivery mask.

Exposure to almost any biological agent can cause dehydration and septic shock. To help prevent this, intravenous solution would be administered to all non-ambulatory patients.

Medical care: Generally, recovery can occur even without treatment. However, complications, should they occur, can be very serious and potentially life threatening. Because this organism shares bacterial characteristics, the infection responds quickly to early treatment with antibiotics such as *tetracycline, doxycycline, co-trimoxazole,* or *rifampin* for endocarditis. In some cases with cardiovascular complications valve replacement may be necessary.

While the disease is not transmitted from person-to-person, strict barrier nursing practices may be needed since only one organism is capable of causing disease.

Vaccine is currently under development.

Protection is possible with *tetracycline* or *doxycycline* within 12 days of exposure.

Supportive Lines of Natural Defense

Use the **Basic Supportive Program** (found on page 89) for your plan of action. Also, consider the following important points about Q Fever that may be useful:

While not life-threatening, Q fever can be a very confusing disease because it comes on as a strong flu. Therefore, it would be wise to keep abreast of what is going on as far as the identification of the disease and the number of people with similar symptoms. Here's where the social line becomes very helpful.

❑ Remember, this disease is not directly contagious. However, caution needs to be exercised, given the fact that it can spread very easily through contaminated materials.

❑ Dogs and cats are vulnerable to this disease.

TULAREMIA
(*Francisella Tularensis*, a gram-negative rod)

Tularemia (deer fly fever, rabbit fever, Ohara's disease in Japan) is an acute infection that is caused by the organism *Francisella tularensis*, and is transmitted by contact with the secretions of infected animals (e.g., wild rabbits), from the bite of a tick, deer fly, or flea that feeds on these animals, or from the ingestion of contaminated water (rare) or undercooked meat (rarely). It may also be contracted by direct contact from the carcass of infected animals via broken skin. Tularemia can be transmitted when bacteria become airborne and are inhaled. There is no evidence of person-to-person transmission.

Any occupation or activity that has contact with susceptible animals is open to infection: hunters, farmers, butchers, fur handlers (the most probable cause), and laboratory workers.

Mechanism of Disease

Once the organism enters the body it localizes to the cells of a functional system (known as the reticuloendothelial system) spread throughout the body that defends against infection and gets rid of debris. From there, the bacteria can spread to the blood and organs. There are four forms of the disease:

- Ulceroglandular (where ulcers develop on the hands and fingers, and the lymph nodes swell at the site of infection)
- Occuloglandular (when eye is touched with infected finger it infects the eye, causing redness and swelling with swollen lymph nodes)
- Glandular (when lymph nodes swell but no ulcers form, probably by ingestion of the organism)
- Typhoidal (can spread to the lungs, and pneumonia can result)

A large drain on the nutrient reserves increases with the progression of the disease.

In humans 10-50 organisms can cause disease when inhaled. The oral route of infection would require millions of organisms to cause disease. The aerosol form would typically cause septicemic typhoidal pneumonia. Those who survive develop lifelong immunity.

Symptoms

It may take from 1-10 days for the symptoms to appear (usually 2-4 days). In general, the onset includes:

- Headaches
- Chills
- Nausea
- Vomiting
- Fever of up to 104 degrees F.
- Severe fatigue or exhaustion
- Profuse sweating
- Within 24-48 hrs an inflamed blister appears at the site of infection—usually on the finger, arm, eye, or roof of the mouth—except in the glandular and typhoid types of the disease.
- Blister rapidly fills with pus and opens to form an ulcer (mostly in the mouth or one of the eyes), around which the lymph nodes may enlarge.
- The *ulceroglandular* form of the disease is the most common, and would manifest the above symptoms except those of the eye and mouth.
- The *occuloglandular* type affects the eye, and is brought on by hand contact with the eye.
- In the *glandular* type the lymph nodes swell but no ulcers form, suggestive of the ingested route of infection.
- The *typhoid* form produces a high fever, abdominal distress, and exhaustion, and, if it infects the lungs, pneumonia may develop.
- Survival rate for those who receive treatment is quite high.

Agent Characteristics as a Weapon
Estimated Level of Attraction
Low 1-2-3-4-5 High

- Availability of information about the agent. **5**
- Ease of performing research, and manipulating agent. **3**
- Ease of manufacture with minimal danger. **1-2**
- Availability of the ingredients. **5**
- Low cost. **4-5**
- Easy to store/house. **5**
- Durability of agent. **5**

- Difficulty for being detected. **5**
- Has a quick rate of action/incubation time. **5**
- Ease of transport. **5**
- Ease of delivery by various methods. **5**
- Ability to inflict widespread harm/death. **1-2**
- Treatable. **1-2**

Assessment

The organism is able to survive long periods of freezing and drying and still remain potent.

The fact that this bacteria can be rendered airborne, and has a rapid onset of infection, is a characteristic that makes it attractive as a weapon. However, culturing the organism in the laboratory can be problematic, because there is a high risk to laboratory workers of being infected from the aerosols. Nevertheless, an experimental non-commercial vaccine does exist and is used by the US Army.

The contamination of water supplies is an unlikely method because it would have to be delivered in large amounts, and it would be destroyed with common chemical treatment; nevertheless it is still a remote possibility.

F. tularensis would most likely be delivered as an aerosol that would cause typhoidal tularemia to the exposed. This would increase the fatality rate beyond the 5-10% normally seen with the naturally occurring form of the disease.

Yet, even with this the lethality factor would remain relatively low. Considering these variables I would estimate the attraction for using this agent to be in the **2-3** range of probability.

Detection and Diagnosis

Diagnostic Tests: Clinical suspicion of infection occurs in those who have contact with the previously mentioned predisposing factors. Infection of the lymph nodes and lungs are difficult to diagnose. Diagnosis is usually confirmed by culturing samples of the ulcers, lymph nodes, blood, or sputum.

However, many labs opt not to risk the chances of culturing this easy-to-catch and virulent organism. Because the disease resembles bubonic plague it is always considered in the diagnosis.

Field Detection: Currently, there are no early warning signs that tularemia is present in the environment or that it may be there at any point in time. Only epidemiological coverage may provide these warnings as a result of hazardous infestation in the general population. Continuous lab testing of food and water supplies is another route of detection, along with the presence and examination of potentially infected animal carcasses.

Tetracore, Inc. has a BTA™ Test Strip for first responders to detect the onsite presence of Tularemia.

Conventional Methods of Care and Treatment

Emergency pre-hospital care would depend on the identification of the condition. First responders would ideally have protective equipment, which consists of a respirator, head and face protection, impervious boots and gloves, and body protective gear. They would:

Perform airway, breathing, and cardiovascular (ABC) checks on site and/or in the ambulance en route to the site of treatment.

Provide adequate ventilation with high flow oxygen with a non-rebreather mask. Such ventilation increases the chances for survival for it reduces the potential for shock.

More serious respiratory conditions (apnea, no breathing) would require incision into the windpipe (trachea) and insertion of a plastic tube (orotracheal intubation) to prevent suffocation, or the use of a bag-valve air delivery mask.

Exposure to almost any biological agent can cause dehydration and septic shock. To help prevent this, intravenous solution would be administered to all non-ambulatory patients

Medical care: The use of masks, gloves, gowns, and measures to isolated patients is observed. Tularemia is treated with antibiotics—*streptomycin, gentamicin,* and *ciproflox-* *acin*—which are injected or taken orally for 5-7 days.

Moist bandages are placed on the ulcers and changed frequently, to help prevent the spread of infection and swelling of the lymph nodes. If abscesses become enlarged they are drained; however, draining them can be risky. In the ocular form the application of warm compresses to the eye and wearing sunglasses helps. Pain relievers are also used.

Patients are monitored with CBC (complete blood count), kidney and liver function tests, and blood cultures. Pulmonary cases are also monitored with chest x-ray.

The survival rate for those who receive treatment is quite high. Even 94 percent of untreated people can survive. Obviously, even an average level of immunity is an important factor. Those who perish are overwhelmed by infection, pneumonia, meningitis (infection of the membrane around the brain and spinal cord), or from peritonitis (infection of the lining of the abdominal cavity). Relapses are uncommon, but can occur with insufficient treatment. Those who survive have immunity to Tularemia

Protection: using *doxycycline,* and *ciprofloxacin* as pro-phylaxis.

Supportive Lines of Natural Defense

Use the **Basic Supportive Program** (found on page 89) for your plan of action. Also, consider the following important points about Tularemia that may be useful:

Even though there is no evidence of person-to-person transmission, this is a highly contagious organism that causes non-life-threatening disease, which has the potential to confuse one at the onset. It is certainly possible for a panic-driven psychology to weaken the immune system and allow this to become a more complicated disorder. Remember how important this line of defense is.

❑ Animals are vulnerable to this disease.

VIRAL WEAPONS

Viruses, miniscule pieces of RNA or DNA wrapped in a bit of protein, float in the atmosphere like tiny time bombs waiting to connect with a living cell in order to become activated. Viruses are sort of half-living equations without a metabolism or capacity to regenerate on their own. Some microbiologists question whether viruses are actually living organisms. Yet these incomplete entities can harm animal, plant, and bacterial cells in various ways:

- They undermine cell function so that the cell eventually dies.
- They alter the biochemistry of the cell to their advantage.

Human diseases that are caused by viruses include the common cold, measles, hepatitis, poliomyelitis, and acquired immune deficiency syndrome (AIDS). The viral agents that are seen as part of the arsenal of WMD are amongst the most powerful pathogens on the planet. Yet there is very little that can be done to conventionally treat the diseases they produce. Most of the medicines are exclusively aimed at bacteria, and have no effect on the viral world. In the midst of this dearth of medicinal options, naturalistic approaches to viral infections have been ongoing for hundreds of years. Have they been successful?

While there is no so-called "hard evidence", there is anecdotal and some scientific evidence that they can be effective. Against Ebola, smallpox, and the like? Again, no one fully knows. However, there is no reason not to use them, for in reality there is no other infallible choice. And, if a virus should emerge, there is no reason why the naturalistic approach cannot be used adjunctively during the course of disease and also during the rehabilitative period for those that overcome it.

NIPAH VIRUS

Nipah virus (in the *paramyxoviridae* family) was first detected in 1999, in Malaysia; because it is a relatively recent discovery much about its pathology is unknown. However, it is believed that it is transmitted through direct contact with the bodily fluids of contaminated pigs (possibly dogs, cats, chickens, and other animals) housed in crowded and unsanitary conditions. Bats have been implicated in the transmission process. It causes a severe, rapidly progressive encephalitis with a high mortality rate.

Mechanism of Disease

Little is known about how it causes disease. However, like all paramyxoviridae viruses, Nipah is likely to possess two membrane proteins that contribute to its virulence. One helps it to attach itself to cell membranes while the other causes it to fuse with the cell.

The protein involved with attachment binds to certain receptors on cells that trigger the clumping of red blood cells (hemagglutination). This disturbs the delivery of oxygen to the tissues.

Furthermore, the protein that triggers red cell clumping is thought to release a biochemical known as *neuroaminidase*, which prevents the aggregation of viral particles to the plasma membrane while the virus is bud-

ding. This prevents the immune system from detecting it during this stage, facilitating the release of viral particles from infected cells. Clinical observations suggest that Nipah virus has a tendency to consolidate in the lungs and brain stem.

During this process, the body draws heavily on its nutrient resources (most likely vitamin C, bioflavonoids, and niacin). If these are undersupplied, in my opinion, further complications are likely.

Symptoms

Nipah virus has an incubation period of 4-18 days. The main clinical symptoms are:

- Pneumonia-like (atypical)
- Fever

- Headache
- Dizziness
- Drowsiness
- Cough
- Shortness of breath
- Vomiting
- Possible reduced level of consciousness.

Other symptoms that may develop are:
- Loss of reflexes
- Lessened muscle tone
- Hypertension
- Rapid heart beat
- Muscle spasms
- Inflammation of the brain (encephalitis) with drowsiness, disorientation, convulsions and coma

Approximately 50-55% of clinically apparent cases die.

Agent Characteristics as a Weapon
Estimated Level of Attraction
Low 1-2-3-4-5 High

- Availability of information on the agent. **1-2**
- Ease of performing research, and manipulating agent. **1-2**
- Ease of manufacture with minimal danger. **1-2**
- Availability of the ingredients. **1-2**
- Low cost. **4-5**
- Easy to store/house. **4-5**
- Durability of agent. **?**
- Difficulty for being detected. **3-4**
- Has a quick rate of action/incubation time. **5**
- Ease of transport. **5**
- Ease of delivery by various methods. **3**
- Ability to inflict widespread harm or death. **3**
- Treatable. **5**

Assessment

Because Nipah can infect through the respiratory system through droplets, it can be converted into a weapon for agroterrorism (affecting animals, especially hog populations), and possibly be used to directly target human populations. Therefore, it would most likely be aerosolized.

Nevertheless, the lack of precise information about the nature of the virus may pose problems for its manufacture into a reliable WMD. Even though the lethality may be high (as much as 55%) it does not appear to be a contagious disease, except from contaminated body fluids and tissue, which would extend its mortality rate. Because of these factors I would estimate its level of attraction, at this time, as a WMD to be within the **2-3** range of probability.

Detection

Laboratory tests can identify it from the blood and infected materials. Typically, it is found as a result of incidental cases based on symptoms and occupational risk (e.g., hog farmers), especially in endemic areas (most likely with a history of occurrence).

Field detection: Currently, there is no means of detecting Nipah virus in the field before it causes infection.

Conventional Methods of
Care and Treatment

Prehospital emergency care: The lack of information on this potentially fatal disease requires that first responders take extreme precaution in helping those who may have contracted the disease. Emergency care would depend on the identification of the condition. First responders would need to have full protective equipment. They would:

Perform airway, breathing, and cardiovascular (ABC) checks on site and/or in the ambulance en route to the site of treatment.

Provide adequate ventilation with high flow oxygen with a non-rebreather mask. Such ventilation increases the chances for survival for it reduces the potential for shock.

More serious respiratory conditions (apnea, no breathing) would require a surgical incision into the windpipe (trachea) and insertion of a plastic tube (orotracheal intubation) to prevent suffocation, or the use of a bag-valve air delivery mask.

Exposure to almost any biological agent can cause dehydration and septic shock. To help prevent this, intravenous solution would be administered to all non-ambulatory patients.

Medical care: Even though the risk of transmission from sick animals to humans appears to be low, and the transmission from person-to-person has not been documented, strict patient isolation measures need to be taken. Infection through broken skin is considered to be possible. Because respiratory secretions contain the virus, inhaling droplets from the infected is a risk.

No drug treatments have yet been proven to be effective for Nipah infection. Intensive supportive care is required. However, the antiviral drug *ribavirin* has been able to reduce the feverishness and the overall severity of the disease.

Supportive Lines of Natural Defense

Use the **Basic Supportive Program** (found on page 89) for your plan of action. Also, consider the following important points about Nipah Virus that may be useful:

- ❏ To prevent in natural settings, use sanitary farming methods, wear protective masks, and hygienically cover broken skin areas.
- ❏ Homeopathic physicians might recommend: (1) During a community alert regarding exposure to bacterial or viral infection, use Arsenicum; and/or (2) Carbo Veg, Arsenicum, Hepar-sulph-cal, Sulphur, Rhus-tox for shock.[137]
- ❏ "Tea and juices of apple, cranberry, grape, pear, prune, and strawberry all seem to help kill viruses. Tannins are usually the active components of these juices."[138]
- ❏ Wild Mountain Oil of Oregano (Super Strength): rub 2-3 drops along the lymphatic areas—especially the groin, neck, and underarms—and along the full length of the spine every 3-4 hours. For sensitive skin dilute with 1 tsp of olive or sesame oil or castor oil (for deeper penetration.) Theoretically, the oil will be absorbed through the skin and kill the virus replicating there. Personally, I consider this skin application to be very important.

---

[137] Note: FDA does not endorse homeopathic remedies for prophylaxis.
[138] Duke, J., previously cited.

SMALLPOX
(*VARIOLA MAJOR*)

Smallpox is an acute, highly contagious infectious disease caused by the poxvirus *variola*. After a global eradication program, the World Health Organization pronounced smallpox eradicated on October 26, 1979, 2 years after the last naturally occurring cased was reported in Somalia. Vaccination is no longer recommended, except for certain laboratory workers. The last known case in the United States was reported in 1949. Smallpox infects only humans, which is one factor that helped in its eradication since no animal could harbor and protect it. Although naturally occurring smallpox has been eradicated, variola virus preserved in laboratories remains a potential source of infection. Smallpox can be acquired as:

- *Variola major* (classic smallpox), which carried a high mortality;
- *Variola minor*, a milder, less virulent strain, that occurred in non-vaccinated persons; and
- *Varioloid*, a mild variant of smallpox that occurred in previously vaccinated persons with only partial immunity.

The smallpox virus is transmitted directly by respiratory droplets from coughs and sneezing, from the dried scales of infected lesions, or indirectly through contact with clothing, linens, and other objects. Possibility of contagion exists during all phases of the disease. Because of this smallpox can produce a considerable epidemic among highly clustered urban populations.

Mechanism of Disease

The virus infects the upper respiratory tract and local lymph nodes, and then enters the blood (primary viremia). Internal organs are infected. Then the virus reenters the blood (secondary viremia) and spreads to the skin. "These events occur during the incubation period, when the patient is still well. The rash is the result of virus replication in the skin, but there may be an immune component as well."[139] Smallpox manifests in two forms in about 10% of the cases:

- A rapidly progressive *malignant form*, which is often fatal within 5-7 days; and
- A *hemorrhagic form*, which comes on as an extremely exhaustive condition during the early stages of the disease and, eventually, develops into hemorrhages in the skin and mucous membranes. Pregnant women are most vulnerable.
- Both forms have a 95-100% probability for being fatal.

All forms contribute to severe nutripenia.

Symptoms

Incubation may take from 7-17 days, after which the following symptoms suddenly appear:

- Sudden onset of chills (and possibly convulsive seizures in children)
- Fever with temperature above 104 degrees F
- Headache
- Backache
- Severe malaise
- Vomiting
- Prostration and occasionally violent delirium
- Stupor or coma
- Within two or so days the symptoms worsen, followed by a period of one or two days of feeling better before a sore throat and cough develop with lesions appearing on the mucous membranes of the oral cavity and respiratory tract.
- In about 5 days, lesions appear on the skin (usually prominent on the face and extremities), and form into pimples that eventually become filled with pus. At this stage the fever will rise again.

---

[139] Levinson, W.; Jawetz, E., previously cited, p. 217.

125

- Within 8-9 days into the illness, scabs will form, become crusty, and fall off, leaving a pigment-free skin.
- Transmission of the disease occurs **only when** the rashes appear until the scabs have completely fallen off.

Agent Characteristics as a Weapon
Estimated Level of Attraction
Low 1-2-3-4-5 High

- Availability of information about the agent. **5**
- Ease of performing research, and manipulating agent. **5**
- Ease of manufacture with minimal danger. **3-4**
- Availability of the ingredients. **5**
- Low cost. **3-4**
- Easy to store/house. **5**
- Durability of agent. **5**
- Difficulty for being detected. **5**
- Has a quick rate of action/incubation time. **5**
- Ease of transport. **5**
- Ease of delivery by various methods. **5**
- Ability to inflict widespread harm or death. **5**
- Treatable. **5**

Assessment

Even though smallpox has been relatively eradicated its potential use as a weapon brings it back on the list of high alert. Tests done by the Army in May of 1965 to evaluate the effectiveness of smallpox as a bioweapon found it to be "an excellent choice"[140] for terrorism. It has a long incubation period of relatively constant duration, which permits the operatives responsible for the attacks to leave the country before the first case is diagnosed. It poses a serious threat because of its 30% mortality rate in unvaccinated persons, while there is no specific therapy. "In the United States, few persons under 27 years of age have been vaccinated."[141] It meets most of the requirements to make it an extremely attractive WMD. Therefore, I would estimate it to be a **5**.

---

[140] Miller, J.; Engelberg, S.; Broad, W., previously cited, p. 60.
[141] PDR Guide to Biological and Chemical Warfare Response. (P. 30.)

Detection

Diagnostic tests: Because of its long absence from the clinical scene many physicians would need to be retrained to diagnose and treat it. Initially, smallpox is identified by the characteristic skin lesions. At one time, the best determination was a culture of the virus that was taken from the aspirate of small blisters and pustules. Significant laboratory tests may include microscopic examination of smears from lesion scrapings, and complement fixation, (complement consists of a group of proteins that function to destroy foreign substances directly or in conjunction with other components of the immune system), to detect virus or antibodies to the virus in the blood.

These tests may not be able to differentiate smallpox from cowpox or monkey pox. Electron microscopy has become the most common and simple method. However, the only method that can precisely diagnose smallpox is PCR (polymerase chain reaction).

Field detection: As far as I know there are no predictive measures short of incidental epidemiological evidence of the general population.

A recent development for on-site testing for first-responders (police, HAZMAT, etc.) has become available for smallpox. The biotech lab, Tetracore, Inc., has produced the **Bio Threat Alert™ (BTA) Test Strip** for biological agents. It is a rapid (1-15 minutes) hand-held on-site screening test.

Conventional Methods of Care and Treatment

Prehospital care: This is a very contagious disease that requires full protection by first responders. Person-to-person transmission occurs from airborne contaminated materials or droplet exposure from coughing, and by contact with skin lesions or secretions. Airway, breathing, and cardiovascular (ABC) checks would be made on site and/or in the ambulance en route to the site of treatment. Ventilation plus intravenous hydration increases the chances for survival and reduces the potential for shock.

Medical care: There is no specific treatment for this disease. Those who contract the disease need to be hospitalized and isolated.

As soon as the diagnosis is made, all suspected cases of smallpox, and people who have had face-to-face contact, should be isolated. Clothing, linens, etc. are removed, bagged and sealed for incineration.

Antibiotics are used to treat the bacterial complications.

Vigorous supportive measures need to be employed to deal with the lesions and arrest the itching of the pustules. Drainage material coming from lesions is highly infective, and precautions need to be taken, especially with the mucous membranes, the eyes, and broken skin.

Copious amounts of water are used to rinse the eyes. Skin is washed with soap and water.

Pain-relieving medications (aspirin, codeine, and possibly morphine) would need to be used.

The patient would be given I.V. infusions, tube feeding to maintain calories, fluids, and electrolytes when swallowing becomes difficult. The administration of *dopamine* or *norepinephrine* is used for hypotension.

Vaccine: Vaccination would be required immediately for all contacts of those exposed, including health care workers. "Within 3 days of exposure to the virus the recommended prophylaxis is immunization with the smallpox vaccine. After 3 days, passive immunization with *vaccinia immune globulin* (VIG) is recommended in addition to immunization with the smallpox vaccine. VIG should be given in conjunction with the vaccine to all individuals who need vaccination but are also at risk of developing vaccine-related complication."[142]

Supportive Lines of Natural Defense

Use the **Basic Supportive Program** (found on page 89) for your plan of action. Also, consider the following important points about Smallpox that may be useful:

Psychological integrity during an incidence of smallpox is perhaps the most important defense one can have. This is a very contagious disease with many social implications. First Aid and Home Caring Skills would be valuable.

Preventative/Specific Lines:
- ❑ Homeopathic physicians might recommend: (1) During a community alert regarding exposure to bacterial or viral infection, use Arsenicum; and/or (2) Variolinum as pr otection against smallpox and, possibly Carbo Veg, Arsenicum, Hepar-sulph-cal, Sulphur, Rhus-tox for shock.[143]
- ❑ If infected, avoid daylight. Keep curtains drawn to help prevent scarring.
- ❑ "Tea and juices of apple, cranberry, grape, pear, prune, and strawberry all seem to help kill viruses. Tannins are usually the active components of these juices."[144]
- ❑ Wild Mountain Oil of Oregano (Super Strength): rub 2-3 drops along the lymphatic areas—especially the groin, neck, and underarms—every 3-4 hours. For sensitive skin dilute with 1 tsp of olive or sesame oil or castor oil (for deeper penetration). Do not rub on skin rashes, but use a small spray bottle in which the oil has been diluted with olive or sesame oil. Theoretically, the oil will be absorbed through the skin and may kill the virus replicating there. Personally, I consider this skin application to be very important.

Pets:
- ❑ Smallpox infects only humans.

---

[142] Arizona Department of Health Services, (4/9/02). Bioterrorism Agent Profiles for Health Care Workers: Smallpox. (P. 2.)

[143] Note: FDA does not endorse homeopathic remedies for prophylaxis.
[144] Duke, J., previously cited.

TICKBORNE ENCEPHALITIS VIRUSES
(Arborviruses)

Tickborne encephalitis viruses are classified under arborviruses (diseases naturally transmitted by ticks and mosquitoes). It is a classification of more than 400 kinds of viruses. These viruses have been typically named for the disease they cause or the place where they were originally identified. The diseases caused by these viruses fall into three clinical categories: 1) encephalitis (inflammation of the brain), 2) hemorrhagic fever (bleeding disorder), and 3) fever with muscle pain, joint pain, and rash (non-hemorrhagic). They range in severity from mild to rapidly fatal. The hemorrhagic fever viruses are covered in a separate section. Here the focus is on viruses that can produce **encephalitis** that have the potential to be used as weapons.

Viruses of medical interest that cause encephalitis in the US are: eastern equine encephalitis virus (EEE), western equine encephalitis virus (WEE), St. Louis encephalitis virus (SLE), California encephalitis virus (CE, however, this disease is most prevalent in the north-central states), Colorado tick fever virus (CTF), West Nile virus (WNV), and the Venezuelan equine encephalitis virus (VEE) occurring in Florida.

Eastern Equine Encephalitis Virus
(Alphavirus of the Togavirus Family)

Of the above mentioned viruses EEE causes the most severe form of disease with a mortality rate approximating 50%. Mosquitoes are the natural transmitters of the virus. They feed off wild-bird reservoirs and pass it on to horses and humans (dead-end-hosts). No antiviral therapy is available. However, there is a vaccine to protect horses but not humans.

Western Equine Encephalitis Virus
(Alphavirus of the Togavirus Family)

While WEE produces a greater incidence of infections than EEE the similar illness it brings on is less severe. The virus is transmitted by mosquitoes feeding off wild-bird reservoirs, mainly in the irrigated farmlands of the western states. No antiviral medication is available for it. Again, there is a vaccine for horses but not for humans.

St. Louis Encephalitis Virus
(Flavivirus of the Flavivirus Family)

The SLE virus is transmitted by mosquitoes, which feed off wild birds (especially English sparrows). It can be found in the southern, central, and western states, including urban areas where the mosquitoes breed in pools of stagnant water. Humans are dead-end hosts. The virus causes a moderately severe form of encephalitis with a mortality rate approximating 10%.

California Encephalitis Virus
(Bunyavirus of the Bunyavirus Family)

While CE virus has been identified with California where it was found in 1952, it prevails in the north central states. A strain of CE virus is also known as La Crosse for the city in Wisconsin where it was isolated. The clinical effects produced by CE can vary from mild to severe, and death is rare.

Colorado Tick Fever Virus
(Orbivirus of the Reovirus Family)

The CTF virus is transmitted by the wood tick (*Dermacentor andersoni*), which feeds off small rodents (eg, chipmunks and squirrels) of the Rocky Mountains. Infections occur mainly in hikers and campers. Prevention focuses on protective clothing and skin inspection for ticks.

West Nile Virus
(Flavivirus of the Flavivirus Family)

The West Nile virus (WNV) originated in Uganda, and it was discovered in North America in 1999, when it caused an outbreak of encephalitis in New York City. Currently, it has spread to 37 states and the District of Columbia. It is mainly transmitted by mosquitoes, which draw the virus from infected birds and then infect animals and humans through bites. While most of the infections have occurred with wild birds, the virus can also infect horses (the most affected by the disease), rabbits, dogs, and cats.

128

In areas with infectious mosquitoes, less than 1% of the people bitten and infected become severely ill. About 12% of the hospitalized cases have been fatal. The most vulnerable are people over 50 years of age and those with compromised immune systems. Recently, there is news about the virus being transmitted through blood transfusions. Most people who contract the virus experience mild, flu-like symptoms, or none at all, and are probably unaware that they have become infected.

Venezuelan Equine Encephalitis Virus
(Alphavirus of the Togavirus Family)
In the natural state infection is transmitted by a wide variety of mosquitoes. It mainly produces infection in horses, mules, and donkeys (Equidae), the natural reservoir of the disease, before it proceeds to humans. The disease is endemic to parts of Central and South America, and Florida. While the spread rate of the disease is close to 90% it produces a 1% fatality rate in adults. However with children, being more susceptible to the disease, it may peak to 20%. With the immune-deficient it may be even higher. Those who survive the encephalitic stage of the disease may develop neurological complications such as brain damage.

Mechanism of Disease

The means of these diseases involve the cytocidal (cell-killing) effect of the viruses together with complications with the immune system. There is a predilection of these viruses for affecting the nerve cells of the brain and central nervous system. Those who recover may develop lifelong immunity.

During the disease process enormous nutrients are depleted, especially vitamin C and bioflavonoids.

Symptoms

Many of these encephalitic diseases present quite similar clinical signs and symptoms.
- Malaise
- High fever
- Tremors

- Chills
- Severe headache
- Sensitivity to light (possible)
- Stiff neck
- Muscular aches and pains
- Nausea and vomiting (possible)
- Sore throat (possible)
- Diarrhea (possible)

After these symptoms subside, further neurological complications may develop such as:
- Personality changes
- Confusion
- Insomnia
- Diplopia (seeing double)
- Convulsions and/or seizures
- Coma
- Paralysis

Agent Characteristics as a Weapon
Estimated Level of Attraction
Low 1-2-3-4-5 High

- Availability of information on the agent. **4-5**
- Ease of performing research, and manipulating agent. **4**
- Ease of manufacture with minimal danger. **3**
- Availability of the ingredients. **3-4**
- Low cost. **4**
- Easy to store/house. **4-5**
- Durability of agent. **5**
- Difficulty for being detected. **5**
- Has a quick rate of action/incubation time. **5**
- Ease of transport. **5**
- Ease of delivery by various methods. **5**
- Ability to inflict widespread harm/death. **3-4**
- Treatable. **5**

Assessment
The two viruses that have more potential for being used by terrorists would be the Eastern Equine Encephalitis Virus (EEE) and the Venezuelan Equine Encephalitis Virus (VEE): the EEE by its high mortality rate, and the VEE by its high attack rate affecting 90% of those who are exposed. Because these diseases can be spread from contaminated blood and body fluids the aerosol method of attack would be the most likely. "VEE could be produced in either a wet or

dried form and stabilized for use in biological warfare."[145]

Questions, personally, still remain about the WNV incidents that initially took place in NYC, and have spread to other states across the country. Did they naturally occur or were they mosquito implants into the environment? We keep thinking aerosol, but mosquito vectors could certainly be a possibility.

"A BW (bio-warfare) attack with virus disseminated as an aerosol would cause human disease as a primary event. With VEE, if Equidae (horses, mules, donkeys) were present, disease in these animals would occur simultaneously with human disease. Secondary spread by person-to-person contact occurs at a negligible rate. However, a BW attack in a region populated by Equidae and appropriate mosquito vectors could initiate an epizootic/epidemic."[146] There is no specific therapy or form of protection. Considering these factors, I would estimate these viruses to have a **3-5** range of attraction.

Detection and Diagnosis

Diagnostic tests: Clinical diagnosis uses: 1) identification through cell culture, 2) direct microscopic identification, 3) serologic procedure to detect rise in antibody titer or the presence of IgM antibody, 4) detection of viral antigens, and 5) detection of viral DNA or RNA in the host's blood or cells.
Clinically, it may be difficult to distinguish these diseases from influenza.

Field detection: Viral diseases are environmentally detected through epidemiological findings and through incidental statistics involving death of reservoir animals (birds, mammals). Currently, there are no field instruments to detect their threatening presence.

Conventional Methods of Care and Treatment

Emergency pre-hospital care would depend on the identification of the condition. First responders would ideally have protective equipment, which consists of a respirator, head and face protection, impervious boots and gloves, and body protective gear. They would:

Perform airway, breathing, and cardiovascular (ABC) checks on site and/or in the ambulance en route to the site of treatment.

Provide adequate ventilation with high flow oxygen with a non-rebreather mask. Such ventilation increases the chances for survival for it reduces the potential for shock.

More serious respiratory conditions (apnea, no breathing) would require a surgical incision into the windpipe (trachea) and insertion of a plastic tube (orotracheal intubation) to prevent suffocation, or the use of a bag-valve air delivery mask.

Exposure to almost any biological agent can cause dehydration and septic shock. To help prevent this, intravenous solution would be administered to all non-ambulatory patients.

Medical care: There is no specific therapy. Strict barrier isolation techniques are used and full protective measures for personnel. Victims receive intensive supportive care. Antibiotics may be used for secondary bacterial infections. Hypochlorite solution is an effective decontaminant against viruses.

Vaccine: No vaccine or antidote is available.

Research/Experimental
An experimental vaccine (TC-83) is being developed.

Supportive Lines of Natural Defense
Use the **Basic Supportive Program** (found on page 89) for your plan of action. Also, consider the following important points about Tickborne Encephalitis Viruses that may be useful:

---

[145] PDR Guide to Biological and Chemical Warfare Response. Thomson Physicians' Desk Reference, (2002): Montvale, NJ. (P. 40.)
[146] Pike, J., Ed., previously cited, p. 15.

- Remember, these diseases are not contagious from person-to person. Recently, however, mother's milk, transplants, and blood transfusions have been in question with West Nile virus.
- Arsenicum is used by homeopathic physicians as a general prophylaxis against all viral diseases.[147]
- "Tea and juices of apple, cranberry, grape, pear, prune, and strawberry all seem to help kill viruses. Tannins are usually the active components of these juices."[148]
- Wild Mountain Oil of Oregano (Super Strength): rub 2-3 drops along the lymphatic areas—especially the groin, neck, and underarms—and along the entire length of the spine every 3-4 hours. Important!
- Homeopathic physicians might recommend taking Aconite or Arnica in any emergency in which exposure has taken place followed by using remedies based on symptoms (see How to Use the 12 Basic Remedies on page 83).

Pets:
- These diseases might affect domestic animals; consider giving 1-4 tablets (depending on size) of **Gary Null's** Pet's Health formula 1-2 times a day.
- And/or, ASAP Solution®: similar to the adult dosages, using plastic eyedropper to administer under the tongue.

---

[147] Homeopathy for prophylaxis is not approved by the FDA.
[148] Duke, J., previously cited.

"Viral hemorrhagic fevers" is the general term used to represent a severe bleeding disease caused by a broad group of viruses. Most notable in this group are: ebola virus, Marburg virus, Lassa fever, hantavirus, Rift Valley fever, yellow fever, Dengue fever, and Congo-Crimean hemorrhagic virus. The viruses in question fall into four distinct families:

1. *arenaviruses* (Lassa fever, and South American hemorraghic fever viruses),
2. *bunyaviruses* (Crimean-Congo hemorrhagic fever, Rift Valley fever, and hantaviruses),
3. *filoviruses* (Ebola and Marburg viruses), and
4. *flaviviruses* (yellow fever, tick-bone encephalitis, Kyasanur Forest, and dengue viruses).

These viruses naturally reside in an animal host (zoonotic) or inside insects (arthropod vectors), and depend on their hosts for replication and survival (usually, rodents, ticks, and mosquitoes). However, the host sources are unclear for the filoviruses, and the Ebola and Marburg viruses.

While hemorrhagic viruses are found over much of the globe, each is associated with a particular host species, and the disease it causes tends to remain in the area where the host lives. Some of these hosts are distributed worldwide, like the rat, and therefore can extend the incidence of transmission, especially where their habitat is disturbed or when their natural predators have been eliminated or reduced.

Some hemorrhagic fever viruses can spread from person-to-person such, for example, as has been seen with Ebola, Marburg, Lassa, and Crimean-Congo cases. Usually, however, transmission is through contact with infected hosts or carriers.

With infected rodents, transmission occurs by contact with urine, feces, saliva, and other body excretions. With insect carriers transmission occurs through piercing the skin, or when a human crushes them. It is possible for infected insects to spread the viruses to animals. Humans can become infected when slaughtering and/or eating the animals.

Ebola Virus

Ebola virus is a member of the *filovirus* family. The non-human reservoir that serves as the source of infection is not known. To date, we know of four outbreaks of Ebola virus with humans. Two have occurred in Sudan (1976, 1979), and two in Zaire (1976, 1995). The virus multiplies quickly and overwhelms the body. It has close to 100% mortality rate, and there are no treatments for it. Since most of the cases arise by secondary transmission through contact with a patient's blood or secretions, prevention is crucial in stemming its spread. No cases have been reported in the United States.

Experimental: Research led by Dr. Maurice Iwu, of the London-based Bioresources Development and Conservation Program in West Africa, has found that flavonoids from the *Garcinia Kola* plant might be effective against the Ebola virus.[149]

Marburg Virus

Marburg virus is a member of the *filovirus* family. Two lesser outbreaks of the Marburg virus occurred in Germany and Yugoslavia in 1967, but were linked to the outbreaks in Africa. Exposure to African green monkeys seems to have been the common source of transmission. Like the spread of Ebola, most of the incidents of the disease took place at inadequate hospital settings without the proper medicines and treatment protocols to avert the disorder. Caretakers and those who have close personal contact are particularly susceptible. Otherwise there is no evidence of person-to-person contagion beyond these

---

[149] From: http://news.bbc.co.uk/1/hi/health/411030.stm. BBC NEWs (Aug. 5, 1999).

conditions. There have been no confirmed cases in the United States.

Lassa Fever Virus

Lassa fever virus is a member of the *arenavirus* (sand-like appearance under the microscope) family. It was first detected in 1969 in the Nigerian town of Lassa. The natural reservoir host for Lassa fever virus is the small rodent *Mastomys*, which sustains a chronic lifelong infection. Transmission to humans occurs from food or water contaminated by animal urine. Secondary contamination also occurs, and is a cause of serious concern amongst family members and caretakers. There's no available vaccine or antiviral treatment. Prevention centers on rodent control and spread of secondary contamination.

Hantaviruses

Hantaviruses are members of the *Bunyavirus* family. Hantaviruses are a group of at least 14 viruses carried by wild rodents (rats, mice, squirrels, beavers, and the like). Awareness of the hantaviruses arose in the U.S. when they were deemed to cause an acute respiratory disease now known as hantavirus pulmonary syndrome (HPS). Previously, these viruses were known to cause a form of hemorrhagic (bleeding) fever with renal syndrome (HFRS) that is endemic, almost exclusively, to the Eastern Hemisphere.

The viruses are excreted in the urine, feces, and saliva of these carriers, which do not have symptoms of the disease. They are transmitted to humans when aerosols (suspension of fine particles or liquid or solid substances in air, gas, as mist, smoke, or fog) contaminated with the virus are inhaled. Bites by infected rodents, exposure through broken skin, or contact with mucous membranes are also possible routes of transmission. Although there have been incidents of apparent person-to-person transmission it has not been confirmed to be common.

Rift Valley Fever

Rift Valley fever virus is a member of the *Phlebovirus* family. The virus is typically found in sub-Saharan Africa. Mosquitoes are the natural transmitters of the disease when they feed off infected domestic animals, which are susceptible to the disease, and often die off in large numbers. In addition to mosquito-borne infections, virus-laden aerosols or droplets can infect human hosts.

Yellow Fever

Yellow fever virus is a member of the *flavivirus* family. The disease is characterized by jaundice (hence its name) and fever. It is transmitted to humans in two ways: (1) by mosquitoes (*Haemagogus* species) that feed off monkeys found in African and South American tropical jungles, and (2) by mosquitoes (*Aedes aegypti*) that breed in the stagnant waters of urban areas and feed off humans. Incubation period after being bitten is 3-6 days.

It is considered to be a severe life-threatening disease. It begins with:
- Sudden onset of fever,
- Headache,
- Myalgia, and
- Photophobia.
- After this initial stage, the symptoms progress to involve the liver, kidneys, and heart.
- Followed by: prostration and shock, accompanied by upper gastrointestinal tract hemorrhage.

"**Diagnosis** in the laboratory can be made either by isolating the virus or by detecting a rise in antibody titer. No antiviral therapy is available, and the mortality rate is high. If the patient recovers, no chronic infection ensues and lifelong immunity is conferred."[150] **Immunization** with a live vaccine is available, conferring protection for about 10 years. However, it should not be given to people with weak immunity or to pregnant women.

Dengue Fever

The dengue virus is of the *flavivirus* family. It is transmitted by the *aegypti* mosquito, which is the same kind that transmits the yellow fever virus. There are two forms of den-

---

[150] Levinson, W. (MD, PhD); Jawetz, E. (Md, PhD), previously cited, pp. 255-6.

gue: (1) the classic form that produces its characteristic muscle, glandular swelling, and bone-joint pains (known as "break-bone fever"), which is rarely fatal; and (2) dengue hemorrhagic fever, which produces a more severe disease with a 10% fatality rate. Like the classic form, this variation begins with influenza-like symptoms, but progresses to shock and hemorrhaging, especially in the gastrointestinal tract and skin. No viral therapy or vaccine is available.

Congo-Crimean Hemorrhagic Fever

Congo-Crimean hemorrhagic fever virus was first isolated in the Congo in 1956, and later, associatively, in Crimea in 1969. It also occurs in the Middle East, the Balkans, the former USSR, and eastern China. In its natural state it is transmitted through tick bites, by crushing an infected tick, or from the slaughter of infected livestock. Little is currently known about the variations of the viral properties over the huge geographic areas in which it is found. It is rarely spread from person-to-person.

Mechanism of Disease

These viruses target the vascular system, causing radical changes in vascular permeability (ability of fluids to pass through the vascular walls). Thrombocytopenia (an abnormal decrease in the production of platelets, small discs circulating in the blood, which aid in the clotting of blood) and leukopenia (an abnormal decrease in the number of white blood cells) are involved with many of these infections. The lack of blood clotting factors plus the leakage of blood through the vascular walls cause the profuse hemorrhaging. The condition is further complicated with the loss of white blood cells, for it compromises immune response. All these factors contribute to the deadliness of these diseases. As the disease progresses, huge amounts of nutrients are consumed by the host as it launches its defense, especially vitamin C and bioflavonoids.

Symptoms

With each type of virus the symptoms may vary, but often display 3-16 days after exposure:

- Marked fever;
- Fatigue;
- Dizziness;
- Muscle aches;
- Weakness;
- Exhaustion.

Severe cases typically show signs usually after 3-5 days of exposure:

- Bleeding under the skin
- Internal organ hemorrhaging;
- Bleeding from orifices like the mouth, eyes, or ears (however, the above mentioned forms of bleeding—the inability of the blot to clot—is often not the cause of death)
- Shock
- Nerve dysfunction
- Coma
- Delirium
- Seizures
- Kidney failure
- Multi-organ failure, which often leads to death

Agent Characteristics as a Weapon
Estimated Level of Attraction
Low 1-2-3-4-5 High

- Availability of information on the agent. **2-3**
- Ease of performing research, and manipulating agent. **3**
- Ease of manufacture with minimal danger. **3**
- Availability of the ingredients. **3-4**
- Low cost. **4**
- Easy to store/house. **5**
- Durability of agent. **?**
- Difficulty for being detected. **5**
- Has a quick rate of action/incubation time. **5**
- Ease of transport. **5**
- Ease of delivery by various methods. **4**
- Ability to inflict widespread harm or death. **5**
- Treatable. **5**

Assessment

While almost any bacterial agent can be freeze-dried and turned into a powder that can be stored for years, there doesn't appear to be a historical precedence of biowarfare with these viruses. There's so little known about how they cause disease. Handling them seems to be very risky business. However, their capacity to inflict harm is great. Considering these factors I would estimate their level of attraction for bioterrorism to be within the **2-3** range of possibility.

Detection and Diagnosis

Diagnostic tests can be made in the laboratory by isolating the virus in a cell culture or by the use of serologic tests to detect the presence of specific antibodies.

Field detection: Presently, no method of field detections exists short of patterns of reported incidents.

Conventional Methods of Care and Treatment

Emergency pre-hospital care would depend on the identification of the condition. First responders would ideally have protective equipment, which consists of a respirator, head and face protection, impervious boots and gloves, and body protective gear. They would:

Perform airway, breathing, and cardiovascular (ABC) checks on site and/or in the ambulance en route to the site of treatment.

Provide adequate ventilation with high flow oxygen with a non-rebreather mask. Such ventilation increases the chances for survival for it reduces the potential for shock.

More serious respiratory conditions (apnea, no breathing) would require a surgical incision into the windpipe (trachea) and insertion of a plastic tube (orotracheal intubation) to prevent suffocation, or the use of a bag-valve air delivery mask.
Exposure to almost any biological agent can cause dehydration and septic shock. To help prevent this, intravenous solution would be administered to all non-ambulatory patients.

Medical care: Previous outbreaks, for instance, of Ebola and Marburg have been suc-

cessfully managed by providing medical isolation of the ill, the use of masks, gowns and gloves, by careful sterilization of needles and syringes, and by proper handling of waste and of the deceased (proper mortuary procedures).

Fresh frozen plasma and packed red blood cells are given to replace severe loss of blood. Cases that develop hypotension are given injections of *dopamine* or *norepinephrine*. Renal failure may require hemodialysis.

Decontamination: Continuous decontamination procedures need to be employed in any area where infection has occurred or is present, using soap and water and/or hypochlorite solution.

Supportive Lines of Natural Defense

Use the **Basic Supportive Program** (found on page 89) for your plan of action. Also, consider the following important points about Viral Hemorrhagic Fever Viruses that may be useful:

Social Line:
- Remember, these diseases are in one form or another very indirectly contagious.
- First Aid and Home Caring Skills would be valuable.

Specific Line:
- Physicians practicing an orthomolecular form of medicine find that these kinds of diseases are similar in dynamics to the onset of scurvy, and therefore emphasize the use of Vitamin C (as the main micronutrient of a health maintenance program) to be taken to bowel tolerance.
- Bioflavonoids 1000 mg 3 times daily with food and/or vitamin C.
- "Tea and juices of apple, cranberry, grape, pear, prune, and strawberry all seem to help kill viruses. Tannins are usually the active components of these juices."[151]
- Homeopathic physicians might recommend the use of Aconite or Arnica if exposure has occurred.

Pets:
- It's not known if domestic animals can contract these diseases. However, the following measures would not be harmful.

---

[151] Duke, J., previously cited.

135

- ❑ Consider giving 1-4 tablets (depending on size) of **Gary Null's** Pet's Health formula 1-2 times a day.
- ❑ ASAP Solution®: similar to the adult dosages, using plastic eyedropper to administer under the tongue.
- ❑ Homeopathic remedies are available for pets. (See Resources for how to get them for your kind of pet.)

Rehabilitation:
- ❑ Relaspse may be possible with these diseases.
- ❑ Continue taking Olive Leaf Extract 2 capsules 3 times daily for 2 months. Afterwards, decrease to 1-2 capsules 2 times daily or less.
- ❑ Continue with the ASAP Solution® 2 times daily.
- ❑ Continue applying Wild Mountain Oil of Oregano (Oreganol would be fine) to skin in lighter amounts 1-2 times daily for 1 month. Thereafter, 1 time daily until full health returns.
- ❑ **AKG Shark Liver Oil** contains substances known as *alkylglycerols* (AKG) that, according to studies[152], are able to stimulate the pr o-duction of platelets, and to enhance immune function. There are diseases caused by biological agents that cause a rapid loss of blood platelets (thrombocytopenia), and shark liver oil with AKGs might prove beneficial. **Dosage:** 5 capsules daily of 200 mg of AKG Shark Liver Oil.
- ❑ **Caution: AKG Shark Liver Oil** Should not be taken in such high doses for over 30 days since it might over stimulate the production of platelets.

---

[152] Reported in: Segala, M. Ed., previously cited, p. 45.

Biological Toxins as Weapons

Biological toxins are produced by or derived from bacteria, plants, and animals. For example, ricin and saxitoxin are derived from plants. Bacterial toxins are produced by bacteria, and do not require the presence of the bacteria to cause harm. Examples of animals are the puffer fish that produce a paralytic poison, or certain insects like the scorpion. In most instances, these substances could be categorized as toxic chemicals. The toxic material itself does not regenerate and pose the contagious potential that bacteria do. Many of these toxins are extremely lethal, and so they are of interest to those with terrorism on their minds.

From a medical perspective, the key method of treatment is the use of antidotes. The naturalistic complement would consider the use of chelators and antioxidants, for toxicity accelerates the formation of free radicals. In many instances, those substances with antioxidant activity circulating in the body can deactivate the toxin before it can create much damage. Both methods would use absorbents like activated charcoal, gastric lavage, and antimicrobials to avert opportunistic infection.

Nevertheless, the amount of time that it takes for these toxins to affect life is very short. Therefore, if no antidote is present at the moment of or soon after exposure, survival will depend on the amount of exposure. Natural therapies would be more useful if the exposure occurs orally, which is certainly a possibility if these toxins were used to poison food and water supplies. Most authorities in the field tend to agree that attacks would occur with the release of aerosols in highly populated areas. If such were the case, the best protection would not depend so greatly on therapeutic interventions but on the preventative, social, and environmental lines of defense.

While there are "convincing" reports of why it is useless to use a protective mask, I somewhat disagree. Consider the unexposed that may need to pass through an exposed area. Knowledge that an attack has occurred would allow them to don their masks and increase their level of safety as they exit the toxic site, and possibly assist others who are in need of help.

BOTULISM
(*Clostridium botulinum* Toxin)

Botulism is often a form of food poisoning due to the toxins produced by the bacterium *Clostridium botulinum*. In addition to being derived from foods it can be contracted through spores entering wounds, or, in infants under 12 months of age, where the ingestion of honey has been highly suspect. These toxins are known to be amongst the deadliest, capable of severely damaging nerves and muscles. In its naturally occurring state it is considered to be a rare disease (at less than 200 cases per year in the United States). It is mostly associated with careless preparation and storage of foods.

"It is becoming more common with the use of microwave cooking, which may not sterilize food completely. Botulism is usually associated with canned food, especially improperly home-canned non-acidic vegetables, such as string beans, sweet corn, beets, asparagus, spinach, and chard. Toxin production is favored when contaminated food is stored at neutral or slightly alkaline Ph at room temperature for 12 to 24 hours away from air, and then not reheated before serving. Improperly stored restaurant foods (potato salad, pot pies, stews, turkey loaf, preserved meat, fish, and milk), have been reported as causes of outbreaks of botulism. Low-acid foods that are not canned, such as salami and other processed meats, depend upon a combination of treatments to inhibit germination of C. botulinum spores and bacterial growth: mild heat treatment, the addition of sodium nitrate and other additives; and refrigeration."[153]

---

[153] Ronzio, R. (1997). Encyclopedia of Nutrition & Good Health. Facts On File, Inc.. New York, NY.

Infant botulism, which in susceptible infants of less than 12 months of age can propagate before the development of the proper intestinal flora (friendly bacteria) which would inhibit it. Unlike food borne botulism, this form results from ingesting spores, which then grow in the intestines and eventually release the toxin. Honey has been implicated in this form of botulism, however in most cases the cause is unknown.

Mechanism of Disease

Botulinum toxin is absorbed from the intestines, or through a wound, or the lungs, and transported by the blood to the space between nerve cells (synapses) where it binds to receptor sites for acetylcholine, a neurotransmitter that acts between cells to control muscle contraction. Occupying these sites, it blocks the release of acetylcholine. This causes a flaccid paralysis of the muscles, which includes those involved in respiration, which is the typical cause of death. The food borne toxin can be fatal in as many as 60% of the untreated.

During this process, tremendous amounts of nutrients, especially antioxidants, are consumed. The detoxification processes performed by the liver will be critically challenged.

Symptoms

Depending on the route of exposure, the incubation period may vary: from 8 to 36 hours after being ingested, 3 or more days from entry through a wound, and up to 72 hours after being inhaled (in 3 known cases). The symptoms may include:

- No fever
- Blurred or double vision
- Drooping eyelids
- Inability to focus on nearby objects
- Pupils of eyes don't constrict (they remain dilated) when exposed to light (**key sign** of botulism versus nerve gas poisoning, which produces constricted pupils).
- Dry mouth
- Difficulty swallowing or speaking, which may lead to inhalation of food and aspiration pneumonia

- General weakness, the muscles of the arms and legs become progressively weaker
- Shortness of breath, the muscles involved in breathing become progressively weaker
- Nausea (in some people)
- Vomiting (in some people)
- The mind, surprisingly, remains clear (since the toxin cannot penetrate the blood brain barrier).
- Heart function is also not impacted (except from the lack of oxygen due to lung paralysis).

Agent Characteristics as a Weapon
Estimated Level of Attraction
Low 1-2-3-4-5 High

- Availability of information about the agent. **5**
- Ease of performing research, and manipulating agent. **5**
- Ease of manufacture with minimal danger. **5**
- Availability of the ingredients. **5**
- Low cost. **5**
- Easy to store/house. **5**
- Durability of agent. **5**
- Difficulty for being detected. **3-4**
- Has a quick rate of action/incubation time. **5**
- Ease of transport. **5**
- Ease of delivery by various methods. **5**
- Ability to inflict widespread harm/death. **2-3**
- Treatable. **4-5**

Assessment

Botulism's potential as a weapon has already been established by experts in the field. All agree that a very low quantity of toxin (1 billionth of a gram) is needed to cause a life-threatening or fatal disorder. It is easy to produce, and it can be incorporated into military weapon systems that would aerosolize the spores. The spores are quite durable and can last a long time. They are also highly resistant to heat, able to survive boiling for several hours. It takes a minute amount of the toxin entering the body by mouth, through the respiratory system, absorption through eyes, or through a break in the skin to cause serious illness. The aerosolized form would most likely be the choice of terrorists. However, the effect would be more localized. This is not a contagious disease. Considering these factors, I would estimate it to have a **3** level of attraction.

Detection and Diagnosis

Diagnostic tests: While usually not cultured, it can be detected in uneaten food or from the patient's serum, using laboratory mice as subjects. Inoculated mice die unless protected by antitoxin. Treatment should not wait for test results.

Field detection: A recent development for on-site testing by first-responders (police, HAZMAT, etc.) is available for botulism. The biotech lab, Tetracore, Inc., has produced the *Bio Threat Alert*™ (BTA) Test Strip for biological agents. It is a rapid (1-15 minutes) hand-held on-site screening test.

Conventional Methods of Care and Treatment

Prehospital emergency care by fully protected first responders would depend on the identification of the condition. Once identified, the use of antidote (needs to be given by physician or trained assistant) and enriching the oxygen supply is key to survival. With botulism, respiratory support is crucial since the cause of death is due to respiratory failure. The use of agents such as **Ipecac** to induce vomiting is **avoided**. Activated charcoal is used to absorb gastrointestinal toxins.

Medical care: Trivalent antitoxin (types A, B, and E) is administered, along with respiratory support.[154] According to Dr. De Lorenzo and Porter "Complete recovery from

even severe botulinum toxicity is possible if respiratory support is initiated and continued until recovery (which can take weeks)."[155]

This aggressive approach might not be possible in a mass casualty situation, but is completely reasonable depending on how many victims the emergency medical system is able to support.

Treatment For Consideration: Hemoperfusion is a method that has been used quite successfully to clear toxins out of the blood stream. Similar to hemodialysis, the patient is hooked up to a machine that draws the blood out and through a special activated charcoal filter and returns it to the body. This method would not be feasible during a mass crisis, but has its applications in smaller situations. At this time, I have no knowledge of how many hospitals or health facilities use this equipment.[156]

Supportive Lines of Natural Defense

Use the **Basic Supportive Program** (found on page 89) for your plan of action. Also, consider the following important points about Botulism that may be useful:

Because the reaction time of these toxins can be quite fast, detection in the field is crucial for survival. Also, the amount of exposure must be taken into consideration, for many would survive when not too close to the point of release.

Psychological Line:
- ❑ Prepare in advance to have the ability to be calm and alert during emergencies by performing the Relaxation Response (or a comparable form of meditation) on a regular basis.

Preventative Line:
- ❑ Cook foods properly. Use caution with microwave ovens.
- ❑ GSE solution to spray foods using 10 drops per pint of water.
- ❑ Charco-Zyme 2-6 capsules with suspicious foods. Note: the aerosol of this toxin could also enter the gastrointestinal system. Avoid

---

[154] Levinson, W.; Jawetz, E. (2000), previously cited, p. 103.

[155] De Lorenzo, R.; Porter, R. Weapons of Mass Destruction: Emergency Care. Prentice-Hall, Inc.: Saddle River, N.J. (P. 75.)

[156] See: Cooney, D. (1995). Activated Charcoal: Antidote, Remedy, and Health Aid. TEACH Services, Inc.: Brushton, NY.

taking activated charcoal together with medications. Separate by at least 2 hours.

❑ Nux-Vomica is a remedy used by homeopathic physicians for basic support during a community alert regarding bacterial or chemical toxins.

Specific Line:

❑ Aconite or Arnica are remedies homeopathic physicians might recommend to be used immediately with actual exposure. Hypericum is a remedy used by homeopathic physicians for any form of paralysis as a subsequent symptom.

❑ Activated Charcoal Formula: 30 grams (3 tbsp) of activated charcoal in 4 ounces of water. Drink as soon as possible after known or suspected ingestion of the toxin. Also, continue to take 250-1000 mg of activated charcoal capsules every 2 hours afterwards for that day. At some point, activated charcoal may bind the stools and cause constipation. To prevent this drink plenty of water.

❑ If medical support is unavailable, an available source of **oxygen** could be life saving.

❑ Iron Chelation with Phytic Acid (IP6): Studies have shown that removal of iron negatively affects the activity of botulism toxin.[157] However, this in itself is not an antidote. Use 2,000-4000 mg with room temperature bottled-or-filtered water only (no juice, etc.) between meals.

❑ Activated Charcoal Formula can be mixed into juice for children. However, it will make the juice black. If vomiting is to be induced it should be done before giving the activated charcoal. If not, it can cause respiratory problems when the charcoal is brought up. Depending on the age of the child one would need to be creative. Dairy products, ice cream and sherbet decrease the absorbing activity of activated charcoal, and should not be given an hour before or after, or at all.

Pets:

❑ Activated charcoal can be mixed into food for pets to absorb ingested toxins. Can also be mixed in water (see above) and given as a slurry, and possibly delivered with a plastic syringe-like dispenser.

Rehabilitation:

❑ Make sure chelation is included in the **rehabilitation** program: Oral Chelation Formula (by Extreme Health or comparable formula) 3 capsules daily near bedtime, + 3 caplets of Age-Less Formula in the morning with food

for adults for 60-90 days. Children ages 2-7 use 1/2 of a capsule (can be opened in juice) near bedtime + 1/2 caplet in the morning with food (can be crushed and placed in food). Children ages 8-13 use 1 capsule near bedtime + 2 caplets of Age-Less Formula in the morning with food. Children ages 13 up can take the adult dose.

---

[157] Alternative Medicine, (January, 2002). Protecting Yourself from Bioterrorism. (P. 17.)

EPSILON TOXIN
(*Of Clostridium perfringens,* a gram-positive rod)

Epsilon toxin is a potent toxin produced by the spore-forming bacterium *Clostridium perfringens,* of which there are five types (A-B-C-D-E). Of the five, B and D produce epsilon protoxin, which, when activated in the intestines of the host, is responsible for a rapid destruction of the local tissue, which is often fatal. The disease is acquired from spores found in the soil. *C. perfringens* is also part of the normal flora of the intestines.

"*C perfringens* can cause disease in most domestic animals and some wildlife, including horses, poultry, sheep, birds, rabbits, goats, hogs, cattle, mink, ostrich, emu, dogs, cats, and others.

Mechanism of Disease

The bacteria produce a protoxin, which must be converted into a toxin in the body. Research[158] into its nature suggests that once it is activated into a toxin, it does not enter the target cell but acts on the surface causing potassium (K+) inside the cell to leak out (disturbing the sodium/potassium balance of cellular respiration). This produces an increase in intestinal permeability, leading to vascular damage and edema in many organ systems such as the brain, heart, lungs, and kidneys. The epsilon toxin is toxic to the nerves in laboratory animals.

"It occurs as a severe, usually fatal form of food poisoning that kills the small intestine. … The trouble starts when the balance of bacteria in the gut is disrupted, giving *C perfringens* a chance to proliferate unchecked."[159]

It is important to note that all five types of *C. perfringens* also produce the *Alpha toxin,* which disrupts intestinal function. Also, the five different strains "…produce a host of toxic proteins; nearly twenty have been described scientifically and there may be more."[160]

C perfringens thrives on oxygen-depleted dead tissue, and it is associated with three distinct disease syndromes: (1) gas gangrene (clostridial myonecrosis: most *Clostridia* species produce large amounts of gas—CO_2 and hydrogen—that cause intense swelling of soft tissues and the release of foul-smelling odor from the wound); (2) deadly inflammation of the mucosal lining of the small intestine (enteritis necroticans); and (3) clostridium food poisoning.

Symptoms

Symptoms of the disease may be subtle before fulminant toxemia develops. Within 6-24 hours of incubation signs of systemic toxicity appear, including:

- Diarrhea
- Dysentery (bowel inflammation and pain)
- Gangrene (wounds)
- Muscle infections
- Confusion
- Tachycardia (rapid heart beat)
- Sweating

Progression of the disease leads to:
- Liver damage
- Damage to skin;
- Edema in many organs such as the brain, lungs, heart, and kidneys.

Agent Characteristics as a Weapon
Estimated Level of Attraction
Low 1-2-3-4-5 High

- Availability of information about the agent. **3**
- Ease of performing research, and manipulating agent. **2**
- Ease of manufacture with minimal danger. **3**
- Availability of the ingredients. **3**
- Low cost. **3**

---

[158] Derived from Internet article: Structural Studies On Epsilon Toxin done at Birkbeck College, University of London by Prof. David Moss, et al.

[159] See: McGinly, S., Clostridium Perfringens: New ways to type strains of deadly bacteria. ECAT, College of Agriculture (part of the 1998 Arizona Experiment Station Research Report.

[160] McGinley, S. (Cited above.)

- Easy to store/house. **4**
- Durability of agent. **5**
- Difficulty for being detected. **5**
- Has a quick rate of action/incubation time. **5**
- Ease of transport. **4**
- Ease of delivery by various methods. **5**
- Ability to inflict widespread harm or death. **4**
- Treatable. **5**

Assessment

Because isolation of the toxin requires a certain amount of sophistication, the spores, in my opinion, would be a more likely choice as a WMD. *C perfringens* strains reproduce by spores that can lie dormant in the soil for many years. An aersol of the spores could be used to contaminate food or be inhaled. It carries high mortality unless therapy begins immediately. There's basically no treatment other than fluid replacement and the alleviation of abdominal cramping. Vaccine is currently not available, and, if the intestinal form is caught early in human victims, surgery is perhaps the only possible treatment

Strains have been reported that are resistant to *penicillin*, *tetracycline*, *erythromycin*, *chloramphenicol*, *metronidazole*, and *clindamycin*.

With the development of PCR assay the epsilon toxin can be isolated from the other toxins. This provides for a purer form of production. Prior to the PCR assay biotyping to identify the toxins was an involved and expensive and inaccurate process.

However, the exact mechanism of disease of the epsilon toxin is still somewhat blurry. How the aerosols would affect the system is not so well known. The nervous system seems to be affected. More is known about the ingestion of the toxin. Even so, I would say that either form has a **3** range of attraction for terrorist activity.

Detection and Diagnosis

Diagnostic tests: This organism has been difficult to pin point with laboratory tests because it "...is so promiscuous in terms of its hosts that it's found wherever there are domestic animals, and it makes a lot of toxins,

and it is almost always lethal."[161] Because of the many toxins produced by the different strains of *C perfringens*, existing laboratory tests produce a lot of false negatives and false positives.

Songer and associates have developed a more accurate singular test—the *multiplex polymerase chain reaction (PCR) assay*—that allows for simultaneous detection of the four major toxins and their genetic configurations. This may lead to the development of a more specific form of vaccination.

Field detection: no current method of detection is available.

Conventional Methods of Care and Treatment

Prehospital emergency care: Extreme caution needs to be exercised by first responders. Emergency care would depend on the identification of the condition. First responders would need to have full protective equipment. Patients are given fluid and respiratory support to prevent shock.

Medical care: Use of protective clothing, gloves, and masks, when in contact with infectious materials. Frequent hand washing is advised. "Clostridial myonecrosis (destruction of muscle tissue) is fatal unless identified and treated early. Hyperbaric oxygen, antibiotics (such as *penicillin*), and removal of necrotic (dead) tissue can be lifesaving."[162]

Note on Disinfectants: 1% sodium hypochlorite solution has a moderate affect on the spores, but they are susceptible to high-level decontaminants (such as glutaraldehyde) with prolonged contact time.

---

[161] Glenn Songer, veterinary scientist in the College of Agriculture at the University of Arizona. Web site: gsonger@u.arizona.edu.
[162] Gladwin, M. (M.D.); Trattler, B. (M.D.). (2002). Clinical Microbiology Made Ridiculously Simple, Edition 3. MedMaster, Inc.: Miami, Fl. (P. 43.)

Surgery: While surgery is not practiced on animal stocks it can save human victims.

Vaccine: none available.

Prophylaxis: none available.

Treatment For Consideration: Hemoperfusion is a method that has been used quite successfully to clear toxins out of the blood stream. Similar to hemodialysis, the patient is hooked up to a machine that draws the blood out and through a special activated charcoal filter and returns it to the body. This method would not be feasible during a mass crisis, but has its applications in smaller situations. At this time, I have no knowledge of how many hospitals or health facilities use this type of equipment.

Supportive Lines of Natural Defense

Use the **Basic Supportive Program** (found on page 89) for your plan of action. Also, consider the following important points about Epsilon Toxin that may be useful:

Because of the rapid onset of symptoms with this disease it is important to keep a level mind while taking care of yourself and seeking medical help. If the condition presents with intestinal complications it may not be possible to take things orally. Detection in the field is crucial for survival. Also, the amount of exposure must be taken into consideration, for many would survive when not too close to the point of release.

Psychological Line:
- ❑ Perform <u>Relaxation Response</u> (or a comparable form of meditation) 1-2 times daily to develop the capacity to be calm and alert during an emergency.

Social Line:
- ❑ <u>Remember, this disease is highly infectious.</u>

Preventative Line:
- ❑ With suspicious food (as soon as possible after suspected ingestion) take 2-6 capsules of <u>Charco-Zyme</u>™ (Atrium, Inc.) with 200 mg of <u>Betaine HCL</u> to absorb and inactivate the bacteria, spores, or toxin. Continue taking every 1-2 hours until the symptoms clear. Ingesting large amounts of activated charcoal may bind the stool and cause constipation. Drink plenty of water to prevent this. Avoid taking activated charcoal together with medicines. Separate by at least 2 hours.

Specific Line:
- ❑ <u>Activated Charcoal Formula with Grapefruit Seed Extract (GSE)</u>: 30 grams (approx 3 tbspns) of activated charcoal in 4 ounces of water to which 10 drops of GSE have been stirred in. Drink as soon as possible. Use as many times as needed, especially when having loose bowel movements.
- ❑ <u>Activated Charcoal Formula</u> can be mixed into juice. However, it will make the juice black. Older children might be able to take the capsules. If vomiting is to be induced it should be done before giving the activated charcoal. If not, it can cause respiratory problems when the charcoal is brought up. Depending on the age of the child, one would need to be creative. Dairy products, ice cream and sherbet decrease the absorbing activity of activated charcoal, and should not be given an hour before or after, or at all.
- ❑ <u>Nux-Vomica</u> is a remedy used by homeopathic physicians for basic support during a community alert regarding bacterial or chemical toxins. <u>Aconite</u> or <u>Arnica</u> are remedies homeopathic physicians might recommend to be used immediately with actual exposure.

Rehabilitation:
- ❑ <u>Circulegs</u>™ (Solaray) 1-2 capsules 2-3 times a day to strengthen blood vessels. <u>Reduce Salt Intake</u>.
- ❑ Make sure to use chelation as part of the rehabilitation program: <u>Oral Chelation Formula</u> (by Extreme Health or comparable formula) 3 capsules daily near bedtime, + 3 caplets of <u>Age-Less Formula</u> in the morning with food for adults for 60-90 days. Children ages 2-7 use 1/2 of a capsule (can be opened in juice) near bedtime + 1/2 caplet in the morning with food (can be crushed and placed in food). Children ages 8-13 use 1 capsule near bedtime + 2 caplets of <u>Age-Less Formula</u> in the morning with food. Children ages 13 up can take the adult dose.
- ❑ Probiotics are very important.

Pets:
- ❑ Activated charcoal can be mixed into pet's food to absorb ingested toxins. Can also be mixed in water (see above) and given as a slurry, and possibly delivered with a plastic syringe-like dispenser.
- ❑ Pets: Use <u>ASAP Solution</u>® to protect against secondary infections: 1/2-1 tsp 3 + times a day, with a plastic eyedropper under the tongue.
- ❑ Probiotics are very important.

RICIN TOXIN
(From *Ricinus Communis*, Castor Beans)

Ricin is a potent cell toxin made quite easily from the mash that remains after processing castor beans (derived from the castor plant) to make castor oil. Poisoning can occur following inhalation, ingestion of contaminated food or water, or from the injection of the toxin into the body.

Mechanism of Action

Ricin toxin directly effects cell metabolism by inhibiting protein synthesis in the cellular factory inside the cell, known as the ribosome. This also impairs the cell's ability to utilize oxygen. Lack of protein synthesis and oxygen (hypoxia) kills the tissue (necrosis), a condition that can spread and cause multiple organ failures.

The ingestion of ricin causes severe lesions in the throat, esophagus, and the stomach and intestines. The inhaled form can cause severe damage to the upper and lower respiratory system.

Symptoms

The time from oral exposure to onset of symptoms can range from less than 1 hour to 12 hours or greater. Eating Castor beans (especially after being chewed) or ricin-contaminated material causes:

- Bloody diarrhea
- Nausea
- Vomiting
- Profuse internal bleeding
- Liver and kidney failure
- Rapid heart beat can also occur
- Circulatory failure

If ricin dust is inhaled the incubation period is approximately from 8 to 24 hours, and can lead to:

- Acute fever
- Cough
- Chest tightness
- Profuse sweating
- Inflammation of upper and lower respiratory system
- Pulmonary edema
- Cyanosis (bluish color of the skin and mucous membranes)
- Hypotension

- Respiratory failure
- Circulatory failure
- Death typically occurs 36-72 hours later, depending on the dose

Injection of ricin would most likely result in:

- Muscle necrosis (death of tissue) at the site of injection
- Probable multiple organ failure
- Death

Agent Characteristics as a Weapon
Estimated Level of Attraction
Low 1-2-3-4-5 High

- Availability of information about the agent. **5**
- Ease of performing research, and manipulating agent. **5**
- Ease of manufacture with minimal danger. **5**
- Availability of the ingredients. **5**
- Low cost. **5**
- Easy to store/house. **5**
- Durability of agent. **5**
- Difficulty for being detected. **5**
- Has a quick rate of action/incubation time. **5**
- Ease of transport. **5**
- Ease of delivery by various methods. **5**
- Ability to inflict widespread harm/death. **2-3**
- Treatable. **5**

Assessment

The relative ease of producing ricin makes it attractive to terrorists. Castor beans are widely available, and the toxin is easy to extract. It can be produced as a liquid, a crystalline form, or freeze-dried to make a powder. Therefore, it can be used to contaminate food or water supplies or delivered into the atmosphere to be inhaled into the lungs. It can also be placed in a warhead. It's not likely that the injectable method is of any major concern.

According to the *PDR Guide to Biological and Chemical Warfare Response*, "Ricin is less toxic than botulinum; a large quantity would be required to cover a significant area."[163] If used as an aerosol it would most likely be a localized event with minimal casualties. The food borne toxin poses a greater threat. Nevertheless, as lethal as it may be, the oral route has a lower rate of toxicity due to poor absorption of the toxin.[164] In the context of other WMD I would estimate that ricin toxin is in the **3-4** level of attraction.

Detection and Diagnosis

Diagnostic tests: Blood or other body fluids can be used for antigen detection with enzyme-linked immunosorbent assays (ELISA).

Field detection: Tetracore, Inc. has developed a *Bio Threat Alert*™ (BTA) test strip for ricin toxin to be used by first responders.

Conventional Methods of Care and Treatment

Prehospital emergency care would depend on the identification of the condition. Secondary aerosols of ricin do not pose a problem for first responders. Nevertheless, first responders would ideally have full protective equipment. Airway, breathing, and cardiovascular (ABC) checks would be made on site and/or in the ambulance en route to the site of treatment.

Given the propensity of respiratory complications from an aerosol attack, priority would be given to maintaining airway and providing adequate ventilation. With ricin, oxygen therapy is crucial, increasing the chances for survival and reducing the potential for shock.

Medical care: Supportive hospital care is required. The emphasis is on preventing respiratory failure and lack of oxygen. Isolation is not required.

Thorough decontamination is required. Because of its complex protein structure (tox-albumin) ricin is susceptible to heat, soap and water, and mild 0.1% hypochlorite solutions.

The use of activated charcoal and gastric lavage would be done for an oral exposure.

Vaccination: Vaccine and antitoxin are not available for treatment of ricin poisoning.

Treatment For Consideration: Hemoperfusion is a method that has been used quite successfully to clear toxins out of the blood stream. Similar to hemodialysis, the patient is hooked up to a machine that draws the blood out and through a special activated charcoal filter and returns it to the body. This method would not be feasible during a mass crisis, but has its applications in smaller situations. At this time, I have no knowledge of how many hospitals or health facilities use this type of equipment.

Research/Experimental

Researchers have identified the key structural and functional regions of this toxin that can be used to protect against the inhalation of ricin aerosol. This may lead to an antidote. Also, a chemically modified ricin has been reported to have the potential of producing a vaccine.[165]

Along these lines, scientists have successfully produced an antiviral protein prepared from the leaves of Pokeweed (*Phytolacca americana*) that blocks the active chain of the ricin toxin from entering the cell.[166] However, I don't recommend taking pokeweed as an antidote, for it is a toxic herb.

Study shows that vitamin C protects against the activity of ricin in vitro (test tubes). [Holtsclaw, S.A.; Clark, C.E. (1977). Ascorbic

---

[163] Published by: Thompson/Physician's Desk Reference. (2002). Montvale, N.J. (P. 25.)

[164] Patocka, J. Abrin and Ricin: Two Dangerous Poisonous Proteins. Department of Toxicology, Military Medical Academy, Hradec Kralove, Czech Republic. E-mail: patocka@pmfhk.cz. (P. 1.)

[165] Poli, M., Rivera, V.R., Pitt, L. Voge, P. Aerosolized specific antibody protects mice from lung injury associated with aerosolized ricin exposure. In: 11th World Congress on Animal, Plant, and Microbial Toxins; 1994; Tel Aviv, Israel.

[166] Irwin, J.: Pokeweed Antiviral Protein, *Pharmac. Ther.* 21, 371 (1983).

145

Acid: effects of ricin intoxicated HeLa cells. Journal of Nutritional Science Vitaminol: 23 (6): 475-80, (Tokyo, Japan).]

Supportive Lines of Natural Defense

Use the **Basic Supportive Program** (found on page 89) for your plan of action. Also, consider the following important points about Ricin Toxin that may be useful:

Because of the rapid onset of symptoms with this disease it is important to keep a level mind while taking care of yourself and seeking medical help. If the condition presents with intestinal complications it may not be possible to take things orally. Detection in the field is crucial for survival. Also, the amount of exposure must be taken into consideration, for many would survive when not too close to the point of release.

Psychological Line:
- ❑ Psychological preparation is important.

Social Line:
- ❑ Remember, this disease is not contagious.

Preventative/Specific Line:
- ❑ Source of oxygen can be life saving.
- ❑ Vitamin C: taken to body tolerance.
- ❑ Activated Charcoal Formula: 30 grams of activated charcoal in 4 ounces of water. Drink as soon as possible after ingestion of the toxin. Note: 1 tbsp of the activated charcoal equals about 10 grams. Also, continue to take 250-1000 mg of activated charcoal capsules every 2 hours afterwards for that day. Avoid taking activated charcoal together with medications. Separate by at least 2 hours.
- ❑ Activated Charcoal Formula can be mixed into juice for children. However, it will make the juice black . Older children might be able to take the capsules. If vomiting is to be induced it should be done before giving the activated charcoal. If not, it can cause respiratory problems when the charcoal is brought up. Depending on the age of the child, one would need to be creative. Dairy products, ice cream and sherbet decrease the absorbing activity of activated charcoal, and should not be given an hour before or after, or at all.
- ❑ With suspicious food take 2-6 capsules of Charco-Zyme™ (Atrium, Inc.), as soon as possible after ingesting, with a glass of water,
- ❑ Prolonged use of absorbents may bind the stools and cause constipation. To help prevent this drink plenty of water.
- ❑ Nux-Vomica is a remedy used by homeopathic physicians for basic support during a community alert. Aconite and Arnica are remedies homeopathic physicians might recommend to be used immediately with actual exposure.

Rehabilitation:
- ❑ Make sure to use Oral Chelation as part of the rehabilitation program.

SAXITOXIN

Saxitoxin belongs to a family of chemically related neurotoxins produced by a species of freshwater and marine algae known as dinoflagellates. Some forms of marine life such as mussels, clams, scallops, and the blue-ringed octopus consume this kind of algae, and the toxin builds up in their system. Humans who ingest them can suffer a life-threatening illness known as paralytic shellfish poisoning.

Mechanism of Action

Absorption of the toxins through the gastrointestinal tract is rapid, producing symptoms within a few minutes. Urinary excretion of the toxin from the system is fairly rapid, and, depending on the dose, those who survive for at least 12-24 hours usually recover. Because of the paralytic effect of the toxin on the nerves it may involve disruption of the neurotransmitter acetylcholine. No medical information exists about the human respiratory route of exposure, but animal experiments suggest that the mechanism of action can be accelerated where death may occur in minutes.

High production of antioxidants may overwhelm the system and lead to additional organ complications.

Symptoms

Initial symptoms include:
- Nausea
- Light-headedness
- Vomiting

Tingling or numbness around the mouth followed by:

- Flaccid paralysis of extremities (can occur 1-12 hours after exposure)
- Respiratory paralysis is the main cause of death

Agent Characteristics as a Weapon
Estimated Level of Attraction
Low 1-2-3-4-5 High

- Availability of information about the agent. **5**
- Ease of performing research, and manipulating agent. **4**
- Ease of manufacture with minimal danger. **3**
- Availability of the ingredients. **5**
- Low cost. **4**
- Easy to store/house. **5**
- Durability of agent. **5**
- Difficulty for being detected. **5**
- Has a quick rate of action/incubation time. **5**
- Ease of transport. **5**
- Ease of delivery by various methods. **5**
- Ability to inflict widespread harm or death. **3**
- Treatable. **5**

Assessment

The Federation of American Scientists consider saxitoxin a potential weapon that could be deployed as an inhalant via a projectile or used to contaminate water supplies. The toxin can also be made into an aerosol. As an aerosol, it would not inflict widespread harm or death, but would certainly produce a degree of panic. Saxitoxin cannot be destroyed by cooking or boiling. However, the severity of the poisoning is diminished if the water used in cooking is not consumed. Water or food contamination is questionable, but possible. Activated charcoal (filter systems, and ingested capsules) can absorb it. It is not contagious. It appears to meet most of the above criteria, and would in my opinion be within the **3-4** range of attraction.

Detection

Diagnosis is typically confirmed by detection of the toxin in food, water, stomach contents or in environmental samples. Considering the small time frame for appropriate action, routine laboratory tests are not usually helpful.

Field Detection is not available.

Conventional Methods of Care/Treatment

Prehospital Emergency Care would depend on the identification of the condition. First responders would ideally have full protective equipment. Airway, breathing, and cardiovascular (ABC) checks would be made on site and/or in the ambulance en route to the site of treatment. Given the propensity of respiratory complications from an aerosol attack, priority would be given to maintaining airway and providing adequate ventilation. Such ventilation increases the chances for survival for it reduces the potential for shock.

Because exposure to almost any biological agent can cause dehydration and septic shock, intravenous solution would be administered to all non-ambulatory patients.

Hospital/Medical Care: Routine emergency care for ingested poisons would be employed. Isolation is not required. Diuresis (increased excretion of urine) may increase elimination of toxin. Severe cases may need intubation and respiratory support.

Supportive Lines of Natural Defense

Use the **Basic Supportive Program** (found on page 89) for your plan of action. Also, consider the following important points about Saxitoxin that may be useful:

Because of the rapid onset of symptoms with this disease it is important to keep a level mind while taking care of yourself and seeking medical help. If the condition presents with intestinal complications it may not be possible to take things orally. Detection in the field is crucial for survival. Also, the amount of exposure must be taken into consideration, for many would survive when not too close to the point of release.

Psychological Line:
- ❑ Psychological preparation is important.

Social Line:
- ❑ Remember, this disease is not contagious.

Specific Line:
- ❑ Source of oxygen can be life saving.
- ❑ Activated Charcoal Formula: 30 grams of activated charcoal in 4 ounces of water. Drink as soon as possible after ingestion of the toxin. Note: 1 tbsp of the activated charcoal equals about 10 grams. Also, continue to take 250-1000 mg of activated charcoal capsules every

2 hours afterwards for that day. Avoid taking activated charcoal together with medications. Separate by at least 2 hours.

- ☐ Activated Charcoal Formula can be mixed into juice for children. However, it will make the juice black. Older children might be able to take the capsules. If vomiting is to be induced it should be done before giving the activated charcoal. If not, it can cause respiratory problems when the charcoal is brought up. Depending on the age of the child, one would need to be creative. Dairy products, ice cream and sherbet decrease the absorbing activity of activated charcoal, and should not be given an hour before or after, or at all.
- ☐ With suspicious food take 2-6 capsules of Charco-Zyme™ (Atrium, Inc.), as soon as possible after ingesting, with a glass of water,
- ☐ Prolonged use of absorbents may bind the stools and cause constipation. To help prevent this drink plenty of water.
- ☐ Nux-Vomica is a remedy used by homeopathic physicians for basic support during a community alert regarding bacterial or chemical toxins. Aconite or Arnica are remedies homeopathic physicians might recommend to be used immediately with actual exposure.

- ☐ Drink lots of water.
- ☐ Use **Thompson's** diuretic formula; follow directions on container.

Rehabilitation:
- ☐ Make sure to use chelation as part of the rehabilitation program: Oral Chelation Formula (by Extreme Health or comparable formula) 3 capsules daily near bedtime, + 3 caplets of Age-Less Formula in the morning with food for adults for 60-90 days. Children ages 2-7 use 1/2 of a capsule (can be opened in juice) near bedtime + 1/2 caplet in the morning with food (can be crushed and placed in food). Children ages 8-13 use 1 capsule near bedtime + 2 caplets of Age-Less Formula in the morning with food. Children ages 13 up can take the adult dose

Pets:
- ☐ Activated Charcoal can be mixed into pet's food to absorb ingested toxins. Can also be mixed in water and given as a slurry, and possibly delivered with a plastic syringe-like dispenser.

STAPHYLOCOCCUS ENTEROTOXIN B

Staphylococcus aureus (a gram-negative cocci) is one amongst several common bacteria that produce toxins that affect the intestines (enterotoxins). It secretes five toxins, identified by the letters A, B, C, D, and E. The A type is the most commonly incurred. Staphylococcus enterotoxin B (SEB) is often associated with food poisoning derived from non-refrigerated meats, dairy, and bakery products. Essentially, most protein foods attract it, especially within a few hours at room temperature. Normally, it affects the intestines, which may result in high morbidity, but is not necessarily fatal. However, when SEB is inhaled, it produces significantly different clinical effects. Even so, the inhaled toxin may also enter the gastrointestinal system and additionally produce its typical effects.

Mechanism of Disease

This toxin acts at the site of exposure as a superantigen, which causes certain white blood cells (known as T lymphocytes) to multiply in huge numbers. This goes on to stimulate the overproduction of cytokines (interleukin-1 and interleukin-2), messengers that mobilize the immune system and inflammation. Consequently, the activity of the immune system becomes abnormally amplified to the point where it may cause the blood vessels to over expand. This causes the excessive release of blood fluids, a precipitous drop in blood pressure (hypotension), and the loss of oxygen to the tissue (hypoxia). As a result, other organ systems will not be able to function. Clinically, these dire events are referred to as septic shock, which is often life threatening.

Symptoms

When SEB is ingested it has an incubation period of 1-8 hours (rarely, yet possible, up to 18 hours), and it produces the following symptoms:

- Intense nausea
- Vomiting
- Cramping and abdominal pain
- Nonbloody diarrhea
- The illness may last for less than 24 hours (usually from 6-10 hours)

The effects of inhaled SEB may manifest from 1 to 6 hours. It typically produces:
- Sudden onset of fever
- Headache
- Chills
- Dry cough
- Difficulty breathing (in more severe cases)
- Chest pain (in more severe cases)
- Recovery usually takes from 1-2 weeks

It's important to note that the symptoms of the oral and inhaled forms of the disease may occur simultaneously.

Agent Characteristics as a Weapon
Estimated Level of Attraction
Low 1-2-3-4-5 High

- Availability of information about the agent. **5**
- Ease of performing research, and manipulating agent. **5**
- Ease of manufacture with minimal danger. **5**
- Availability of the ingredients. **5**
- Low cost. **5**
- Easy to store/house. **5**
- Durability of agent. **5**
- Difficulty for being detected. **5**
- Has a quick rate of action/incubation time. **5**
- Ease of transport. **5**
- Ease of delivery by various methods. **5**
- Ability to inflict widespread harm or death. **1**
- Treatable. **1**

Assessment

Obviously, this is an incapacitating disease. One might wonder why it's considered a possible WMD. A small amount of toxin is needed to cause illness. It can be easily aerosolized. It is very stable, and it is very soluble in water, quite resistant to temperature fluctuations (can tolerate boiling for several minutes). In the freeze-dried form it can be stored for over a year. SEB can cause widespread damage, multi-organ system failure,

and can produce shock followed by death in very high doses. However, aerosol exposure is not usually lethal but has incapacitating effects, which can produce a profound immobilizing illness that may last as long as 2 weeks. Large amounts would need to be released as an aerosol and in water to make any significant impact. Food sources would be the most likely target.

Another feature it has for use as a weapon is the "invisibility factor" in that it will not be easily detected as a biowarfare incident, allowing the perpetrators to render the target population weak and incapable of resisting a more life-threatening follow-up event. Considering these factors, I would estimate SEB to be within **2-3** range of attraction as a WMD.

Detection and Diagnosis

Diagnostic tests: Often laboratory tests are not required. SEB can be confused with a number of other gastroenteritis diseases. However, SEB can be confirmed with enzyme-linked immunosorbent assays (ELISA) of tissue or body fluids. Elevated erythrocyte (red blood cell) sedimentation rate (the rate that red blood cells settle in still plasma to the bottom of a test tube) is also a possible indicator. Nasal swabs are useful for detection of exposure to the aerosol form of SEB within a 12-24 hour period. Radiographs are used to reveal a high exposure to aerosolized SEB.

Field detection: In the US the epidemiological evidence is scanty because cases of normal exposure are so mild that patients rarely seek treatment. Currently, no field detection methods are available. The toxin cannot be detected by the senses.

Conventional Methods of
Care and Treatment

Emergency pre-hospital care would depend on the identification of the condition. First responders would ideally have protective equipment, which consists of a respirator, head and face protection, impervious boots and gloves, and body protective gear. They would:

Perform airway, breathing, and cardiovascular (ABC) checks on site and/or in the ambulance en route to the site of treatment.

Provide adequate ventilation with high flow oxygen with a non-rebreather mask. Such ventilation increases the chances for survival for it reduces the potential for shock.

More serious respiratory conditions (apnea, no breathing) would require a surgical incision into the windpipe (trachea) and insertion of a plastic tube (orotracheal intubation) to prevent suffocation, or the use of a bag-valve air delivery mask.

Exposure to almost any biological agent can cause dehydration and septic shock. To help prevent this, intravenous solution would be administered to all non-ambulatory patients.

Medical Care is basically supportive, and it involves the administration of intravenous fluids for those who are dehydrated.

Patients with pulmonary symptoms require treatment with humidified oxygen, and steroids for pain control.

Significant exposure may need intubation (the passage of a rubber tube into the larynx to deliver air to the lungs) and assisted ventilation with high levels of oxygen.

The effectiveness of steroids has not been confirmed. Antibiotics have also not proven effective against SEB.

For diarrhea and abdominal pain, *paragoric* or *Lomotil* may be used. However, evidence that *Lomotil* may prolong bacterial infections may influence against its use.

Contamination is possible, but contagion is not. Protective hospital-grade masks can provide protection against inhalation of SEB.

Vaccine/Antidote: None available.

Supportive Lines of Natural Defense

Use the **Basic Supportive Program** (found on page 89) for your plan of action. Also, consider the following important points about Staphylococcus Enterotoxin that may be useful:

Social Line:
- Remember, this disease is not contagious.

Preventative Line:
- Taking Charco-Zyme™ (Atrium, Inc.) 2-4 capsules with suspicious foods might offer protection from absorbing the toxin. (Not to be taken at the same time with medications. Separate by at least 2 hours.)
- Food-borne SEB can be prevented by properly storing dairy and meat products, and by the thorough cooking of meat products.

Specific Line:
- Activated Charcoal Formula can be mixed into juice for children. However, it will make the juice black. Depending on the age of the child, one would need to be creative. Dairy products, ice cream and sherbet decrease the absorbing activity of activated charcoal, and should not be given an hour before or after, or at all.
- Take 1 tsp of acidophilus powder + 1/2 tsp of Inner Strength (Ethical Nutrients or comparable product) in warm water 3-6 times daily. Especially important when taking any form of antimicrobial (synthetic or natural). KidZyme™ or FloraBear For Kids™ can be given to children.
- Lung support: Oregacyn™ (North American Herb and Spice Co.) 1-2 capsules every 4-6 hours with or without food. Also, Oreganol™ (Wild Mountain Oil of Oregano), a few drops may be rubbed on chest as extra support for lung health.
- Ginger tea to alleviate nausea. Ginger candy available in health food stores can be given to children.

Pets:
- Activated charcoal can be mixed into pet's food to absorb ingested toxins. Can also be mixed in water and given as a slurry, and possibly administered with a plastic syringe-like dispenser.

TRICHOTHECENE MYCOTOXINS

Trichothecene mycotoxins (T2) form a diverse group of more than 100 compounds produced by fungus molds (of the genus *Fusarium*). T2 grows on certain agricultural products—corn, wheat, and barley—which, when consumed by animals, produces a disease known as moldy toxicosis poisoning. Exposure to animals and humans occurs from ingesting contaminated food, contact with the skin, in chemotherapy, and from the inhalation of aerosols.

The diverse nature of these mycotoxins can affect many organ systems, the effects of which can resemble the damage done by radiation, or the burn of nitrogen mustard. Serious damage occurs mainly to the gastrointestinal tract, the lymphatic system, and the red-blood-cell producing process in the bone marrow.

These toxins have been implicated in the bio-war incidents known as "yellow rain" in Laos, Cambodia, and Afghanistan.

Mechanism of Action

These toxins are potent inhibitors of protein and nucleic acid (DNA) synthesis. Consequently, affected cells cannot grow and develop. Therefore, wherever cell division is most rapid (such as with the skin, mucous membranes, gastrointestinal tract, and bone marrow), its action would be more quickly noticed as initial symptoms.

Symptoms

Symptoms have been documented to occur within minutes to 2-4 hours after exposure. Contact with the skin produces the following symptoms at the site of exposure:

- Itching
- Redness
- Painful skin lesions
- Burning skin
- Dead skin tissue (necrosis)

Exposure to the eyes causes:

- Redness
- Tearing
- Pain
- Blurry vision

Exposure to the upper respiratory tract causes:

- Nose pain
- Throat pain
- Nasal discharge
- Nosebleed

Exposure to the lower respiratory tract causes:

- Cough
- Difficulty breathing
- Wheezing
- Chest pain
- Bloody sputum

High exposure causes:

- Light headedness
- Shortness of breath

- Rapid onset of hemorrhage
- Incapacitation and death

Ingestion of the toxin causes a condition known as *alimentary toxic aleukia* characterized by:

- Ulcerative inflammation of the mucous membranes of the throat and gastrointestinal tract
- Hemorrhage
- A marked reduction or absence of white blood cells and/or platelets
- Depletion of bone marrow.

Because T2 affects the cell nucleus (as occurs with exposure to radiation), survivors may develop a radiation-like sickness with:

- Fever
- Nausea
- Vomiting
- Diarrhea
- Reduced white blood cells and/or platelets
- Bleeding
- Blood infection
- Recovery may take several weeks to months.

Agent Characteristics as a Weapon
Estimated Level of Attraction
Low 1-2-3-4-5 High

- Availability of information about the agent. **5**
- Ease of performing research, and manipulating agent. **?**
- Ease of manufacture with minimal danger. **3-4**
- Availability of the ingredients. **5**
- Low cost. **5**
- Easy to store/house. **5**
- Durability of agent. **5**
- Difficulty for being detected. **4-5**
- Has a quick rate of action/incubation time. **5**
- Ease of transport. **5**
- Ease of delivery by various methods. **5**

- Ability to inflict widespread harm or death. **3**
- Treatable. **5**

Assessment

T2 has a subversive history of use as a bio-warfare agent, and therefore there is a supportive technology. Employed as a weapon, T2 could produce exposure through inhalation, contact, and through ingestion of contaminated food and water. This potential range of exposure broadens the potential kinds of effects it may have. T2 is very stable under high temperatures, and meets most of the criteria of attractiveness, but, as with most toxins, it would not inflict widespread harm because it is not contagious and would have a localized effect. Therefore, I estimate it would register a **3-4** on the scale of attractiveness.

Detection

Diagnostic Tests: T2 has a long "half-life" in the system and can be detected up to 28 days after exposure.

Field Detection: "T2 exposure can be hard to differentiate from mustard agent poisoning. However, mustard agents have a characteristic odor and are readily detected by field tests. Mustard has a slower onset of action, taking several hours to produce symptoms."[167]

Conventional Methods of Care and Treatment

Emergency pre-hospital care would depend on the identification of the condition. First responders would ideally have protective equipment, which consists of a respirator, head and face protection, impervious boots and gloves, and body protective gear. They would:

Perform airway, breathing, and cardiovascular (ABC) checks on site and/or in the ambulance en route to the site of treatment.

Provide adequate ventilation with high flow oxygen with a non-rebreather mask.

Such ventilation increases the chances for survival for it reduces the potential for shock.

More serious respiratory conditions (apnea, no breathing) would require a surgical incision into the windpipe (trachea) and insertion of a plastic tube (orotracheal intubation) to prevent suffocation, or the use of a bag-valve air delivery mask.

Exposure to almost any biological agent can cause dehydration and septic shock. To help prevent this, intravenous solution would be administered to all non-ambulatory patients.

Medical Care: There is no antidotal therapy for T2 mycotoxins. Supportive measures should begin within 5-60 minutes. It should focus on thorough decontamination (hypochlorite solution is effective).

Saline solution should be used to decontaminate the eyes. Soap and water wash can significantly diminish localized effects of the toxin on the skin. Decontaminated patients require no special isolation measures.

Respiratory distress should be treated with oxygen, aerosolized beta-agonists (*albuterol*), and if necessary, intubation and mechanical ventilation. Skin lesions should be dressed with dry gauze.

Hypotension and shock are treated with intravenous fluids such as saline, administration of *dopamine* or *norepinephrine* for unresponsive patients. Blood transfusion to replace platelets and white blood cells may be necessary.

Vaccination/Prophylaxis: There is no vaccine or prophylaxis available.

Research/Experimental

The Federation of American Scientists report[168] that ascorbic acid (400-1200 mg, per kilogram of body weight, of vitamin C), administered intravenously, worked to decrease the lethality of T2 in animal studies, but has not been tested in humans.

---

[167] De Lorenzo, R., Porter R., previously cited, p. 77.

[168] Pike, J. Ed., previously cited, p. 14.

They also report, that "While not yet available for humans, administration of large doses of monoclonal antibodies (antibodies produced in a laboratory from a single clone of B lymphocytes) directed against T2 and metabolites have shown prophylactic and therapeutic efficacy in animal models."

The above-mentioned research on the use of ascorbic acid (vitamin C) is in keeping with the claims made by a group of ortho-molecular physicians, regarding the clinical administration of this vitamin, intravenously and orally, to reduce toxic load in patients.[169]

Supportive Lines of Natural Defense

Use the **Basic Supportive Program** (found on page 89) for your plan of action. Also, consider the following important points about Trichothecene Mycotoxins that may be useful:

Because of the rapid onset of symptoms with this disease it is important to keep a level mind while taking care of yourself and seeking medical help. If the condition presents with intestinal complications it may not be possible to take things orally. Detection in the field is crucial for survival. Also, the amount of exposure must be taken into consideration, for many would survive when not too close to the point of release.

Psychological Line:
- ❑ Psychological preparation is important.

Social Line:
- ❑ Remember, this disease is not contagious.

Preventative Line:
- ❑ With suspicious food take 2-6 capsules of Charco-Zyme™ (Atrium, Inc.), as soon as possible after ingesting, with a glass of water.
- ❑ Nux-Vomica is a remedy used by homeopathic physicians for basic support during a community alert regarding bacterial or chemical toxins.
- ❑ Considering the damaging effect that T2 has on the cell nucleic acids (DNA, RNA), I would add to my daily preventative program 60-120 mg of Co-Q-10 (coenzyme-Q-10) during an alert. This enzyme has been shown to protect the DNA/RNA of cells (especially, in the energy-producing mitochondria within the cell), and for cell integrity in general.[170]

Specific Line:
- ❑ Source of oxygen can be life saving.
- ❑ Activated Charcoal Formula: 30 grams of activated charcoal in 4 ounces of water. Drink as soon as possible after ingestion of the toxin. Note: 1 tbsp of the activated charcoal equals about 10 grams. Also, continue to take 250-1000 mg of activated charcoal capsules every 2 hours afterwards for that day.
- ❑ Activated Charcoal Formula can be mixed into juice for children. However, it will make the juice black. Older children might be able to take the capsules. If vomiting is to be induced it should be done before giving the activated charcoal. If not, it can cause respiratory problems when the charcoal is brought up. Depending on the age of the child, one would need to be creative. Dairy products, ice cream and sherbet decrease the absorbing activity of activated charcoal, and should not be given an hour before or after, or at all.
- ❑ Prolonged use of absorbents may bind the stools and cause constipation. To help prevent this drink plenty of water.
- ❑ Aconite or Arnica are remedies homeopathic physicians might recommend to be used immediately with actual exposure.

Rehabilitation:
- ❑ Make sure to use chelation as part of the rehabilitation program: Oral Chelation Formula (by Extreme Health or comparable formula) 3 capsules daily near bedtime, + 3 caplets of Age-Less Formula in the morning with food for adults for 60-90 days. Children ages 2-7 use 1/2 of a capsule (can be opened in juice) near bedtime + 1/2 caplet in the morning with food (can be crushed and placed in food). Children ages 8-13 use 1 capsule near bedtime + 2 caplets of Age-Less Formula in the morning with food. Children ages 13 up can take the adult dose

Pets:
- ❑ Activated Charcoal can be mixed into pet's food to absorb ingested toxins. Can also be mixed in water and given as a slurry, and possibly delivered with a plastic syringe-like dispenser.
- ❑ Homeopathic physicians might recommend the remedy Nux Vomica to protect against the exposure to toxins.

---

[169] See bibliographic entry for Robert Cathcart, M.D.
[170] Life Extension Magazine (Collector's Edition 2002), Mitochondria hold the key to cellular life and death. (P. 109.)

CHEMICAL WEAPONS

As the complexity of a WMD becomes simpler, its reaction time increases. And so it is with the chemical WMD. However, there are trade offs. Chemical agents are not contagious, and, as lethal as many are, their effects are determined by the proximity and amount of exposure. Not to diminish the value of a single life, large amounts would be needed to affect large populations. While they may be delivered on warheads, the necessary equipment and detection of such intent would add to the complexity of doing so, and therefore would reduce the level of attraction.

Blister/Vesicants

Blister agents (also known as vesicants) cause burns and/or large blisters by direct contact with skin, the mucous membranes of the eyes, and the respiratory system when inhaled. They have historically been used by the military during war, both to produce casualties and to hamper fighting efficacy by forcing troops to wear cumbersome protective gear. Although blister agents can be lethal in certain concentrations, they generally incapacitate the victim. Blister/vesicant agents include:

- **Mustard Gas** (H)
- **Sequi Mustard**
- **Sulphur Mustard** (HD)
- **Nitrogen Mustard** (HN-1, HN-2, HN-3)
- **Mustard/Lewisite** (HL)
- **Lewisite-1** (L-1, L-2, L-3), (an arsenical vesicant)
- **Ethyldichloroarsine** (ED)
- **Methyldichloroarsine** (MD)
- **Phenodichloroarsine** (PD)
- **Phosgene Oxime** (CX)

Mustard agents include the nitrogen mustards (HN-1, HN-2, HN-3), sulfur mustards (H, HD), and mustard-lewisite (HL). They consist of oily liquids that can range from a pure colorless state to pale yellow to dark brown. They can be identified as having a faint odor of mustard, onion, garlic, or horseradish. Mustard agents are slightly soluble in water and may endure for long periods at the site of exposure. Contrary to its name, mustard gas is actually a liquid, not likely to change into a gas at ordinary temperatures.

What distinguishes mustard agents from the other vesicants is the time it takes for symptoms to develop. Mustard agents have a delayed reaction time (which may take hours), but **Lewisite** and **phosgene oxime**, for example, bring on immediate symptoms to the exposed area. Phosgene oxime is more soluble in water. In addition to its quick reaction time, Lewisite also presents the dangers of **arsenic poisoning**.

Of the entire group of vesicants, the most feared are the sulphur mustard (HD) and the nitrogen mustards (HN-2) due to their stability, persistence at the site of exposure, and their effect on attacking the eyes, skin, and respiratory system. However, the treatment protocols for vesicants are essentially the same, except for a few variations with the non-mustards.

Mechanism of Harm

Essentially, vesicants cause chemical reactions that destroy skin and mucous membranes. One of the characteristics of vesicants that contribute to their harmfulness is that they are slightly soluble in water. This makes it very difficult to use water to clear them off the skin. Absorbents and chelators need to be used. Vesicants are particularly more active in warm environments.

154

In certain concentrations, vesicants can be absorbed into the body and the blood to cause systemic complications. Mustard can affect the blood-forming process in the bone marrow and become life threatening weeks after exposure. On the other hand, phosgene oxime does not affect the bone marrow.

A longer-term effect of mustards is the possible formation of lung cancer (by altering the structure of the nucleic acid DNA). Lewisite compounds also have complications related to arsenic poisoning, which can create systemic problems more quickly than mustards.

Of the vesicants, mustards bind to cellular glutathione, a peptide that is a major free radical scavenger. This leads to the depletion of glutathione and to a cascade of dire intracellular events such as: the inactivation of enzymes, the loss of calcium homeostasis, lipid rancidity, cellular breakdown, and cell death. Mustards can also evoke a decrease in the numbers of certain white blood cells and immune proteins.

Symptoms

After exposure, mustards may take hours before their effects are noticed. This delay increases the danger, as the victim may remain in the area with contaminated clothing on, which will increase the level of exposure. The non-mustard compounds react with the tissue more quickly. Environmental temperature, body sweat, wet skin, and individual sensitivity to the chemical are additional factors that contribute to the severity of symptoms. In general, exposure to liquid or vaporized vesicants produces the following symptoms:

Eyes: (The vesicant may be transferred from the hands when rubbing the eyes.)
- Pain
- Bloodshot eyes
- Swelling
- Lesions (with severe exposure of 1-3 hours)
- Temporary blindness (with severe exposure)

- Permanent blindness is very rare.

Skin:
With mild exposure:
- Skin irritation
- Redness

Itching, which may be intense with higher exposure:
- Burns (deeper when produced by Lewisite)
- Blisters, which are not painful (except with Lewisite), but feel tight and uncomfortable
- Note: **Phosgene oxime** does not cause blistering even though it is corrosive to the skin and mucous membranes
- Most sensitive areas are: face, armpits, genitalia, neck, skin between fingers, and the nail beds
- Blisters are full of a clear slightly-yellow liquid
- Blisters are delicate and may be ruptured by contact with bandages, linen, bed surface, etc.
- Blisters eventually slough off and give way to a suppurating necrotic wound that may be susceptible to infection
- Fluid from blisters does not create more blisters
- Deep burns and loss of entire skin (more likely to occur on the penis and scrotum).
- Regeneration of tissue is slow (weeks to months)
- Future scarring and fragile skin are possible.

Respiratory Tract:
- Nasal discharge
- Burning pain in throat and hoarseness of voice
- Dry cough (possibly painful) followed by copious expectorations
- Throat spasms
- Difficulty breathing
- Infection of lower airways is likely, which can lead to bronchial pneumonia in about 2 days

- If dose has been exceedingly high, the person may die in few days from pulmonary complications, bacterial infections, and impaired immune response

Gastrointestinal Tract:
- Nausea
- Vomiting (may be blood stained)
- Pain
- Diarrhea (may be blood stained)
- Anorexia
- Exhaustion

General Symptoms (Regardless of the Route of Exposure):
- Headache
- Nausea
- Vomiting
- Gastrointestinal pain
- Convulsions (with high exposure)
- Unconsciousness (with high exposure)
- Heart irregularities
- Heart failure (possible)

Agent Characteristics as a Weapon
Estimated Level of Attraction
Low 1-2-3-4-5 High

- Availability of information about the agent. **5**
- Ease of performing research, and manipulating agent. **5**
- Ease of manufacture with minimal danger. **5**
- Availability of the ingredients. **5**
- Low cost. **5**
- Easy to store/house. **5**
- Durability of agent. **5**
- Difficulty for being detected. **2-3**
- Has a quick rate of action/incubation time. **5**
- Ease of transport. **5**
- Ease of delivery by various methods. **3-4**
- Ability to inflict widespread harm/death. **1-2**
- Treatable. **4**

Assessment

The use of blister agents by terrorists would most likely be a localized target, depending on the extent of dispersion. The vaporized form would be particularly attractive. Consequently, Sulphur mustard (HD) would be favored, followed by phosgene oxime and Lewisite. Phosgene oxime is a severe, potentially lethal irritant to the respiratory system in low concentrations. Lewisite presents immediate systemic problems since it is a form of arsine. Being easy to manufacture, vesicants are a common component in countries with chemical weapons.

Vesicants can penetrate not only cell membranes but also a great number of materials such as wood, leather, untreated rubber, plants, etc. They can be manipulated to be extremely persistent in cold and temperate climates, rendering them difficult to remove by decontaminating procedures. The localization of potential incidents, the low lethality factor, and the increased sophistication with chemical detection would, in my opinion render these agents as a **3** level of attraction.

Detection

Diagnostic Tests: There is currently no effective medical test to determine if one has been exposed to vesicants.

Field Detection: Most of these agents can be identified as having a faint odor of mustard, onion, garlic or horseradish. However, this is not a reliable indicator. Once launched, it may take hours before their effects are noticed (except for Lewisite and phosgene oxime).

The <u>SAW MINICAD mk II</u>, is a small portable chemical agent detector that will alert of the presence of trace levels of blister/vesicants in the environment. <u>Dräger</u> has developed chemical detection systems for all (over 1000) chemical WMD.

Conventional Methods of
Care and Treatment

Prehospital Emergency Care: Protection from these agents can be achieved only with full protective gear. The respirator mask protects against eye and lung damage. To protect from skin contact a **rubber chemical suit is required**. The eyes, skin, and lungs are the most vulnerable organs.

The site of exposure may remain contaminated for days or even weeks, and therefore one must abandon the area until it has been decontaminated. Time is of the essence to reduce the harmful effects, which can take place within minutes. Victims must be removed as soon as possible into fresh air, and clothing needs to be removed. **Ordinary clothing provides little or no protection against these agents.**

If eyes are affected, they must be decontaminated with uncontaminated water. A low-pressure source of water such as from a hose or from a container is suitable.

Mustards must not be removed off the skin with plain water because this spreads the reaction. Water may only be used on the eyes.[171] Certain chemical absorbing powders (e.g., Fuller's earth) or a chemical decontamination kit are used to remove the vesicant. "In the case of thickened mustard, where the usual procedure is inadequate, the agent may be scraped off with a knife or similar hard object.

This may be followed by wetting the surface with a cloth drenched in an organic solvent, e.g., petrol (**unleaded gasoline**) and subsequent application of the usual decontaminating procedure. If water is available in abundant amounts these procedures should be followed by copious washing."[172]

Note: chlorination is ineffective against phosgene oxime; alkalis[173] are best.

Medical Care focuses on the eyes, skin, respiratory system, and gastrointestinal system. Generally, metabolic status is watched and maintained with oxygen, fluid and electrolyte replacement.

Eyes: For painful eyes, local analgesics are avoided, for they can produce damage to the cornea. Instead, systemic analgesics (narcotics) are favored.

Antibacterial preparations are applied to avert secondary infections and scarring of the cornea.

Sterile saline solutions are used for excessive secretions. Sterile petroleum jelly is applied under the eyelids to prevent sticking. Eyelids may be forced open to show patients they are not blind. Bandages are avoided since they produce ocular pressure. Instead, dark or opaque goggles are used. The application of citrate, vitamin C eye drops, and topical steroids may be used.

Skin: More extensive decontamination follows. Vesicants may be transported into wounds by pieces of clothing. These wounds should be examined using a non-touch technique to extract any fragments. The removed cloth should be placed in a bleach solution to remove the mustard vapor **hazard of secondary gases**.

Wounds are irrigated using a solution containing 3000-5000 ppm (parts per million) of free chlorine (dilute solution) for approximately 2 minutes, then irrigated with saline solution. Such irrigation should not be performed when situated on the abdominal or thoracic cavities, nor with intracranial head injuries. Serious wounds are dressed.

Calamine lotion or *corticosteroids* in solution or even water are used to relieve itching. Ointments and creams are avoided due to possible infection.

Skin infection is an important problem. The formed roof on blisters may or may not be removed (depending on the physician) to decrease secondary infection. Antibiotics may be used. Sepsis from mustard lesions is surprisingly low.

Respiratory System: Mild exposure and injury usually require no treatment. *Codeine* may be used for cough. Inflammation of the upper respiratory tract may be relieved with inhalation of warm vapor or a nebulized cool mist. For severe injuries with bacterial pneumonia appropriate antibiotic therapy is used.

---

[171] Emergency Medicine: Part III, Chapter 3, Vesicant (Blister Agents). Derived from the Internet. (P. 3.)
[172] Emergency Medicine (cited above. P. 3.)
[173] Alkali are base substances such as found in soap.

Prophylaxis: There are currently no drugs to prevent the effects of vesicants on the skin and mucous membranes.

Antidote: There are no specific antidotes for mustards. With **Lewisite**, the antidote is *dimercaprol* to displace the arsenic bound to enzymes. *Dimercaprol* eye ointment may be effective if applied within 20 minutes of exposure. It is used on the skin, after any other lotion has been cleared off, to chelate the harmful chemicals. (*Dimercaprol* is chemically incompatible with *silver sulphadiazine*.)

Supportive Lines of Natural Defense

Use the **Basic Supportive Program** (found on page 89) for your plan of action. Also, consider the following important points about Blister/Vesicants that may be useful:

Because of the rapid onset of symptoms with this disease it is important to keep a level mind while taking care of yourself and seeking medical help. If the condition presents with intestinal complications it may not be possible to take things orally. Detection in the field is crucial for survival. Also, the amount of exposure must be taken into consideration, for many would survive when not too close to the point of release.

Psychological Line:
- Psychological preparation is important.
- Remember, this disease is not contagious. However, in helping others, care needs to be exercised because vesicants linger at the site of exposure and on the victims.
- Source of oxygen can be life saving.
- With blister/vesicants there are common fears associated with the physiological effects
- Fear of death, though **recovery is often the case**.
- Fear of blindness, **though blindness is rare**.

Social Line:
- Portable Emergency Gas Mask would be useful for protecting eyes and respiratory system from exposure to vesicants. In the event that Lewisite is used, its immediate harsh effect on the lungs would be a signal to don a mask to significantly reduce exposure. **However,** vesicants can penetrate the material of a mask, unless it is made of vesicant-proof materials.
- Ordinary clothing does not protect against these agents; only certain NBC (nuclear, biological, chemical) suits designed for this purpose would.
- Ideally, a **full gas mask** (covering eyes, nose, and mouth), and **gloves** should be worn when decontaminating a victim. There's a possibility of secondary toxic gases being released from wounds in which might have contaminated clothing and/or debris in them.

- **Important:** (1) a source of decontaminated water to wash eyes (e.g., bottled water; remember, **don't use plain water on the skin since it will spread the reaction**), (2) sprinkle an absorbent powder, like a 1 lb bag Chickpea Flour (to increase absorption mix in 1 cup of Activated Charcoal) per person, to help draw the chemical off the skin, (3) use a plastic or wooden tongue depressor to scrape off the surface vesicant (or similar object such as the back of a plastic knife, etc.

- After decontaminating the eyes, consider using swim goggles with children to isolate the eyes from being inadvertently touched while decontaminating the skin.

- **Also:** "Talcum powder and/or flour are excellent means of decontamination of liquid agents. Sprinkle the flour (e.g., chickpea or other kind, ideally mixed with activated charcoal, see above) or powder liberally over the affected skin area, wait 30 seconds, and brush off with a rag or gauze pad. (Note: The powder absorbs the agent, so it must be brushed off thoroughly. If available, protective gloves should be used when carrying out this procedure."[174]

- **0.5% Hypochlorite Solution** is used on the skin, **avoiding the eyes**. (Add 1/2 gal of household bleach to 5 gal of water.) Wear rubber gloves, and apply with large sponge or spray bottle. Avoid getting in eyes.

- **5% Hypochlorite Solution** is used to decontaminate all garments and equipment (**except the mask**). (Add 48 ounces of **calcium hypochlorite** powder[175] to 5 gals of water.) Make sure you wear rubber gloves, and **avoid** breathing in the fumes.

- **Rinse off** with copious amounts of water such as from a shower or garden hose.

- Professional decontamination kits are available for vesicants or when the nature of the chemical is unknown. (See Resources.)

Environmental Line:
- Vesicants are not natural compounds; they are not being used in industrial processes.

---

[174] United States Department of State, Bureau of Diplomatic Security. Responding to A Biological or Chemical Threat: A Practical Guide.

[175] Calcium hypochlorite powder is used to purify pools. It has a longer shelf life than liquid bleach, but is very concentrated and potentially toxic if not used correctly.

- The only way they would enter the environment is through accidental (not likely) or intentional release.
- They do not easily go into water, and the amount that does breaks down quickly. Because of this decontamination of an exposed site is very important.
- They are more stable in soil, but break down within days; may take longer during colder weather.
- They do not leach into ground water from the soil. (Phosgene oxime is probably the exception.)
- They do not build up in animal or human tissue, breaking down and being detoxified rather quickly.
- Vesicants are not likely to be used in homes or apartments. However, this should not be discounted.
- Consider the work environment to see where protective measures can be used against aerosol of vesicants. For example, the barring of access to air conditioning ducts, etc. Perhaps, rapid emergency exhaust ventilation to extract vapors out into a neutralizing medium (e.g., absorbent powder) and to reduce concentration.
- Tunnels used for mass transportation are likely targets. Warning system and portable mask would be useful.
- Placing a vesicant agent detector such as the SAW MINICAD mk II in a strategic area to provide warnings, and/or hooking up to exhaust system to turn it on. Dräger has developed gas detection systems for over 1000 noxious chemicals.
- Ideally, decontamination of clothing, objects, and water should be done professionally using special formulas that break down the vesicant molecules safely.

Focus on the Preventative Program:
- Continue with the general nutrient support, and add the following.
- Vitamin C (ascorbate powder, tablets, or capsules) 1000 mg in 1/2 to 1 cup of water every hour to bowel tolerance. Then cut back until stools firm up, and continue with that dose divided over a 24-hour period. The buffered form (calcium ascorbate) is best with disorders that produce diarrhea because pure ascorbate can overly aggravate this condition), use 2,000-5,000 mg every 4 hours. Important detoxifier, for collagen repair, and all-around healing agent.
- MSM (methyl sulfonyl methane) 500 mg for every 30 lbs of weight, divided into equal doses with food, 1-2 times daily. Excellent to support tissue repair.

- Vitamin E (mycelized) 400 IU 3 times daily with food.
- Zinc 50 mg 2 times daily with food (not to exceed 100 mg from combined sources). Important for wound healing. In severe cases could be taken up to 200 mg.
- Vitamin A (mycelized) 5,000 I U 3 times daily (not to exceed 50,000 IU per day, or not more than 10,000 IU if you're pregnant; up to 100,000 may be taken under the supervision of a physician). Can be added to room temperature drinks.

Rehabilitation:
- Continue with the preventative nutrients.
- Focus is also on supporting cell-membrane integrity.
- The inhalation of the mist of Lavender Essential Oil (food grade) 3-6 times daily could have a beneficial effect on the caustic damage to the respiratory system. If possible, consider using a nebulizer* with 4-5 drops of the oil in 1/2 ounce of water. Use eyedropper to fill the cup and breathe in intermittently until the supply is used up.
- Homeopathic physicians might recommend the following:
- Homeopathic Arsenic 7c has been shown to speed up the elimination of toxic doses of arsenic. Boiron Laboratories in France conducted experiments on the action of homeopathic remedies for toxic chemicals. "One involved radioactive traces to study the effect of homeopathic arsenic on the accumulation and elimination of toxic doses of arsenic from poisoned rats. The results indicate that Arsenic 7c does indeed speed up the elimination of toxic does of arsenic."[176] This might be us eful against Lewisite poisoning.
- Homeopathic remedies against mustard compounds also seem promising. "A well controlled trial was conducted during World War II in London and Glasgow where different homeopathic remedies were used in the prevention and treatment of mustard gas burns (Patterson, 1944). A reanalysis of the data using current statistical methods demonstrated the value of homeopathic therapy."[177]
- Lavender Essential Oil (food grade) may be very effective to relieve burns since vesicants are conventionally treated similarly to thermal

---

* May require a physician's prescription to obtain. Check local and federal laws.

[176] Manning, C.; Vanrenen, L., (1988). Bioenergetic Medicines East and West: Acupuncture and Homeopathy. North Atlantic Books: Berkeley, CA. (P. 83.)

[177] Manning, C., Vanrenen, L.. cited above. (P. 84.)

burns. Lavender is famous as a natural remedy for burns. It has anti-inflammatory properties, which help with pain. I would use it periodically as a light topical spray.

- ❑ ASAP Solution® may be sprayed on blisters, its antimicrobial properties may also help with secondary bacterial infection.
- ❑ Breathing exercises such as **Pranayama** will help to restore respiratory health.

Pets:

- ❑ Vesicants pose a special problem on animal's fur. Use the above-mentioned absorbents (if necessary cut off the fur around the affected area), and decontaminate, muzzling the pet so it won't be licked off before rinsing.

- ❑ Since vesicants can endure after adhering to hard surfaces, paws are vulnerable. Decontaminate them to make sure.
- ❑ ASAP Solution®: similar to the adult dosages (perhaps using plastic eyedropper to administer under the tongue). For reducing secondary infections.
- ❑ Consider consulting with a veterinarian that provides homeopathic remedies that may be useful with your type of pet in these situations.
- ❑ Consider giving 1-4 tablets (depending on size) of **Gary Null's** Pet's Health formula 2 times a day for rehabilitation.

BLOOD AGENT: ARSINE

On the CDC list, the chemicals arsine (SA), cyanogen chloride (CK), hydrogen chloride, and hydrogen cyanide (AC) are classified as blood agents. However, only arsine has a dire effect on red blood cells. The others do not. The cyanogens (CK, AC) affect cellular metabolism, and hydrogen chloride is a tissue corrosive. **So here I will address only arsine**. The others will be addressed in separate sections under Cyanogens, and Hydrogen Chloride.

Arsine is a highly toxic, colorless gas with a mild garlic odor. It is soluble in water, and slightly soluble in alcohol and alkalies.[178] When nascent hydrogen is generated in the presence of arsenic, or when water reacts with a metallic arsenide, arsine evolves. The gas is heavier than air and will tend toward the ground and settle in lower places. **It is extremely flammable.**

"Most cases of arsine poisoning have been associated with the use of acids and crude metals, one or both of which contained arsenic as an impurity. Ores contaminated with arsenic can liberate arsine when treated with acid. Arsine is commercially produced for use in organic synthesis and the processing of solid state electronic components."[179]

The majority of reported cases of accidental arsine poisoning occur in industrial settings, especially in the smelting and refining of metals. "However, there are many other situations where exposures to lethal concentrations of the gas have been reported, including galvanizing, soldering, etching, and lead plating operations. Arsine can be produced by fungi (especially in sewage) in the presence of arsenic. The renewed interest in coal as a source of energy causes concern for a possible increase in the number of exposures to arsine, because coal contains considerable quantities of arsenic."[180]

Even though it has been considered for use in the battlefield during the two world wars there is no record of it ever having been used militarily. Other compounds of greater toxicity were found more attractive (such as lewisite). Also, it is **highly flammable** (reacts violently with oxidizing agents such as chlorine, nitric acid, and fluorine) and poses problems in the manufacturing process. Yet it cannot be ignored as a potential terrorist weapon.

---

[178] Alkali are base substances such as found in soap.

[179] US Department of Health and Human Services (DHHS)– National Institute for Occupational Safety and Health (NIOSH) – Publication No. 79-142.

[180] DHHS – NIOSH, cited above.

Mechanism of Action

Inhaled arsine is rapidly distributed throughout the system. It combines with hemoglobin and causes massive red blood cell hemolysis (rupture of red blood cells). This compromises the delivery of oxygen to the tissue, which can lead to widespread lack of oxygen to the cells. Liver and heart complications can occur from the direct effect of arsine on these organs.

With severe exposure, the products emanating from the breakdown of the red blood cells and hemoglobin will clog the kidneys, causing a reduction in the amount of urine formed, sometimes to the point of complete blockage of urine formation. This often leads to kidney failure and death. However, prior to the use of **hemodialysis** as a treatment, arsine poisoning of the kidneys produced 100% fatalities. With hemodialysis, mortality rates do not exceed 25%.

Long-term or repeated exposure can lead to cancer. Arsine may remain in the tissue after a person has recovered, and it would be wise to undergo a period of detoxification.

Symptoms

While the effects of arsine may begin within 30-60 minutes, the initial symptoms may appear 2-24 hours after exposure. Initially:

- Victims may appear well
- Have red staining on the membrane of the eyes
- Produce a garlic odor in the breath
- Lower quality blood agents may create a bitter almond smell or taste. Otherwise they are odorless.
- Develop a headache
- Become thirsty
- May start shivering

As the red blood cells begin to rupture the victim experiences:

- Generalized weakness
- Abdominal pain
- Muscle cramps
- Dizziness
- Difficulty breathing
- Nausea and vomiting may occur

After 4-6 hours after exposure:
- Bloody urine (light to dark red)

After 12-48 hours after exposure:
- Jaundice (yellow discoloration of the skin and whites of the eyes)
- Bronze-like discoloration of the skin may be apparent if the exposure has been severe.

Agent Characteristics as a Weapon
Estimated Level of Attraction
Low 1-2-3-4-5 High

- Availability of information about the agent. **5**
- Ease of performing research, and manipulating agent. **5**
- Ease of manufacture with minimal danger. **2-3**
- Availability of the ingredients. **5**
- Low cost. **5**
- Easy to store/house. **5**
- Durability of agent. **5**
- Difficulty for being detected. **3-4**
- Has a quick rate of action/incubation time. **5**
- Ease of transport. **4-5**
- Ease of delivery by various methods. **3-4**
- Ability to inflict widespread harm/death. **2-3**
- Treatable. **3**

Assessment

Even though arsine has not been favored in the battlefield, it can be placed in small containers for release in highly populated areas. Its volatility will cause it to disperse rather quickly in open areas, but not so in enclosures. Use in ventilated tunnels or moving vehicles will disperse the arsine, thereby reducing the lethal concentration and number of victims. The same would be true for ventilation systems. However, the difficulty and dangers in manufacture and handling, and its low, unpredictable lethality rate contribute to it not being high on the terrorist list of needs. If it were to be used at all it would most likely occur in highly populated enclosures. Therefore, I would estimate it to be in the **2-3** range of attraction.

Detection and Diagnosis

Diagnosis: First signs of ruptured red blood cells can be picked up by the amount of free hemoglobin in the plasma by drawing blood and spinning the hematocrit tube in the centrifuge. Urine dipstick can also be used. Blood arsenic levels can be assessed to confirm the level of toxicity.

Field Detection is possible with the use of a Dräger Civil Defense System unit for 8 chemical substances, which includes blood agents. Building on the Drager Gas Detection Sytems, the new MAXxess systems have a full range of over 1000 noxious chemicals that can be detected.

Conventional Method of Care and Treatment

Prehospital Emergency Care: Full protection would be required for first responders to a site where arsine has been criminally released. Victims would need to be immediately removed from the site of exposure to where there is fresh air and/or are given high flow oxygen. **They must be kept in a half-upright position.**

While the inhaled gas would be the most likely occurrence, contact with the liquid form could produce frostbite and redness to the eyes and the skin. Both must be rinsed with plenty of preferably warm water (hose, shower) for a **maximum of 30 minutes**. Clothing is not removed. Contact lenses are removed after rinsing.

Medical Care: At the hospital or clinic, humidified oxygen support would continue to compensate for the reduction in red blood cells.

Procedures such as the administration of large volumes of IV fluids to increase the flow of urine are employed to prevent kidney failure and hypotension. It is important to alkalinize (using sodium bicarbonate) the urine to avert kidney damage. Low doses of *dopamine* may be used to preserve blood flow to the kidneys.

Hemodialysis would be used in patients with acute renal failure. **Chelating agents** to remove arsine from the system **are avoided** since the focus is on dealing with the hemoly-sis and not the removal of arsine. Blood exchange may be required to replace destroyed red blood cells.

Supportive Lines of Natural Defense

Use the **Basic Supportive Program** (found on page 89) for your plan of action. Also, consider the following important points about Arsine that may be useful:

With arsine, the emphasis initially is less on the specific line than the other lines, especially the social and the environmental supportive lines of defense.

Psychological Line:
- Perform the Relaxation Response (or a comparable form of meditation) 1-2 times daily or as needed to quell fears and develop calmness in the midst of perceived danger. Previous development is an advantage. During an attack one would think of cues such as a word, image, etc., that would elicit the response.

Very Important:
- **Seek medical help.**
- Never give anything by mouth to an **unconscious person**.
- Remember, this condition is not contagious.
- Physical movement or exertion can aggravate the effects of arsine poisoning. While it's important to move away from an exposed site find a place to rest in order not to deplete your available oxygen. (Another important reason to access a calm state of mind.)
- Emergency items that would be most useful with arsine are: (1) Portable Emergency Gas Mask, (2) A portable supply of Oxygen, (3) a Cellular Telephone, (4) Water, (5) Soap.
- As far as I know, there are no verified natural antidotes for arsine poisoning.
- **Arsine is extremely flammable**. Avoid sparks or flames of any kind. Don't turn on electrical devices. Don't spend time turning things off. Exit the site of exposure into fresh air as soon as possible.
- A Portable Emergency Gas Mask should be worn as soon as one suspects or knows of an attack in one's area.

Environmental:
- Because the reaction time of arsine can be quite fast, detection in the field is crucial for survival. Also, the amount of exposure must be taken into consideration, for many would survive if not too close to the point of release.
- Arsine is heavier than air and will settle close to the ground and in low-lying areas. If possible, move up to a higher area.
- Arsine is a gas at room temperature. Therefore, ingestion is not likely.

- ❑ <u>Dräger Detection</u> equipment is available to detect arsine.
- ❑ Detector might be connected to high power exhaust system to draw arsine out into a neutralizing chamber or safe atmosphere. "Most chemical and biological agents that present an inhalation hazard will break down fairly rapidly when exposed to the sun, diluted with water, or dissipated in high winds."[181]

Pets:
- ❑ The faster metabolism of dogs, and especially cats, may make them more vulnerable to the effects of blood agents.
- ❑ Consult with a holistic veterinarian for antidotes and/or homeopathic remedies for pets.
- ❑ Homeopathic animal practitioner might recommend <u>Arsenicum</u>
- ❑ Consider giving 1-4 tablets (depending on size) of **Gary Null's** <u>Pet's Health</u> formula 2 times a day for rehabilitation.

Rehabilitation:
- ❑ Return to the preventative program.
- ❑ Reduce high potassium foods and supplements for about 2 weeks if blood work has shown it to be high during medical treatments. Use diuretic herbs, like in the <u>Thompson</u> formula, to help excrete it.
- ❑ <u>Oral Chelation Formula</u> (by Extreme Health or comparable formula) 3 capsules daily near bedtime, + 3 caplets of <u>Age-Less Formula</u> in the morning with food for adults. Children ages 2-7 use 1/2 of a capsule (can be opened in juice) near bedtime + 1/2 caplet in the morning with food (can be crushed and placed in food). Children ages 8-13 use 1 capsule near bedtime + 2 caplets of <u>Age-Less Formula</u> in the morning with food. Children ages 13 up can take the adult dose.
- ❑ <u>Hair Analysis for Arsenic</u> to monitor lingering traces of the toxin in the tissue.
- ❑ Drink plenty of water. Frequent sips throughout the day are best.
- ❑ <u>Sweat Therapy</u> 2-3 times weekly (afterwards drink electrolyte-rich fluids).
- ❑ Homeopathic physicians might recommend the use of <u>Homeopathic Arsenic 7c</u>, which has been shown to speed up the elimination of toxic doses of arsenic. Boiron Laboratories in France conducted experiments on the action of homeopathic remedies for toxic chemicals. "One involved radioactive traces to study the effect of homeopathic arsenic on the accumulation and elimination of toxic doses of arse-

nic from poisoned rats. The results indicate that Arsenic 7c does indeed speed up the elimination of toxic doses of arsenic."[182]

---

[181] United States Department of State, Bureau of Diplomatic Security. Responding to A Biological or Chemical Threat. A Practical Guide.

[182] Manning, C., Vanrenen, L., previously cited, p. 83.

CHOKING/LUNG/PULMONARY DAMAGING

As the category implies, these agents aim to disrupt the respiratory system and thereby incapacitate and, secondarily, do bodily harm through asphyxiation. In addition to their toxic characteristics, many of these agents were used by the military as "smoke screens" to prevent surveillance of strategic weapons and maneuvers. Pulmonary agents include **phosgene (CG)**, the representative agent of this group, other halogen compounds, and various nitrogen-oxygen compounds. During WWI, phosgene was used in combination with chlorine, another pulmonary agent.

However, these compounds were not deemed suitable for military use. Nevertheless, each agent has certain characteristics that warrant specific attention. While the disruption of the pulmonary system is common to these agents, each may have distinct symptoms upon exposure.

Usually Non-Life Threatening

Sulfur Trioxide-Chlorosulfonic Acid

Sulfur Trioxide-Chlorosulfonic Acid (FS), also known as sulfuric oxide, is a colorless liquid, which can exist as ice, fiberlike crystals, or gas. When atomized into the atmosphere it rapidly absorbs water and forms white fumes and sulfur acid. Because of its unpractical corrosiveness, military use has been discontinued.

Sulfur Trioxide-Chlorosulfonic Acid is so irritating that those who are exposed quickly flee from the source of exposure. They typically complain of:
- Cough
- Aches or soreness just beneath the breastbone (sternum)
- Burning sensation in eyes, nose, mouth, and throat
- Blurry vision and photophobia (inability to tolerate light) may also be reported

If inhaled exposure is severe enough:
- Explosive cough
- Shortness of breath
- There may be complaints of prickling sensation of exposed skin, which could be the prelude to a pending chemical dermatitis
- Usually the victims remain without symptoms for up to 6 hours.

Red Phosphorous

Red Phosphorous (RP) provided an adequate screen for tanks in the battlefield. Upon being inhaled and exposed to water vapor in the respiratory tract, a mixture of phosphorus acids is formed which produces relatively mild irritations to the upper airways. No human deaths have been attributed to exposure to RP. Red Phosphorous exposures produce complaints of:
- Eye, nose, and throat irritation with mild exposure
- Severe exposure can produce an explosive persistent cough
- Most often these symptoms resolve once the individual is removed from the source of exposure
- If the person has had contact with unoxidized phosphorous, they may show patches of redness on the skin, and painful chemical burns

Teflon and Perfluroisobutylene

Teflon and Perflurorisobutylene (PHIB) form a particle mass of fumes that when inhaled causes an extremely rapid toxic effect on pulmonary tissue. Pulmonary edema may result within 5 minutes. Even mild exposure can produce inflammation. Intense exposure can lead to hemorrhagic inflammation of the lungs.

Teflon and Perfluroisobutylene produce clinical complaints that resemble the symptoms of influenza. Approximately 1-4 hours after exposure the person complains of:
- Malaise
- Fever (possibly to 104° F)
- Chills
- Sore throat
- Sweating
- Chest tightness

- These symptoms usually resolve within 24-48 hours after being removed from the source

Perfluroisobutylene

Perflurorisobutylene (PHIB) appears to be the main cause of toxicity in particulates released from Teflon fumes. Even a low amount of the inhaled, ultrafine, particles initiate a severe inflammatory response.
(See Teflon and Perfluroisobutylene for symptoms.)

Titanium Tetrachloride

Titanium Tetrachloride (FM) is a colorless-to-pale yellow liquid that produces white fumes. It is used as military screens and has a strong odor. Contact with water, amongst other compounds, transforms it into hydrochloric acid (an irritating corrosive). When these fumes make contact with the skin, mild and transient irritation occurs which subsides within 24 hours. When mixed with water it can produce deep burns.

"Although several industrial exposures have occurred with FM liquid and smoke, only 1 death has been reported. This was a worker who accidentally was splashed over his entire body with liquid FM. He died from complications resulting from inhalation of FM fumes and overwhelming super infection."[183]

Potentially Life Threatening
Chlorine Gas

Chlorine gas is a greenish-yellow, noncombustible gas at room temperature and atmospheric pressure. Its moderate solubility in water would explain its effect on the moist qualities of mucous membranes of the upper and lower respiratory tract. This affinity would prolong the effects of the inhaled gas for at least several minutes. The density of the gas causes it to settle in lower levels (ground level, basements, etc.). Gas masks offer full protection.

---

[183] Daniel T Smith, MD, Lung-Damaging Agents, Toxic Smokes, p.7.

Chlorine gas exposure has immediate effects such as:
- Acute inflammation of the conjunctiva (membrane of eyes), nose, pharynx, trachea, and bronchi
- Irritation leads to localized edema and pulmonary congestion
- Hypoxia (lack of oxygen to tissue) can occur within minutes or hours, and its persistence can lead to death.

Typical symptoms may vary. Such as:
- Cough
- Shortness of breath
- Chest pain
- Burning sensation in throat area
- Nausea and/or vomiting
- Eye irritation
- Choking
- Muscle weakness
- Dizziness
- Abdominal discomfort
- Headache

Diphosgene

Diphosgene (DP, trichloromethylchloroformate) attacks lung tissue directly, causing pulmonary edema (excessive accumulation of fluid in the lung tissue). As a solution to avert protection by gas masks for soldiers, chlorine was replaced with DP by combining chloroform with phosgene. This combination **destroyed the gas filters**.

It is a colorless gas. In ventilated areas DP rapidly vaporizes into phosgene and chloroform. The chloroform does not reach levels sufficient to cause toxicity even when up close. DP is heavier than air and settles to lower lying areas. However, DP is cumulative because the body can't detoxify it.

Like phosgene, DP is characterized by a delayed pulmonary edema. Doses of 1-10 ppm can cause upper respiratory irritation. Doses greater than 25 ppm can be rapidly fatal. Because DP has a low-water solubility **significant amounts need to be inhaled before symptoms appear.**

Various symptoms can develop:
- Irritation of eyes and skin

- Chest discomfort with low concentrations
- Lacrimation (tears) and irritation of eyes and skin with somewhat higher exposure;

With high exposure:
- Pulmonary edema
- Respiratory failure
- Hypotension
- Death

Nitrogen Oxide

Nitrogen Oxide (NO) forms a nitrite when inhaled, causing a drop in blood pressure and cellular hypoxia (lack of oxygen). Unlike DP, NO **can cause rapid death** (with severe exposure) without the formation of pulmonary edema.

Nitrogen Oxide may produce, with mild exposure, the following symptoms:
- Upper airway and eye irritation, such as itching or burning eyes
- Cough
- Shortness of breath
- Fatigue
- Chest tightness
- Throat tightness
- Nausea
- Vomiting
- Vertigo
- Drowsiness
- Possible loss of consciousness

With severe exposure three phases are typical.
In the first phase:
- Intense respiratory syndrome
- Severe cough
- Shortness of breath
- Rapid onset of pulmonary edema, which could be aggravated by physical exertion
- If patient survives this phase, spontaneous remission occurs within 48-72 hours

Second phase:
- Can last from 2-5 weeks and is relatively uneventful
- A mild residual cough with malaise
- Some lingering shortness of breath

Third phase:
- Symptoms may recur 3-6 weeks after exposure
- More acutely severe exposures can cause immediate death from respiratory spasm or asphyxia.

Phosgene

Phosgene (CG) gas produces a white cloud that, in low concentrations, smells like newly mown hay. In high concentrations, it produces an irritating and somewhat suffocating pungent odor. It can directly damage the lungs. Although it hasn't been deployed militarily since 1918 it continues to be used in industrial processes (e.g., vinyl chloride; fire extinguishers, and during arc welding procedures). Inhalation can cause an inadequate delivery of oxygen to lung tissue, and death.

Phosgene produces the following dose-dependent symptoms:
At low concentrations:
- Red inflamed eyes
- Mild cough
- Shortness of breath

At moderate concentrations:
- Cough
- Wheezing
- Chest discomfort

Runny nose at high concentrations:
- Tearing
- Pulmonary edema within 2-6 hours
- Respiratory spasms, which may cause sudden death
- If victim survives 24-48 hours prognosis is generally favorable

Zinc Oxide

Zinc Oxide (HC) is amongst the most acutely toxic of the military smokes and obscurants, afflicting the upper respiratory tract, where it acts much like a corrosive irritant.

Zinc Oxide mild exposure can cause:
- Nose, throat, and chest irritation
- Cough
- Some nausea

With moderate exposure:

- May show rapid clinical improvement from above symptoms within 6 hours
- 24-36 hours later symptoms may worsen, especially shortness of breath
- All this eventually clears, but significant lung damage may persist **with a low availability of oxygen**

High, prolonged exposure may result in sudden early collapse and death. However, if severe exposure does not prove immediately lethal, the individual may experience:

- Hemorrhagic ulcerations of the upper airway
- Accompanied with severe coughing and bloody secretions
- Followed by death within hours

Agent Characteristics as a Weapon
Estimated Level of Attraction
Low 1-2-3-4-5 High

- Availability of information about the agents. **5**
- Ease of performing research, and manipulating agent. **5**
- Ease of manufacture with minimal danger. **4-5**
- Availability of the ingredients. **5**
- Low cost. **5**
- Easy to store/house. **5**
- Durability of agent. **5**
- Difficulty for being detected. **2-3**
- Has a quick rate of action/incubation time. **5**
- Ease of transport. **4**
- Ease of delivery by various methods. **3**
- Ability to inflict widespread harm or death. **3**
- Treatable. **3-4**

Assessment

The military use, dating back to World War I, aimed at causing death by severely damaging the lungs. Since large concentrations were required to make them effective, they're not generally considered practical in conventional forms of warfare. Blistering and nerve agents have largely replaced many of the pulmonary agents.

Therefore, it's not likely that these would be weapons of choice for terrorists. But because these chemicals (or their constituents) are extensively used in manufacturing processes the plants that house them and the vehicles that transpor them could be targets of sabotage. In

this regard some caution needs to be exercised.

New, very accurate real-time detection devices increase early warning possibilities. Because of the increased vigilance in the chemical industry the likelihood of phosgene being used as a WMD is probably in the **2-3** range of possibility.

Detection

Diagnostic Tests: urine analysis using GCMS (gas chromatography mass spectrophotometry).

Field Detection: Dräger devices are able to detect of all these agents.

Conventional Methods of
Care and Treatment

Emergency: The emergency medical treatment of choice uses phosgene as the representative agent. Full protective equipment is required with these agents.

Initial priority is given to the airway, breathing, and circulation (ABC) status. According to De Lorenzo and Porter, "The other pulmonary agents share similar properties and give similar symptoms. Emergency treatment for all agents in this class is the same."[184]

Accordingly, mild pulmonary agent exp osure manifests with the common mild symptoms of shortness of breath, wheezing, and cough. More severe symptoms involve pulmonary edema, severe shortness of breath, loud harsh breathing, and airway obstruction.

One key point in dealing with these cases is realizing that the initial symptoms may lead to a serious condition within a few hours, especially with exertion. Therefore, **rest is an important component** in the field treatment of these exposures. Exerting oneself by walking and doing other activities is discouraged, unless absolutely necessary.

Mild symptoms require the use of a beta-agonist (*Albuterol*) delivered by a nebulizer using a mouthpiece mask, or through an en-

---

[184] Previously cited, p. 66.

dotracheal tube, oxygen, and rest. The treatment may need to be repeated every twenty minutes up to three times, or every three to four hours during long transports. More severe cases require airway management, and positive pressure ventilation.

Supportive Lines of Natural Defense

Use the **Basic Supportive Program** (found on page 89) for your plan of action. Also, consider the following important points about Lung Damaging Agents that may be useful:

With these agents, the emphasis, initially, is less on the specific line than the other lines, especially the social and the environmental supportive lines of defense.

Psychological Line:

❑ Perform the Relaxation Response (or a comparable form of meditation) 1-2 times daily or as needed to quell fears and develop calmness in the midst of perceived danger. Previous development is an advantage. During an attack one would think of cues such as a word, image, etc., that would elicit the response.

Very Important:

❑ **Seek medical help.**

❑ Never give anything by mouth to an **unconscious person**.

❑ Remember, this condition is not contagious.

❑ Ingestion is not likely.

❑ Antidotes are not available.

❑ An available supply of oxygen could be life saving.

❑ Physical movement or exertion can aggravate the effects of these toxins. While it's important to move away from an exposed site, find a place to rest in order not to deplete your available oxygen.

❑ Important emergency items: (1) Portable Emergency Gas Mask, (2) A portable supply of Oxygen, (3) a Cellular Telephone, (4) Water, (5) Soap.

Homeopathy:

❑ Homeopathic physicians might recommend Arsenicum Album 30C and/or Carbolicum Acidum 30C one dose every 15 minutes, up to six doses, until person stabilizes.[185]

Consult with a homeopathic physician about these and other possibilities.

Preventative Line:

❑ "As with most toxic inhalations, severity of the disease and presentation are related to the concentration of the smoke or fumes, length of time of exposure, manner in which the exposure is delivered, and underlying health of the exposed individual."[186]

❑ Alpha Lipoic Acid has shown promise in experimental models to prevent chemical poisoning.[187] Consider taking 300 mg of sustained release 2-3 times daily between meals at least 30 minutes before food with water.

Environmental:

❑ These chemicals are heavier than air and will settle close to the ground and in low-lying areas. If possible, move up to a higher area.

❑ A Portable Emergency Gas Mask should be worn as soon as one suspects or knows of an attack. Also, use if necessary to traverse a known exposed area.

❑ Dräger equipment is able to detect these agents.

❑ Detector might be connected to high power exhaust system to draw the aerosol out into a neutralizing chamber or safe atmosphere. "Most chemical and biological agents that present an inhalation hazard will break down fairly rapidly when exposed to the sun, diluted with water, or dissipated in high winds."[188]

Pets:

❑ The faster metabolism of dogs, and especially cats, may make them more vulnerable to these agents.

❑ Consult with a holistic veterinarian for antidotes and/or homeopathic remedies for pets.

❑ Consider giving 1-4 tablets (depending on size) of **Gary Null's** Pet's Health formula 2 times a day for rehabilitation.

Rehabilitation:

❑ Consider having Lung Kichadi 2-3 times a week.

❑ Oral Chelation Formula (by Extreme Health or comparable formula) 3 capsules daily near bedtime, + 3 caplets of Age-Less Formula in the morning with food for adults. Children ages 2-7 use 1/2 of a capsule (can be opened in juice) near bedtime + 1/2 caplet in the morning with food (can be crushed and placed in food). Children ages 8-13 use 1 capsule near bedtime + 2 caplets of Age-Less Formula

---

[185] See: Nauman, E.; Derin-Kellog, G. (2000). Homeopathy 911. Kensington Publishing Corp.: New York, NY. (P. 133.)

[186] Smith, (M.D.) D. (June 11, '01). Chemical, Biological, Radiological, Nuclear and Explosive: Lung-damaging Agents, Toxic Smokes. eMedicine Journal: Vol 2, No. 6. (P. 5)

[187] Natural Medicines Comprehensive Data Base, previously cited, p. 41.

[188] United States Department of State, Bureau of Diplomatic Security. Responding to A Biological or Chemical Threat: A Practical Guide.

in the morning with food. Children ages 13 up can take the adult dose.

❑ Clear Lungs (Blue Label) formula would be useful.

Cyanogens

Cyanogen is a very toxic, colorless gas prepared in the laboratory by heating mercury (II) cyanide. It has a pungent biting odor, and it is soluble in water, ethanol, and ether. However, cyanogens **are not combustible**. Cyanogens are cyanide-based chemicals, such as Cyanogen chloride (CK), and hydrogen cyanide (AC). Of the two, CK is widely used by industry in the U.S. in the making of fertilizers, in mining, and in metal work. Therefore, industrial accidents are more likely to produce CK toxicity cases than those from AC. With some minor differences, all cyanogens produce similar toxic mechanisms.

Mechanism of Action

Poisoning can occur by inhaling the vapor, or by ingesting contaminated food or water, or when the liquid is absorbed through the skin. Cyanogens disturb the body's cellular metabolism. When cyanogens enter the body they liberate cyanide molecules into the blood stream, which are distributed to the tissues.

Once inside cells, they bind to the enzyme a3, which disrupts the oxygen processes that take place in the mitochondria (which provide the body's principal source of cellular energy). As a consequence, oxygen is not available to be used for energy. This has a rapid hypoxic effect on organ systems that are very dependent on oxygen supply such as the brain and heart. Because of this, cyanogens, in *high concentrations* (especially the less volatile CK), can have lethal effects within 6-8 minutes, especially when exposure occurs in poorly ventilated enclosures.

Even though the body can excrete small amounts of cyanide, large exposures overwhelm the detoxification process and thereby reduce potential treatment time. All toxins also produce a cascade of free radicals into the system, which further aggravate the detoxification and healing processes.

Symptoms

Symptoms related to cyanide poisoning must take the level of exposure into consideration.

With low doses:
- Pulmonary mucous discharges
- Lacrimation (tears)
- Runny nose

With moderate exposure, onset of symptoms takes several minutes, except for immediate irritant effects.
- Rapid breathing (brief)
- Rapid heart beat
- Feelings of anxiety or apprehension
- Vertigo
- Nausea and/or vomiting

High levels of exposure:
- Loss of consciousness within 30-60 seconds
- Convulsions
- Paused or very slow breathing within 2-3 minutes
- Heart failure within 6-8 minutes

Agent Characteristics as a Weapon
Estimated Level of Attraction
Low 1-2-3-4-5 High

- Availability of information about the agent. **5**
- Ease of performing research, and manipulating agent. **5**
- Ease of manufacture with minimal danger. **2-3**
- Availability of the ingredients. **5**
- Low cost. **5**
- Easy to store/house. **3-4**
- Durability of agent. **5**
- Difficulty for being detected. **4-5**
- Has a quick rate of action/incubation time. **5**
- Ease of transport. **5**
- Ease of delivery by various methods. **5**
- Ability to inflict widespread harm/death. **3-4**
- Treatable. **3-5**

Assessment

Because of the high industrial use of CK, a terrorist act would most likely involve the transport of this chemical in densely populated areas. Because this may take precise knowledge of the transport of these chemicals, and with the current level of vigilance in the industry, I would estimate this agent to have a **2-3** level of attraction.

Detection and Diagnosis

Diagnostic Tests: Levels of cyanide in whole blood samples.

Field Detection: <u>Dräger</u> systems can detect the presence of cyanogens in the environment.

Conventional Methods of Care and Treatment

Emergency Care: Full protection against chemical agents is required for all first-responder personnel. Emergency care with exposure to cyanogens needs to occur as soon as possible. One hundred percent (100%) oxygen needs to be given (endotracheal intubation if available) and respiratory support with a bag-valve mask. Humidified oxygen is better for those with airway irritation. **Immediately after**, antidotal therapy is mandatory.

According to established emergency-care procedures, antidoting using intravenous (IV) is done in two stages:

1. The use of *sodium nitrite*, followed by
2. introduction of *sodium thiosulfate*.

The nitrite converts the hemoglobin in the blood to methemoglobin, which then binds and removes the cyanide from the cytochrome a3. Finally, a nontoxic compound is formed, and excreted in the urine.

These two compounds are available in the **Pasadena (formaly Lilly) Cyanide Antidote Kit** for use with IV. If IV is not available an ampule of *amyl nitrite* is broken for the patient to inhale (it can be crushed into gauze and inhaled or broken and placed under an oxygen mask).

Hyperbaric Oxygen Therapy

Hyperbaric oxygen (HBO) may be considered for patients with cyanide toxicity. Hyperbaric oxygenation involves the use of specially designed chambers that permit the delivery of 100% oxygen (by a professionally trained person) at an atmospheric pressure that is three times the normal level. This causes more oxygen to be absorbed by the blood. HBO has been used to treat cyanide poisoning with some success. While I'm not aware of any extensive human studies, animal studies are encouraging. Ivanov showed in 1959 that HBO restored normal activity of the brain in mice poisoned with cyanide.[189] In 1966, Skene demonstrated a drop in mortality from 96% to 20% in a group of mice treated with HBO.[190]

Supportive Lines of Natural Defense

Use the **Basic Supportive Program** (found on page 89) for your plan of action. Also, consider the following important points about Cyanogens that may be useful:

With these agents, the emphasis (initially) is less on the specific line than the other lines, especially the social and the environmental supportive lines of defense.

Psychological Line:

- Perform the <u>Relaxation Response</u> (or a comparable form of meditation) 1-2 times daily or as needed to quell fears and develop calmness in the midst of perceived danger. Previous development is an advantage. During an attack one would think of cues such as a word, image, etc., that would elicit the response.

Very Important:

- **Seek medical help.**
- Never give anything by mouth to an **unconscious person**.
- <u>Remember, this condition is not contagious</u>.
- <u>Ingestion</u> is not likely.
- **Antidotes are available** but need to be used soon after exposure.

---

[189] Ivanov, K.P: Effect of increasing oxygen pressure on animals poisoned with potassium cyanide. Farmakol. Toksik. 1959: 22:468-479.

[190] Skene, W.G.; Norman, J.N.; Smith G.: Effect of hyperbaric oxygen in cyanide poisoning. Proceedings of the Third International Congress on Hyperbaric Medicine. 1966:705-710.

- An available supply of oxygen could be life saving.
- Physical movement or exertion can aggravate the effects of these toxins. While it's important to move away from an exposed site, find a place to rest in order not to deplete your available oxygen.
- **Important**: (1) Portable Emergency Gas Mask, (2) A portable supply of Oxygen, (3) a Cellular Telephone, (4) Water, (5) Soap. Training by a professional health care provider on how to use the **Pasadena Cyanide Antidote Kit.**

Homeopathy:
- Homeopathic physicians might recommend Arsenicum Album 30C and/or Carbolicum Acidum 30C one dose every 15 minutes, up to six doses, until person stabilizes.[191]

Consult with a homeopathic physician about these and other possibilities.

Preventative Line:
- "As with most toxic inhalations, severity of the disease and presentation are related to the concentration of the smoke or fumes, length of time of exposure, manner in which the exposure is delivered, and underlying health of the exposed individual."[192]
- Alpha Lipoic Acid has shown promise in experimental models to prevent chemical poisoning.[193] Consider taking 300 mg of timed (sustained) release 2-3 times daily between meals at least 30 minutes before food with water.
- Co-Q-10 (coenzyme-Q-10) has a protective effect on the mitochondria.

Environmental:
- These chemicals are heavier than air and will settle close to the ground and in low-lying areas. If possible, move up to a higher area.
- A Portable Emergency Gas Mask should be worn as soon as one suspects or knows of an attack. Also, use if necessary to traverse a known exposed area.
- Dräger equipment is able to detect these agents.
- Detector might be connected to high power exhaust system to draw the aerosol out into a neutralizing chamber or safe atmosphere. "Most chemical and biological agents that present an inhalation hazard will break down fairly rapidly when exposed to the sun, diluted with water, or dissipated in high winds."[194]

Pets:
- The faster metabolism of dogs, and especially cats, may make them more vulnerable to these agents.
- Consult with a holistic veterinarian for antidotes and/or homeopathic remedies for pets.
- Consider giving 1-4 tablets (depending on size) of **Gary Null's** Pet's Health formula 2 times a day for rehabilitation.

Rehabilitation:
- Consider having Lung Kichadi 2-3 times a week.
- Oral Chelation Formula (by Extreme Health or comparable formula) 3 capsules daily near bedtime, + 3 caplets of Age-Less Formula in the morning with food for adults. Children ages 2-7 use 1/2 of a capsule (can be opened in juice) near bedtime + 1/2 caplet in the morning with food (can be crushed and placed in food). Children ages 8-13 use 1 capsule near bedtime + 2 caplets of Age-Less Formula in the morning with food. Children ages 13 up can take the adult dose.
- Clear Lungs (Blue Label) formula would be useful.
- GABA (gamma-aminobutyric acid) to help restore what was lost through exposure. Use 500-1000 mg 1-3 times a day between meals with a 8-10 oz glass of water only.

---

[191] See: Nauman, E.; Derin-Kellog, G. (2000). Homeopathy 911. Kensington Publishing Corp.: New York, NY. (P. 133.)

[192] Smith, (M.D.), D., previously cited, p. 5.

[193] Natural Medicines Comprehensive Database (updated 6-3-02). (P. 41.)

[194] United States Department of State, Bureau of Diplomatic Security. Responding to A Biological or Chemical Threat: A Practical Guide.

Nerve agents are among the deadliest chemical compounds known. They were developed during WWII, yet they were never actually used. They are **liquid** under most weather conditions, but, when aerosolized by an explosion or atomizer, they can be rendered into a vapor **denser than air**. Nerve agents are classified as:

- **GB** (sarin) is colorless with no odor.
- **GD** (soman) is colorless with a fruity or camphor odor.
- **GA** (tabun) is colorless to brownish with a fruity odor of almonds.
- **GF** (characteristics undetermined)
- **VX** is amber colored and odorless.

The **G agents** don't persist in the atmosphere for long and remain dangerous only for hours. The **"V" types** can persist for days and even weeks.

Mechanism of Action

The toxic effects of nerve agents are produced by blocking the action of acetylcholinesterase (AchE), which is responsible for breaking down the neurotransmitter acetylcholine (ACH). The role of ACH is to excite or turn "on" smooth and skeletal muscles via the nerve synapses (gaps between nerves). When ACH is blocked, the muscles over-activate, for it is AchE that turns them "off."

The net effect on muscles in a perpetually activated state is at first uncontrolled and un-coordinated contraction of the fibers. In a matter of minutes, the muscles become fa-tigued and stop working. Death from respiratory muscle failure is the typical result.

Symptoms

Nerve agents can enter through the skin, lungs, mouth, and eyes. They **rapidly penetrate** the skin and all surface mucous membranes. Depending on the amount of exposure, nerve agents produce any or all of the following symptoms within 30 minutes to 18 hours:

- A runny nose
- Chest tightness
- Pinpoint pupils (miosis)
- Nausea
- Vomiting
- Diarrhea
- Altered vision
- Difficult breathing
- Drooling
- Profuse sweating
- Cramps
- Involuntary release of saliva, tears, stomach contents, urine, and feces.
- Muscle twitches and spasms
- Flaccid paralysis
- Coma

It's very likely that an aerosol attack would not only enter through the lungs but also land on the skin. Very small droplets can cause symptoms.

Agent Characteristics as a Weapon
Estimated Level of Attraction
Low 1-2-3-4-5 High

- Availability of information about the agent. **5**
- Ease of performing research, and manipulating agent. **5**
- Ease of manufacture with minimal danger. **3-4**
- Availability of the ingredients. **5**
- Low cost. **5**
- Easy to store/house. **5**
- Durability of agent. **5**
- Difficulty for being detected. **3-4**
- Has a quick rate of action/incubation time. **5**
- Ease of transport. **5**
- Ease of delivery by various methods. **3-5**
- Ability to inflict widespread harm/death. **3-4**
- Treatable. **3-4**

Assessment

The technology used to manufacture nerve agents is not very complex, and many rogue nations have this capability. Because of their lethality and ease of manufacture they would be attractive to terrorists. Like most other chemical WMD, they would be stored in munitions (shells, rockets, and bombs), but they could also be stored in a canister and made into a crude bomb by attaching an explosive device. The liquid and the vapor are harmful.

An event would be localized, such as in a highly populated building or a subway. The effect would not be wide spread, and those not near the release would most likely survive. However, because of the lethality factor it would cause much fear. Nevertheless, the attractiveness to terrorists may very well be in the **3-4** range.

Detection

Diagnostic Tests: Because of the rapid onset of the agent, symptoms and assessment of the site of exposure are used diagnostically.

Field Detection: Dräger equipment is available to detect nerve agents.

Conventional Methods of Care and Treatment

Emergency Care: Full protective gear is required by first responders.
Victims:
- Are immediately moved to fresh air
- Are monitored for respiratory distress
- May have clothing, and jewelry, contact lenses, etc., removed (with skin exposure)
- If affected, eyes are irrigated with copious amounts of **0.9% saline solution** or **plain water** (room temperature) for 15 minutes
- Are decontaminated several times with **0.05% Hypochlorite Solution** followed by copious rinse with water
- Or, **Skin Decontaminating Kit** (consisting of pads impregnated with *Ambergard 555* ion-exchange resin and activated charcoal) is rubbed over affected skin, and discarded
- Are then given two antidotes: *Atropine*, and *Pralidoxime*.

Atropine works by blocking the action of excess ACH (acetylcholine) in the receptor sites. **Pralidoxime** works by breaking the bond between the nerve agent and AchE (acetylcholinesterase). Pralidoxime **only works** if the bond has not become permanent, which could occur over a period of minutes to hours.[195]

Administration of **atropine** is **done first**:
- Intravenously (IV), intramuscularly (in the outer thigh muscle or buttock, right through clothing if necessary), or if necessary, the endotracheal route is acceptable.
- With early symptoms, **self administered** (if trained to do so), if emergency help is not available.[196]
- In measured increments[197]

Administration of **pralidoxime** follows in the same manner.

Without medical treatment, the heart rate drops and breathing stops, resulting in death.

Supportive Lines of Natural Defense

Use the **Basic Supportive Program** (found on page 89) for your plan of action. Also, consider the following important points about Nerve Agents that may be useful:

With these agents, the emphasis, initially, is less on the specific line than the other lines, especially the social and the environmental supportive lines of defense.

Psychological Line:
- ❏ Perform the Relaxation Response (or a comparable form of meditation) 1-2 times daily or as needed to quell fears and develop calmness in the midst of perceived danger. Previous development is an advantage. During an attack one would think of cues such as a word, image, etc., that would elicit the response.

Very Important:
- ❏ **Seek medical help.**
- ❏ Never give anything by mouth to an **unconscious person.**

---

[195] Some nerve agents are said to "age,, within minutes to hours and become resistant to the effects of pralidoxime.

[196] One must be trained by a qualified health care professional to do this.

[197] For dosages see: PDR Guide to Biological and Chemical Warfare Response, by Thomson/Physicians' Desk Reference.

- ❑ Antidotes are available but need to be used soon after exposure.
- ❑ Remember, this condition is not contagious.
- ❑ The steps mentioned above in the Conventional Methods of Protection and Treatment are essential for survival.
- ❑ Training in the use of these antidotes would be advantageous.

Emergency Items:
- ❑ Emergency items: (1) Portable Emergency Gas Mask, (2) full protective gear, (3) A portable supply of Oxygen, (4) a Cellular Telephone, (5) Water, (6) Soap.

Preventative Line:
- ❑ "As with most toxic inhalations, severity of the disease and presentation are related to the concentration of the smoke or fumes, length of time of exposure, manner in which the exposure is delivered, and underlying health of the exposed individual."[198]
- ❑ Alpha Lipoic Acid has shown promise in experimental models to prevent chemical poisoning.[199] Consider taking 300 mg of timed (sustained) release 2-3 times daily between meals at least 30 minutes before food with water.

Environmental Line:
- ❑ These chemicals are heavier than air and will settle close to the ground and in low-lying areas. If possible, move up to a higher area.
- ❑ These agents are not flammable.
- ❑ A Portable Emergency Gas Mask should be worn as soon as one suspects or knows of an attack. Also, use if necessary to traverse a known exposed area.
- ❑ Nerve agents can penetrate though the lungs, skin, mouth and eyes. Therefore, full protective gear is required (not allowing skin to be exposed).
- ❑ Dräger Detection equipment is available to detect nerve agents.
- ❑ Detector might be connected to high power exhaust system to draw the aerosol out into a neutralizing chamber or safe atmosphere. "Most chemical and biological agents that present an inhalation hazard will break down

fairly rapidly when exposed to the sun, diluted with water, or dissipated in high winds."[200]

Specific Line:
- ❑ As far as I know, there are no verified natural antidotes for nerve agents.
- ❑ **Avoid** using the herbal extract **Huperzine A** (and products that contain it) since it's an AchE (acetylcholinesterase) inhibitor.
- ❑ **Homeopathic physicians might recommend Arsenicum Album 30C and/or Carbolicum Acidum 30C one dose every 15 minutes, up to six doses, until person stabilizes.[201]**
- ❑ Seek advice from a homeopathic physician.

Pets:
- ❑ The faster metabolism of dogs, and especially cats, makes them very vulnerable to nerve agents.
- ❑ Consult with a holistic veterinarian for antidotes and/or homeopathic remedies for pets.
- ❑ Consider giving 1-4 tablets (depending on size) of **Gary Null's** Pet's Health formula 2 times a day.

Rehabilitation:
- ❑ Consider having Lung Kichadi 2-3 times a week.
- ❑ Oral Chelation Formula (by Extreme Health or comparable formula) 3 capsules daily near bedtime, + 3 caplets of Age-Less Formula in the morning with food for adults. Children ages 2-7 use 1/2 of a capsule (can be opened in juice) near bedtime + 1/2 caplet in the morning with food (can be crushed and placed in food). Children ages 8-13 use 1 capsule near bedtime + 2 caplets of Age-Less Formula in the morning with food. Children ages 13 up can take the adult dose.

---

[198] Smith, D. MD. eMedicine Journal, June 11, '01, Vol. 2, No. 6. Chemical, Biological, Radiological, Nuclear and Explosive: Lung-damaging Agents, Toxic Smokes. (P. 5)
[199] Natural Medicines Comprehensive Database, previously cited, p. 41.

[200] United States Department of State, Bureau of Diplomatic Security. Responding to A Biological or Chemical Threat: A Practical Guide.
[201] See: Nauman, E.; Derin-Kellog, G. (2000). Homeopathy 911. Kensington Publishing Corp.: New York, NY. (P. 133.)

VOMITING AGENTS

Vomiting agents were used during World War I with the primary goal of getting enemy troops to remove their protective masks and make them vulnerable to other toxic chemicals. They can also be used to help control riots. While there are reports that these agents were used in various countries to suppress rioting, there is no documented evidence of its occurrence. In the United States, vomiting agents have never been used against civilians. The method of delivery would be the aerosol route.

The following chemicals are classified as vomiting agents:

- **Diphenylchlorasine** (DA)
- **Diphenylcyanoarsine** (DC)
- **Diphenylaminearsine** (DM, Adamsite)

Mechanism of Action

The primary route of exposure would be the respiratory system. However, exposure can also occur by ingestion and/or absorption through the skin. These agents work as irritants to the mucous membranes of the eyes, respiratory system, and the gastrointestinal system. On initial exposure, vomiting agents are irritants. This irritation is delayed for several minutes after contact. Systemic signs and symptoms subsequently follow the initial irritation, which persist for several hours afterwards. Pre-existing health status can affect the intensity of the exposure.

Symptoms

Symptoms vary with amount of exposure. Even though these agents aim to incapacitate, high levels of exposure **can be lethal**. Typical clinical symptoms are:

- Eyes: reddening of the eyes, tearing (lachrymation), involuntary contraction of the eye lids
- Nose: excessive nasal discharge, sneezing, swelling of the mucous membranes, and edema
- Throat: swelling of the mucous membranes, and edema
- Lungs: excessive coughing, wheezing, extended expiratory phases, and fast breathing
- Heart: fast heart beat
- Abdomen: hyperactive bowel sounds, intestinal cramps, vomiting, and diarrhea

- Skin: redness and edema at the site of contact
- Mental: depression of central nervous system, brief lapses of consciousness (due to lack of oxygen), and possible death (with significant exposure)

Agent Characteristics as a Weapon
Estimated Level of Attraction
Low 1-2-3-4-5 High

- Availability of information about the agent. **5**
- Ease of performing research, and manipulating agent. **5**
- Ease of manufacture with minimal danger. **5**
- Availability of the ingredients. **5**
- Low cost. **5**
- Easy to store/house. **5**
- Durability of agent. **5**
- Difficulty for being detected. **3-4**
- Has a quick rate of action/incubation time. **5**
- Ease of transport. **5**
- Ease of delivery by various methods. **2-3**
- Ability to inflict widespread harm or death. **1**
- Treatable. **1**

Assessment

While many of the signs point to the likelihood that vomiting agents would be attractive to terrorists, the all-important lethality factor is missing. Therefore, it's not likely that terrorists would be attracted to vomiting agents except to incapacitate or get people with protective masks to take them off. However, this would need to be a highly coordinated effort. With the current scenario, these agents could possibly be used to create confusion and panic, since during the early phases of an emergency response the toxin's identification would be unknown and the information could be misleading and inaccurate. However, the likelihood of using them is probably within the **1-2** range of attraction.

Detection

Diagnostic Tests: presence of the chemical in urine using GCMS (gas chromatography mass spectrophotometry).

Field Detection: Dräger systems would be capable of detecting vomiting agents in the field.

Conventional Methods of Care and Treatment

Emergency Care: First responders would have full protection. No antidotes are available. Medical emergency personnel would provide supportive care and focus on relieving irritant and systemic effects.

Medical Care: Medication would involve the use of antiemetics (to relieve nausea and vomiting) such as *Prochlorperazine* (Compazine), *Promethazine* (Phenergan), *Droperidol* (Inapsine), *Metoclopramide* (Reglan, Clopra, Maxolon). These are blockers of **dopamine activity**.

If these drugs are not effective, 5-HT3 receptor antagonists would be used to block **seratonin activity**. This category of drugs would include: Ondansetron (Zofran), Dolasetron (Anzemet), and Granisetron (Kytril).

Bronchodilators would be used such as Albuterol (possibly delivered via nebulizer). For cases with eye exposure the drug *Cyclopentolate* (Cyclogyl, AK-Pentolate) might be chosen to help relax the muscles of the eye.

Most patients recover within the first few hours and suffer no further toxicity. Complications such as with corneal burns, acute bronchospasm, or brain injury need more extensive hospital care.

Supportive Lines of Natural Defense

Use the **Basic Supportive Program** (found on page 89) for your plan of action. Also, consider the following important points about Vomiting Agents that may be useful:

While vomiting agents do not usually pose a serious health risk, they do have psychological consequences when the nature of the chemicals involved are unknown. Therefore, the psychological, social, and rehabilitative lines might be more emphasized in this instance.

Psychological Line:
- ❑ Perform the Relaxation Response (or a comparable form of meditation) 1-2 times daily or as needed to quell fears and develop calmness in the midst of perceived danger. During an attack, it would be advised to think of the cue word, thought, or image that would elicit the Relaxation Response. Previous development is an advantage. The following preparatory suggestions might be helpful.
- ❑ **With exposure, avoid** the use of substances that increase the level of **seratonin**. These would include: 5-HTP (5-hydroxytryptophan), SAMe, and St. Johns Wort. Also, substances that increase the level of **dopamine**, such as Velvet Bean.

Very Important:
- ❑ Never give anything by mouth to an unconscious person.
- ❑ Remember, this condition is not contagious.
- ❑ No Antidotes are available.
- ❑ Exposure can also occur by ingestion and/or absorption through the skin.
- ❑ Emergency items: (1) Portable Emergency Gas Mask, (2) A portable supply of Oxygen, (3) Clothing to cover as much of exposed skin area as possible (4) a Cellular Telephone, (5) Water, (6) Soap.

Important to Remember:
- ❑ Release of vomiting agents outdoors is not likely, for they will dissipate in the atmosphere. If such is the case, move away from the cloud towards fresh air.
- ❑ Release in a building, perhaps the air system, is more likely. Quickly don Portable Emergency Gas Mask, and leave the building into fresh air.
- ❑ A Portable Emergency Gas Mask should be worn as soon as one suspects or knows of an attack. Also, use if necessary to traverse a known exposed area.
- ❑ These agents are not flammable.

Detection:

- ❏ Dräger detection equipment is capable of alerting one to the release of these agents in the environment.
- ❏ Detector might be connected to high power exhaust system to draw the aersol out into a neutralizing chamber or safe atmosphere. "Most chemical and biological agents that present an inhalation hazard will break down fairly rapidly when exposed to the sun, diluted with water, or dissipated in high winds."[202]

Specific Line:

- ❏ Drink 1-3 cups daily of fresh Ginger Tea. Helps with nausea and vomiting. Or, add 30 drops of tincture of ginger into 4 oz of warm water and drink 1-3 times a day until symptoms clear. Any form of ginger would be immediately helpful.
- ❏ Soft sweetened ginger candy or pellets can be given to children if the tea is not accepted.
- ❏ Drink electrolyte-rich fluids (e.g., squeeze juice of 1/4-1/2 lemon into glass of room temperature water, with a pinch of salt) to replace electrolytes (sodium, potassium, calcium) lost in the vomitus.

Homeopathy:

- ❏ Homeopathic physicians might recommend Arsenicum for severe nausea, vomiting, and abdominal pain.

Pets:

- ❏ Follow similar procedures for humans to physically protect against the fumes of vomiting agents.
- ❏ Prepare in advance and have ready a Ginger Glycerite formula for dogs and cats to alleviate vomiting. "Loosely fill a pint jar with coarsely chopped fresh ginger root. Fill the jar to the top with vegetable glycerine, which is available in some health food stores. Leave the jar in a warm room for six weeks or longer, shaking it every few days. Glycerine has a sweet taste and viscous consistency that most dogs and many cats find palatable."[203] **Dose:** about 1/2 tsp per 20 pounds of body weight on empty stomach. Can be mixed in favorite food, if necessary. Might be more palatable to finicky cats if mixed with some Valerian Root.
- ❏ Consider giving 1-4 tablets (depending on size) of **Gary Null's** Pet's Health formula 2 times a day for rehabilitation.

Rehabilitation:

- ❏ Continue with the preventative program.
- ❏ For lingering lung congestion, consider using the Chinese formula Clear Lungs (Blue Label) or Oregacyn 1-3 times a day.

---

[202] United States Department of State, Bureau of Diplomatic Security. Responding to A Biological or Chemical Threat: A Practical Guide.

[203] Puotinen, C J, previously cited, p. 151.

NUCLEAR WEAPONS

Nuclear threats involve: the **detonation** of a nuclear bomb, varying in size and level of energy, and the **dispersion** of radioactive materials (such as from a device like the "dirty bomb") or due to the explosive impact of a nuclear reactor or containers used to transport nuclear waste materials. Each kind of threat poses similar yet different kinds of hazards.

Mechanisms of Action

Energy

Energy is released when the bonds holding elements together are broken or rearranged. The breaking of strong bonds releases more energy than weaker ones. Molecular bonds are weaker than those of the atom. The atomic bonds are weaker than those of the nucleus (protons, neutrons, etc.).

The Release of Energy From Regular Explosives

Regular explosions are caused by breaking or changing the chemical bonds of certain molecules, producing a kinetic form of energy experienced as heat.

Energy Released From Nuclear Bonds

Nuclear energy is generated when the bonds inside the center of the atom (the nucleus) are broken and rearranged. Because nuclear bonds are much stronger than chemical bonds they release much more energy when broken. As a result, two kinds of nuclear reactions can be produced: *fission* and *fusion*.

Fission

Fission reactions are produced when a large unstable nucleus is broken into many smaller and somewhat more stable nuclei, producing a chain reaction. This reaction was the basis of the nuclear weapons of World War Two, and is used to generate power.

Fusion

On the other hand, fusion is the process where smaller atoms are fused into heavier ones. Fusion generates much more energy than fission but requires tremendous levels of heat to set off a chain reaction. This is a very unstable reaction. While scientists have not been able to control this reaction for producing usable domestic energy, it can be created for destructive purposes, considering that fusion is much more powerful than fission.

Unlike fission reactions, detonation of a fusion device additionally creates an **electromagnetic burst or pulse** that does not directly affect humans but can wreak havoc on all kinds of electrical equipment (telephones, radio/TV transmission, motors, computers, etc.).

Radiological Dispersion

Radiological dispersion is produced when a less-than-nuclear kind of explosion causes radioactive material to be dispersed into the environment. Technically, the so-called "dirty bomb" is a radiological dispersion device. It would be made of radioactive waste by-products from nuclear reactors (or other sources) wrapped in conventional explosives. When exploded, it would not cause a chain reaction, but would spew the harmful radioactive particles into the atmosphere.

An attack on a nuclear power plant by a military missile or a large commercial jet could produce the effects of a huge radiological bomb. In such a scenario, the explosive impact on the plant would have the potential to spread the contained radioactive material into the environment.

An explosive would also need to be employed to destroy containers carrying radioactive materials in order to release them into the environment. However, in this case, it would involve a moving target.

Effects

In any case, injury and death can be caused by any or all of the following: direct radiation, blast effects, thermal burns, and radioactive fallout.

Radiation

Radiation is a general term to describe the process by which any form of energy is propagated through space and matter. There are different kinds of radiation produced by high-energy particles-or-rays[204] that emerge from a nuclear reaction. Radiation causes damage to living organisms when it *ionizes* or changes the electron structure of the atoms that comprise its cells. This is known as *ionizing radiation.*

- **Alpha** is a relatively weak particle/ray that can traverse only inches of air, and is stopped by clothing and the surface of the skin. It is a product of fallout, and when inhaled or ingested can cause serious harm.

- **Beta** radiation is a low-speed and a low-energy particle/ray, with a minimal capacity to penetrate air, clothing, and the skin. A thin sheet of aluminum is able to completely block beta radiation. However, beta is faster and can penetrate deeper than alpha particles. It is a common product of fallout decay, which can be a serious hazard to anyone who inhales contaminated air or ingests contaminated water or food. With prolonged exposure, beta radiation can also cause the skin and mucous membranes of the eyes to burn.

- **Gamma** rays (waves) are the most powerful and damaging since they can travel up to a mile in open air and are capable of penetrating all but the most dense of materials. X-ray and *gamma* radiation are similar in nature but occur through different processes.

- **Neutron** radiation is also a very powerful and damaging particle. However, since it rarely extends beyond the site of the nuclear reaction, its greatest threat is within that region.

- **Radioactive iodine 131** (Radioiodine) is also a major constituent of both nuclear bomb explosion and the dispersion of radioactive materials. It can be carried by wind for hundreds of miles. Radioiodine targets the thyroid gland, which can lead to cancer.

With detonation, injury from direct radiation occurs briefly, for a minute or so after the blast, and, later on, from fallout of radioactive material. Therefore, serious injury from direct radiation is limited. Most of the injury and mortality comes from the blast and thermal effects.

This is true for most large nuclear weapons, but not so for weapons based on radiological dispersion, like the "dirty bomb", where the effects of radiation are greater than those of the blast and thermal burn.

Also, **gamma** radiation poses the most danger from the release of radioactive material emanating from the sabotage of a nuclear reactor (or radioactive material being transported).

"While these exposures are not as intense as the radiation exposure associated with an uncontrolled chain reaction, they can result in severe and life-threatening injury to persons **near the source** of radiation."[205]

Fallout

The explosive force of a 5-megaton bomb, for instance, may produce a crater of up to 1 mile wide with a depth of 100 feet. Millions of tons of pulverized matter are drawn up into the fireball. This material is rendered radioactive, carried by the wind, and eventually falls back into the environment. This is known as fallout.

While all nuclear explosions produce fallout, more fallout debris occurs when the detonation is closer to the ground. This fall-

---

[204] Alpha and beta radiation can manifest either as particles or as rays (consisting of waves). However, gamma radiation consists only of electromagnetic waves of extremely short wavelength.

[205] De Lorenzo, R.; Porter, R., previously cited, p. 87. (Emphasis mine.)

out can be life threatening at considerable distances from the epicenter of the explosion.

Weather conditions strongly influence the spread of the fallout. Rainfall can have a significant influence on the way in which radiation is distributed, since rain will carry contaminated particles to the ground, forming "hot spots" where it falls.

"But fallout doesn't come out of the sky like a gas and seep into everything. It can best be described as a fine to coarse sand carried by the winds. Because the wind direction varies at different heights above the ground, it is not possible to judge from the ground where the fallout will settle. It can settle in irregular patterns hundreds of miles from the explosion."[206]

The radioactive material may thusly spread from a few miles near the site of the blast to around the world. The most hazardous radiation (larger, heavier particles) **falls within forty-eight hours** in close proximity to the blast.

Blast Effects

Blast effects would occur from the detonation of an atomic bomb, and not from a radiological dispersion device. The blast effects are the result of a shock wave of overheated air radiating outward from the epicenter at about 160 + miles per hour. The magnitude of the blast depends on an optimum height above ground level (called overpressure). This sudden change in air pressure can crush objects and topple structures such as trees, utility poles, and buildings, creating an additional source of injury. It will also turn debris into harmful missiles. The shock wave eventually diminishes as it travels away from its center. The following chart provides an approximation of its effects.

Blast Energy Effects
(Approximate Distances In All Directions From The Center)

Weapon	Initial Rad[207]	Physical Injury	Burns
5 Meg[208]	11 Km[209]	22.5 Km	70 Km
1 Meg	2.2 Km	4.5 Km	14 Km
100 Kil[210]	1.7 Km	2 Km	6 Km
10 Kil	1 Km	2 Km	1 Km
1 Kil	0.7 Km	0.5 Km	0.5 Km

Thermal Effects

The intense heat radiating from the blast of an atomic explosion is usually responsible for most of the injuries. "The heat rays from the explosion travel at the speed of light, about 186,000 miles per second. It can start fires up to 20 miles away. Many fires are caused when the heat pulse comes through a window to set fire to curtains, paper, clothing and furniture."[211]

The flash of visible light, preceding the blast by several seconds, will produce temporary blindness in those looking in the direction of the explosion.

"Skin burns result from higher intensities of light, and therefore take place closer to the point of explosion. First degree, second degree and third degree burns can occur at distances of five miles away from the blast or more. Third-degree burns over 24 percent of the body, or second-degree burns over 30 percent of the body, will result in serious shock, and will probably prove fatal unless prompt, specialized medical care is available. The entire United States has facilities to treat 1,000 or 2,000 severe burn cases. A single nuclear weapon could produce more than 10,000."[212]

"While thermal injury is the most prevalent from nuclear weapons, it is the easiest

---

[206] Bruce Beach, 11 Steps to Survival…

[207] Radiation.
[208] Equals 5 million tons.
[209] One kilometer is approximately 5/8 of a mile. Three miles is about 4.83 kilometers.
[210] Equals 1000 tons.
[211] Beach, Bruce, Nuclear War Survival Skills.
[212] CBSNews.com, Anatomy of a Nuclear Blast, p. 1.

injury to shield against. Any opaque object between the fireball and victim captures the energy. White or light colored clothing reflects much of the heat energy. The burn involves only the surface facing the detonation, but heat energy may ignite clothing or building materials, resulting in a flame burn."[213]

Exposure to Radiation and Related Injury

We are constantly immersed in a cosmic sea of harmless amounts of radiation coming from stars, our sun, and the earth. It provides us with light, heat, and sound. However, the radiation coming from a nuclear incident is many times more concentrated than the natural sources of radiation.

While thermal burns contribute to most of the injury incurred with a nuclear detonation, ionizing radiation poses different kinds of injuries and challenges because it has the potential to alter the atoms comprising the DNA in the cell's nucleus. Two types of injury occur as a result of exposure to certain levels of radiation: *acute* (immediate), and *chronic* (delayed).

The measure of the amount of radiation in the environment (or absorbed by a person) is expressed in various, sometimes confusing terms. The following terms, while not exhaustive, are commonly used in clinical settings.

- The *Roentgen* (R) measures the amount of radiation in the atmosphere.
- The *sievert* (Sv) is the amount of radiation (based on a quality factor) that is actually absorbed by any tissue or substance.
- The *gray* (Gy) is similar to the *sievert*.
- 1 *gray* and the *sievert* are equal to 100 *rad* (radiation absorbed dose).

Biochemical individuality is an important variable when it comes to how people will be affected by similar levels of radiation. This means that other factors, such as genetics and level of health, are involved that may alter the vulnerability of the cells. Radiation affects one by the amount being emitted and the duration of exposure.

As radiation travels through the body tissue, it can damage certain vital organ systems more seriously than others. The most sensitive in this regard are the **bone marrow**, followed in descending order by the **blood, bowel, skin,** and **nervous** and **cardiovascular systems.** Which systems will be affected depends on how much radiation a person absorbs (Rad).

Radiation Absorbed Dose (Rad) & Effects

Gy/Rad	Possible Symptoms
0.3 Gy/30 Rad:	General feeling of malaise plus probable psychosomatic implications related to fear and anxiety. This level of exposure is thousands of times higher than the peacetime standards. May have negative effects on children, pregnant women, and the immune compromised.
0.5 Gy/50 Rad:	Malaise with no fatalities.
2-3 Gy/200-300 Rad:	Illness similar to the effects of chemotherapy: such as nausea, vomiting, weakness, and hair loss. Possibly affecting the production of red blood and immune cells in the bone marrow, where these cells are produced (affected by 2-10 Gy=200-1000 Rad).
	The bone marrow is viscous material filling the spaces inside certain bones. "It is known as myeloid tissue and is essential in the manufacture and maturation of red blood cells, most white blood cells, and plate-

[213] De Lorenzo, R., Porter, R., cited above, p. 89.

lets."[214] Disruption of this regenerative function reduces the available number of these cells, thereby compromising the delivery of oxygen to tissue.

Disruption of the formation of platelets can lead to clotting disorders.

Symptoms are most severe 6-12 hours after exposure, followed by a symptom-free period of 24-36 hours, during which the regeneration of red blood and immune cells is further compromised, leading to opportunistic infections. "The radiation dosage necessary to damage the bone marrow and blood cells is generally survivable if not complicated by other injuries."[215]

Gy/400 Rad: Affects the bowel (gastrointestinal system): Symptoms affecting the intestinal system are a sign that large doses of primary and secondary forms of radiation (from the ingestion of water and foods contaminated by **alpha** and **beta** particles) have taken their toll on the tissue. These symptoms usually appear within a few hours after exposure, and prior to those from bone-marrow complications. The damage limits the capacity of cells of the bowel lining to regenerate. Early on, one will experience:
Nausea
Loss of appetite
Possible vomiting
Loose or watery stools
Loss of fluids
Malaise

As the condition advances, the loss of fluid causes severe dehydration
As the bowel lining deteriorates, malnutrition occurs
Hemorrhaging and perforation may occur

6 Gy/600 Rad +: Seems to be the border line of almost certain fatality for bone marrow and gastrointestinal complications.

30 Gy/3000 Rad: Such high levels of radiation effect the nerve cells, especially the brain, which become inflamed, causing: Initial symptoms of nausea, vomiting, exhaustion, followed by:
confusion,
incapacitation,
tremors (shaking),
possible coma,
and a **sensation of "being on fire".**
Fatal within a few hours.

Note: Radiation damages exposed skin and leaves a reddening effect. This may also be due to thermal flash burn produced by an atomic explosion. Ordinarily, this is not a life threatening condition but may be a sign of high doses of **beta**, **gamma**, and **neutron** radiation that occur concomitantly with the above-mentioned gastrointestinal complications.

Agent Characteristics as a Weapon
Estimated Level of Attraction
Low 1-2-3-4-5 High

- Availability of information on the agent. **3-5**
- Ease of performing research, and manipulating agent. **1**
- Ease of manufacture/minimal danger.**1-2**
- Availability of the ingredients. **2-4**
- Low cost. **2-3**
- Easy to store/house. **2-4**

---

[214] Mosby's Medical, Nursing, and Allied Health Dictionary (Sixth Edition).
[215] De Lorenzo, R.; Porter, R., cited above, p. 90.

- Durability of agent. **5**
- Difficulty for being detected. **2-3**
- Has a quick rate of action/incubation time. **5**
- Ease of transport. **3-4**
- Ease of delivery by various methods. **3**
- Ability to inflict widespread harm/death. **5**
- Treatable. **3-5**

Assessment

Attack with a large megaton bomb delivered in a warhead, or by other means, seems less likely. The magnitude of such an attack would probably be the work of a nation state, and certainly traceable to the source. The nuclear retaliation would be a severe penalty, which is a considerable deterrent.

However, a relatively small bomb of about 15-kilotons, detonated in a large city, could kill hundreds of thousands of people. To make such a bomb one would need fissile material such as enriched uranium or plutonium.[216] The highly enriched uranium or plutonium needed to produce such a bomb is hard to come by. Even governments sympathetic to the terrorist cause might think twice before supporting such an endeavor, considering that it may boomerang on the government provider. It would need to be purchased on the black market or stolen.

There is some suspicion that fissile material could become available, or that an existing weapon such as the Russian "suitcase" nuclear bomb (each weighing about 60 lbs, about the size of a small refrigerator) might be in the wrong hands.[217] However, one vigilant source on these issues reports that: "The prevailing judgment among Western experts is that Russia may have lost track of the paper trail for any number of bombs, but

that the bombs themselves probably have been dismantled or tucked away in storage, rather than having been stolen."[218]

Most experts agree that the relative ease of obtaining radioactive waste to fashion a **radiological device** using conventional explosives would seem more attractive to terrorists trying to maintain a low profile. "In the United States, radioactive waste is located at more than 70 commercial nuclear power sites in 31 states. Enormous quantities also exist overseas—in Europe and Japan in particular. Tons of wastes are transported long distances, including between continents (Japan to Europe and back)."[219]

The so-called "dirty bomb" (or a source of radiation dispersed by explosives) is one of several likely scenarios in a highly populated city. This would restrict the affected region, but its effects would contaminate the area for a considerable period of time, and have crippling effects on the local health and financial resources. While such a device will not produce much structural damage the ionizing radiation could be a serious problem.

Another possibility is the sabotage of a nuclear power plant. An explosion will not take place, but melt-down could damage the reactor and the containment structure. This may lead to a release of radioactive steam or vapor that will affect the immediate area and communities downwind of the toxic cloud, which could be relatively small, or worldwide. This would require an attack by a powerful explosive missile or a large commercial jetliner to the plant, currently not a very likely possibility. But, it should not be discounted.

An assault on radioactive materials being transported—for medical use, weapons development, industrial use, or storage—is yet another possibility. Radioactive materials are usually shipped in small quantities in

---

[216] Note: "Terrorists could easily make an atomic bomb from MOX fuel, says a confidential report—exclusive from New Scientist Magazine, 30 May 2001.,, See radmeters4u.com article, p 5.

[217] A compact and lightweight, attaché-size, nuclear bomb was secretly built by the US in the 1970's. It was carried (inconspicuously) by a government passenger on an airline flight from coast to coast during the 1980's. Lay knowledge of the whereabouts of this technology is unknown.

[218] CDI Terrorism Project (Oct. 1, 2001). What if the Terrorists Go Nuclear? http://www.org/terrorism/nuclear-pr.cfm. (P. 2-3.)

[219] CDI Terrorism Project, cited above, p. 1.

leak-and-crash-proof containers. As a highly protected moving target, this scenario seems less likely than the dirty bomb. Again, it should not be easily discounted.

In spite of all this, the level of vigilance has increased dramatically since 9/11. Considering the increased methods of surveillance by local, federal, and concerned international authorities, involving greater intelligence and more portable and sensitive detection devices at the ports and in the field, the likelihood of such an attack seems to fall within the **2-3** range of possibility, even though the level of attraction may remain high.

Detection

Radiation cannot be detected by the senses. It cannot be seen, smelled, tasted, or felt. Therefore, detection devices can increase one's chances for survival. They are also useful in determining treatment. It is important to know the amount of contamination in the immediate environment, and the amount of radiation absorbed by an individual. Detection instruments include survey meters and dosimeters.

- **Survey meters** (Geiger Counters) are designed to detect the levels of radiation in the environment. They should be able to detect the full range of radiation, beyond those required for peacetime levels.
- **Dosimeters** are designed to measure the total amount of accumulated radiation to which the body has been exposed over a period of time.
- **Survey-Dosimeters** are units that combine the measurements of survey meters and dosimeters (such as the **Gamma Scout**, which would provide subtle readings, in terms of *micro sieverts*[220], of tissue exposure over time).

Field Detection: The use of x-ray machines and gamma-and-neutron detectors are available to authorities for use in strategic sites in the field to find hidden nuclear weapons. Small hand-held Geiger counters are also available to law enforcement personnel.

Conventional Methods of Response And Treatment

Emergency responders will wear full protective gear (which may not protect them from gamma particles), and, following a local and federal command-structure[221], they would be involved in search and rescue operations, triage (evaluating the degree of injury—physical trauma, radiological effects, burns, etc.—to each victim, and responding accordingly), initial treatment, and transport of victims.[222] Depen ding on the extent of the damage to the environment and injury, special sheltered medical treatment sites would be set up. At these sites, victims would be decontaminated with soap and water. Full protective gear would need to be worn by the caretakers.

Medical Care:[223]
- Those who are caring for patients exposed to radiation need to take precautionary measures to protect themselves from radioisotopes (particles ionized from the atom) emitted from the radiation in the patient's body, bandages, and excrements.
- Caretakers should wear disposable protective clothing, including caps, masks, and shoe covers.

---

[220] A millionth of a sievert.

[221] Most likely stemming from the Office of Homeland Defense.
[222] For a more detailed professional account of this process see: De Lorenzo, R., Porter, R., (2000). Weapons of Mass Destruction: Emergency Care. Prentice-Hall, Inc.: Upper Saddle River, NJ.
[223] For a more detailed professional account of this process and drug-dosage guidelines see: Sifton, D., Ed., (2002). PDR® Guide to Biological and Chemical Warfare Response. Thomson/Physicians' Desk Reference®: Montvale, NJ.

- Further decontamination with soap and water.
- **Radiation exposure:** "Radiation illness develops slowly. It cannot be spread to other people. Except for temporary nausea shortly after exposure, evidence of serious effects from radiation may only appear after an interval of from a few days to three weeks. A combination of loss of hair, loss of appetite, increasing pallor, weakness, diarrhea, sore throat, bleeding gums and easy bruising indicate that the individual requires medical attention. Nausea and vomiting may be caused by fright, worry, food poisoning, pregnancy and other common conditions."[224]
- Radiation illness is essentially treated with rehydration, antibiotics, and *sodium iodide* or *potassium iodide or potassium iodate* to protect the thyroid gland.
- All vomitus, feces, urine, and metal clothing parts are saved for radiological analysis to determine level of exposure.
- Care of wounds from **blunt trauma** (injuries from objects set in motion by the blast), using standard care for these types of injuries.
- Treatments for **pressure trauma** to the lungs, which can lead to swelling, fluid accumulation, and low oxygen delivery to the tissue, require administration of 100% oxygen and other lung resuscitation procedures. Ear and bowel injuries require supportive care.
- Patients with **thermal burns** are given fluid replacement, bone marrow revitalization treatments, and antibiotics (opportunistic infection is a primary threat).

- Those with **bone-marrow deficiency** would be treated with *filgrastrim* (G-CSF, Neupogen) until the absolute neutrophil count (ANC) normalizes.
- For **hypotension** fluid levels are maintained, and *dopamine* or *norepinephrine* may be given to increase the blood pressure.
- Those suffering from **seizures** are given *benzodiazepines* or *barbiturates* as required.
- All patients are monitored with complete blood counts (CBC) with differential, platelets, and electrolytes (sodium, potassium, magnesium, etc.).

Suggestions for Natural Defense

Psychological Line: "The more one knows about the strange dangers from nuclear weapons and about the strengths and weaknesses of human beings when confronted with the dangers of war, the better chance one has of surviving. Terror, a self-destructive emotion, is almost always the result of unexpected danger. Some people would think the end of the world was upon them if they happened to be in an area downwind from surface bursts of nuclear weapons that sucked millions of tons of pulverized earth into the air. They might give up all hope if they did not understand what they saw. People are more likely to endure and survive if they learn in advance that such huge dust clouds, particularly if combined with smoke from great fires, may turn day into night as have some volcanic eruptions and the largest forest fires.

People also should expect thunder to crash in strange clouds, and the earth to shake. The sky may be lit with the flickering purples and greens of "artificial auroras" caused by nuclear explosions, especially those that are miles above the earth."[225]

---

[224] Bruce Beach, 11 Steps to Survival, available on the Internet at www.ki4u/survival/doomsday.htm.

[225] Cited from Cresson Kearny's Nuclear War Survival Skills (Chapter 3: Psychological Preparations).

With the psychological line of defense the aim is to reduce or, better yet, transform fear and panic states of mind into useful states of mind. Negative states have a dire effect on immune response and on the ability to make sound judgments during a nuclear incident. The following suggestions might be helpful to prepare:

- Perform the Relaxation Response (or a comparable form of meditation based on one's personal belief system) 1-2 times daily or as needed in order to develop a relatively calm (habituated) state of mind during such an incident. It is important to remember that during such a threat there is always a level of pressure that can be turned into **eustress** (positive stress) rather than **distress** (negative stress).
- Learn as much as you can about what a nuclear attack entails and what practical steps can be taken. Avoid obsessing about it. Also, there are many misconceptions about the effects of a nuclear attack.
- Aroma Therapy with lavender essential oil
- 5-HTP (5-hydroxytryptophan) 200-300 mg 1-3 times daily between meals at least 45 minutes before food with room temperature or cool non-protein drink (no caffeinated drinks) to increase the calming neurotransmitter seratonin, as a possible anti-depressive. Adults only.
- GABA (gamma-aminobutyric acid) 500-1000 mg 1-3 times daily between meals at least 30 minutes before food with a room temperature or cool non-protein drink (no caffeinated drinks), to help reduce anxiety (worry and nervousness about what might happen). Adults only.

- Melatonin 3-18 mg 1/2 to 1 hour before bedtime with water if you have difficulty getting deep sleep. Adults only.
- Beautiful Calming Impressions are food for the soul.
- **Trust** in your Divinely given power to heal.

Social Line: A nuclear terrorist attack would most likely come as a surprise. Therefore, a prepared social line of defense is of paramount importance. The key elements for empowering this line are:

- Other people: "The very best thing that a survival minded person can do, after preparing themselves an equipped place of refuge, and developing their own survival skills, is to associate themselves with other skilled survivalists. No person can know everything, and almost everyone can contribute something. Agricultural, medical, mechanical, communicator, you name it, all skills will be needed."[226]
- Consider starting a **Neighborhood Defense Support Group** in your community. Feeling the concern and camaraderie of people provides that inner sustenance that helps people cope with the most pressing issues of our time. Set up an agenda based on the topics in this book, as a start. Invite speakers from various relevant organizations. Pick a starting date. Find a place to meet (home, apartment, church, school, public meeting hall, etc.) Find a simple way to broadcast the event. Let the news media know. Keep a record of the meetings. This is one of the best examples of using the social line. The key areas that need to be discussed are as follows:

Oregon Institute of Science and Medicine: Cave Junction, OR.

[226] From: Bruce Beach's You Will Survive Doomsday, available on the Internet (http://www.ki4u/survival/doomsday.htm).

Preparedness

- **Knowledge of nuclear threats** as covered in this book and/or other publications, videos, lectures, discussion sessions, etc.
- **Know the local resources:** It is important that your local municipality have a plan for a nuclear emergency. And it is just as important that you know that plan. This might include:
- Details of how health, police, public utilities, fire and other emergency services will operate.
- Evacuation plans involving traffic arrangements to reception areas and medical facilities in nearby communities.
- **Create a plan for you and your family.**
- Synchronize your personal and family survival plan with the one established in your area.
- The best way to arrive at a workable plan that will be remembered is to practice it.

Communication

- **Warning signal:** every country, community, etc. has an emergency warning signal. It is important to know what it is. When the Attack Warning sounds, you must take protective action.
- **Portable radio** is necessary to keep in touch with news regarding the event and emergency advisories. The ideal portable radio is a battery operated or a wind-up one. I prefer the wind-up version because it would not require replacing the worn out batteries. There are versions that use both. (See Resources.)
- If you don't have a portable radio, turn up the volume of your house radio or TV so that it can be heard in your shelter. If away from home you are forced to take emergency shelter and are near a radio-equipped vehi-

cle, turn up the volume and open all of the vehicle's doors or windows.

- Radio broadcasts will give instructions and advice. These might include:
- Location of nuclear explosions causing local fallout.
- Information about the parts of the country to be affected by fallout.
- Length of time before fallout is likely to reach specific communities or areas. Ways to increase fallout protection. Supplies to take to your fallout shelter. Whether it is safer to stay in your community or area, or to go to other areas free of danger.
- Advice on when to leave shelters and for how long until danger from radioactive contamination diminishes. Requests for help in rescue operations, such as rescue, firefighting and medical assistance. Advice on conservation of food, water and fuel. How to keep warm when power is off and the weather is cold.
- **CB-Radio (Citizen Band)** might be useful to maintain communication between people in a confined area.
- **Telephone:** Avoid using. This keeps the lines of communication open for government responders dealing with the incident. If necessary, the phone should be used sparingly to share vital information.

Shelter, Equipment, Supplies

- **Structural needs** against blast, fire, and fallout: (See Environmental Line below.)
- **Equipment and Supplies:** During a nuclear incident the production and distribution of available food stocks may be curtailed for several days or even weeks. One may need to stay in a shelter for as long as 14 days.
- Those who need to evacuate the larger cities would be dependent

largely on the resources available in safe towns. It is recommended that every person should have emergency supplies to meet their personal and family needs for at least 14 days.

- Whether you choose to evacuate or take shelter locally, a road map is indispensable (to know where the hot spots are) for safe travel.
- See Resources for a complete listing of equipment and supplies.

Fire Fighting and Prevention

- Do you **know** the recommended fire precautions?
- Do you, or anyone in your family, know how to fight small fires?
- **Water:** Can an emergency supply of water be obtained quickly for fire fighting?
- **Fire extinguishers:** Which ones are appropriate? How can they be used?

Nutritional Needs

During a nuclear incident it is necessary to take certain nutrient supplies that would last for at least 14 days.

- **Water** is crucial for survival. How can water be stored? How much would be needed? How can contaminated water be purified? (See the Environmental and the Specific Line below for details.)
- **Food**: Which ones? How much per person? How to safely store. (See the Specific Line below for recommendations.)
- **Air**: Without proper amounts of good air, life can only last for minutes. How can one ensure the quality of the air while in a shelter? (See the Environmental Line below.)

Fitness

- **Exercise** is important, especially when confined to a relatively small space in a shelter. Avoid vigorous exercise that will expend large amounts of energy and consume more oxygen. Stretching, yoga, wall

pushups, and the like are good to keep the muscles in tone, and reduce the tension and anxiety of being "pent up".

Hygiene

- **Bathing** may or may not be possible during a nuclear attack. One may use Grapefruit Seed Extract (GSE) solution in spray bottles (**never use on eyes**) to cleanse and freshen hands and face, underarms, and private areas. Dry with paper towels. This minimizes the use of water, which should have priority for drinking and cooking.
- Your limited supply of water will have to be rationed and used only for essential purposes. If you have enough warning time before the arrival of fallout, fill your bathtub, all available buckets and pans with water. Remember that there is an emergency supply in your hot water tank.
- **Washing utensils** should be kept to a minimum if water supply is limited. Paper plates might be a good choice. If hard plates are used, GSE solution could again be used to decontaminate and wipe clean with paper towel. The same goes for knives, forks, and spoons.
- **Waste:** Personal cleanliness in crowded shelter conditions is important to you and your family. The problems of garbage and human waste disposal can be solved even if fallout keeps you in the shelter. Put all your garbage in tightly covered garbage pails. After using your emergency toilet, you should tie human waste in waterproof plastic (polyethylene) bags and place them in the garbage pail. Store a 14- day supply of the plastic bags. When deemed safe, you may risk leaving the shelter for a few minutes for es-

sential tasks. Then, when your garbage container is filled, move it out of the shelter.

- If your area is free of fallout but is without sewage services, bury human waste and garbage in the ground. Dig the pit deep enough so that the waste will be covered by at least two feet of earth.
- Keep a soft broom in the shelter for tidying it up.

First Aid and Nursing Skills

- This is perhaps one of the most important and humanitarian aspects of the Social Line of Defense. (For more details go to the chapter The Five Supportive Lines of Defense, under the Social Line section.)

Medical Supplies

- First aid medical supplies are required if anyone should get injured or sick during a nuclear incident. (A complete listing is provided in Resources.)

Preventative Line: The purpose with this line is to take whatever preventative measures are possible to minimize the harmful effects of a nuclear attack. Some suggestions are:

- The use of **Potassium Iodide (KI)** and/or **Potassium Iodate (KIO3)** (see the Specific Line below) to protect against the uptake of radioactive iodine by the thyroid gland; best 48 hours or less before exposure. When KI or KIO3 is taken after exposure the protective effect is less and decreases more rapidly with insufficient dietary iodine. "For example, KI administration 2 and 8 hrs after 131-I (radioiodine) intake yields protective effects of 80% and 40%, respectively, with iodine-

sufficient diets, but only 65% and 15% with iodine-deficient diets."[227]

- Therefore, maintain sufficient (100-225 mcg) daily dietary sources of iodine by taking 1-2 **Kelp** tablets daily with meals and/or eating foods that are rich in iodine—asparagus, garlic, lima beans, mushrooms, salt-water fish, sesame seeds, soybeans, spinach, summer squash, Swiss chard, and turnip greens. Of course, iodized and sea salt are sources of iodine also. **Caution:** Some foods **when eaten raw** can block the absorption of iodine in the thyroid gland. These include: Brussels sprouts, cabbage, cauliflower, kale, peaches, pears, spinach, and turnips. Those with under active thyroid should avoid these foods. Also, **excessive** use of iodine (750 + mcg) can block the secretion of thyroid hormone (thyroxin).

Environmental Line: Here we revisit the environmental issues related to nuclear incidents.

Facts About Radioactive Fallout

- A nuclear explosion causes both immediate radiation and residual radiation.
- **Immediate radiation** is given off at the time of the explosion. It is dangerous only within two or three miles. If you were near the explosion without adequate protection and managed to survive the effects of blast and fire, you could still be seriously affected by immediate radiation.
- **Residual radiation** is given off by the radioactive particles left as "fallout" after the explosion.

---

[227] Zanzonico, P.; Becker, D., Effects of Time of Administration and Dietary Iodine Levels on Potassium Iodide (KI) Blockade of Thyroid Irradiation by 131-I From Radioactive Fallout. Health Physics Journal, Volume 78, June 2000.

- If a nuclear weapon is exploded on or near the ground, danger from radioactive fallout is greatest.
- Factors that determine exposure to radiation are: 1) distance, 2) the kind of material between one and the fallout, and 3) the length of time one remains within the fallout area.
- The radioactivity in fallout weakens rapidly in the first hours after an explosion. This weakening is called "decay".
- After seven hours, fallout has lost about 90% of the strength it had one hour after the explosion. After two days it has lost 99%; in two weeks 99.9% of its strength is gone. Nevertheless, if the radiation at the beginning were high enough, the remaining 0.1% could be dangerous.
- One should stay in the shelter until radiation has been measured and you have been told over the radio that it is safe to come out.
- The most effective protection is to place some heavy material between one and the fallout. The heavier the material the better.
- Many common materials give excellent protection. The following materials will stop 99% of radiation:
  16 inches of solid brick
  16 inches of hollow concrete blocks filled with mortar or sand
  2 feet of packed earth, 3 feet if loose
  5 inches of steel
  3 inches of lead
  3 feet of water

Shelter

- Shelter against a nuclear attack involves the creation of a space that will provide shielding from blast effects, fire, and radioactive particles coming from all directions. Protection from blast effects and fire can only be accomplished by distance or from a properly built shelter (ideally three feet below ground level).
- Large cities may already have these in place. However, in more rural settings, they may need to be privately built. There are many do-it-yourself manuals for guidance, and there are other sources for having one built.[228]
- It is important to provide your family and yourself with a shelter. But what kind of shelter? This is a decision you must make yourself after studying the problem. Study your shelter requirements in the same way that you would study accident or fire insurance. Decide upon the degree of protection you want for your family and yourself. Shelter is your insurance against something you hope will not happen, so that if it does, you will be protected.

Questions Regarding Shelter

- Have you decided where you will take shelter if you're not at home when the attack occurs?
- Will you try to get home?
- Will your family know what to do if you are not at home?
- Is there a shelter plan for your children at school?
- Will protection there be better than in your home? Does everybody in your family know your survival plan?
- Do you want them to try to get home?
- In thinking about what you will do or where you would go, you might consider leaving your home to find shelter elsewhere.

Know How to Take Shelter

- Remember, with a detonation the flash of light will precede the blast

---

[228] See Nuclear Shelters in Resources.

by seconds.

- If possible, shield your eyes from the flash of an explosion.
- Move away from windows.
- Lie down and protect yourself from flying glass and falling debris.
- If you are away from home take protective cover immediately.
- If you are driving, stop and take protective cover, or if you are only a few minutes from a safe area, proceed and take protective cover there.

Improvised Protection Against Blast

- One can quickly improvise a barrier to protect oneself from objects propelled by the blast. As soon as the warning signal sounds, build a lean-to (bed springs or boards) against a workbench or heavy table (preferably in the basement), and pile mattresses on it and at the ends.
- If you are **in the open** and there is a ditch or culvert within easy, quick reach (away from buildings that might fall), lie face down in it and cover your face with your arms.
- After the blast and heat of the explosion, find protection against fallout, which will come down later. (Don't forget your battery-powered radio and cell phone).

Improvised Protection Against Fallout

You may not have a fallout shelter when warning of approaching fallout is broadcast. Here are some tips on how to increase your protection in a basement, a crawl space, or in a closet. The amount of protection you can build will depend on how much time you have available until fallout arrives.

- You can improvise a small emergency shelter in the basement by using furniture, doors, dressers, workbench and other materials.
- Select a corner of the basement (if possible away from windows) in which to build your shelter.
- Remove inside house doors from hinges to use over supports (such as cabinets, chests, desks, etc. able to bear a heavy load) to make a roof.
- Place bricks, concrete blocks, sand-filled drawers or boxes, books or other dense items on the roof to help reduce radiation penetration.
- Around the sides and front of your shelter build walls of similar dense materials to provide vertical shielding.
- A small cabinet or dirt-filled box as may be used as a crawl-in entrance, which can be closed behind you.
- On the floor above the corner of the space you select as your shelter area, pile similar heavy objects you may have available.
- Remember, the heavier (or denser) the material that surrounds you the greater the protection.
- Block basement windows with bags filled with earth or use bricks, concrete blocks, books or even bundles of newspaper. In winter, use packed snow.
- On the outside around the shelter pile earth, sand, bricks, etc.
- If your home has no basement or crawl space, build your emergency shelter as close to the center as possible (farthest away from the outer walls and roof). Perhaps in a hall or clothes closet.

Know How to Prevent and Fight Fires

Many believe that a nuclear explosion would incinerate an entire city. This is not necessarily true. The heat from the fireball lasts about 10-15 seconds and would ignite curtains, clothes, furniture and paper, etc. within a certain range. Many of these fires can be put out with water and extinguishers (portable and automatic). If each survivor were able to put out a small fire quickly, mass fires could be avoided.

- Fallout will not start coming down for about 30 minutes, providing a period of time when fire fighting can take place.
- During this half hour, survivors should inspect their houses and put out all the small fires they can.
- Do not rely on the fire department to extinguish these fires as they will be occupied by major events.
- You should have fire extinguishers in your home and place of work.
- In an emergency, create a water supply for fire fighting in pails, bathtubs, washtubs, etc., since the established water supply system may not be operable.
- To learn more, attend any emergency fire fighting classes held in your area.

Fire Prevention

- Prepare for emergency by preventing accumulations of trash and rubbish in and around the home. This would include dry leaves and grass, lumber, boxes, cardboard cartons, old unused furniture, bales of newspapers, etc. Keep waste and garbage in covered containers.
- The shaking and twisting of buildings and homes due to blast waves may break utility inlets at the point they enter the structure. This may allow gas or fuel oil to flow into basements creating a severe hazard. **Do not smoke, strike a match, or use a lighter, or use a lit candle to light your way into a darkened basement.** Gas or oil vapors may be present and a violent explosion and fire may result.
- To lessen the danger of fires and ex-

plosions, follow local instructions about shutting off utility services when the warning signal sounds. If you have a coal-burning furnace, or a wood-stove, extinguish it or at least be sure to close all fuel and draft doors.
- Close curtains, shutters, or blinds on all windows and remove furniture from window areas.

Fire Fighting Tips

To stop a fire from spreading:

- Take away its fuel.
- Get the burning material out of your home.
- Take away its air. Smother it with a blanket, wet if possible, or a rug.
- Cool it with water, earth, sand or fire extinguisher.

Gas, Oil, Electrical Fires

- **Gas fire:** Make sure the gas is shut off and then try to extinguish anything still burning.
- **Oil fires:** Make sure the supply is shut off then smother the fire with earth, sand, rugs or other heavy materials. Don't use water.
- **Electrical fires:** Make, sure the electricity is shut off then put out the fire. Don't use water if the power is still on. Use a fire extinguisher rated for electrical fires.

How to Get Rid of Radioactive Dust

Fallout is like fine, potentially imperceptible sand. To remove the danger, remove the sand.

- If you suspect that your clothes have fallout on them, remove your outer clothing before you come inside your home and leave it outside. Don't shake these clothes inside the house or shelter. You would only scatter the fallout grit and create unnecessary danger to others. If you have water, wash thoroughly, particularly exposed skin and hair. But do not scrub your skin as this might rub in the radioactive particles.

- Exposure to fallout does not make you radioactive.
- Fallout on your clothing or body would expose you and those close to you to radiation. If you suspect you have been exposed to fallout, you will not be a danger to others if you carefully get rid of your outer clothing outside the shelter and wash.
- Even if you are stricken with radiation sickness, this sickness is not contagious.

Air

"One of the general misconceptions regarding fallout and fallout shelters is that the air itself may become radioactive. This is simply not true. Those with a little learning will then say "Ah, yes, but it will contain radioactive particles of fallout". That is true, but a properly designed air intake, even for an expedient shelter, will cause most of the particles to drop out of the airflow before the air enters the shelter. Should the number of particles suspended in the air be a problem, an expedient filter, such as a damp sheet hung in the air intake passageway, will do an adequate job of filtering the air."[229]

Decontamination of Water

Water that has been exposed to nuclear radiation but has not been contaminated by fallout particles is safe for human consumption, unless spoiled by some other manner. Also: "Water in covered containers and from underground sources will be safe. Water into which fallout particles have fallen may become unsafe to drink for a while, because radioactive iodine dissolves in water. Water that is collected from rooftops or other flat areas into cisterns, tanks, or other reservoirs, may have much higher concentrations of radioiodine than other sources of water if there is a rainfall shortly after fallout has arrived. Rivers and streams that are fed mostly by water from the surface rather than from underground springs may also become contaminated by radioiodine if there is a rainfall in the first few days after fallout arrives. Water in large, deep lakes, reservoirs, and rivers may be safe to drink (although it could still be unsafe due to other pollutants) within several hours or days after fallout has arrived, because of dilution of the radioiodine into large volumes of water.

The radioiodine problem will almost completely disappear in any water after a few weeks due to natural radioactive decay. The quantity of the radioactive iodine of greatest concern will become half as much every eight days (the half-life is eight days).

"Radioisotopes that have dissolved in water cannot be removed by boiling or settling. The water can be purified by special filtering or chemical processes, one method being the filtration of water through several inches of soil or clay (not sand). Water filtered through soil must be disinfected either by boiling or by adding chemicals such as chlorine or household iodine."[230] Water can also be purified using Grapefruit Seed Extract.

Decontamination of Foods

Most foods will not be harmed by even the most intense radiation. The danger lies in ingesting or inhaling the radioactive particles.

- A simple dust mask can prevent inhalation.
- Fallout involves alpha, beta, and gamma particles that present as tiny imperceptible bits of dust that can be washed (under flowing water) off foods with a natural covering—eggs, bananas, potatoes, oranges—or those that have been stored in tightly

[229] Beach, B. (1980). You Will Survive Doomsday: http://www.ki4u.com/survive/doomsday.htm. (P. 7.)

[230] Federal Emergency Management Agency, CPG 2-6.4 (September 23, 1983). Radiation Safety In Shelters.

sealed containers or factory packaging.

- Ensure that hands have been thoroughly cleansed before handling food (especially under nails).

Specific Line: Here we focus on what natural measures can be taken to support the protective and healing processes of the body threatened by nuclear radiation. The normal food supply would need to altered to meet the demands of the incident. Certain other precautions also need to be taken, especially to protect the thyroid gland. Antioxidant/detoxification of free radicals is another possibility to defend against the damage to tissue that can be caused by radiation. Focus is also on supporting cellular integrity (especially DNA) and repair.

14 Days Emergency Food Supply

These are suggested items and amounts for each adult for 14 days in a shelter (on page 208). Check off the items as you stock them in the shelter and mark the purchase date on them. Food stored for emergency use should be used and replaced at least once a year.

Since most of your food will be in tightly covered containers (cans, bottles, plastic, boxes), it will all be safe to eat or drink if you wash the containers.

- Food, if it is unspoiled and free of grit or dust, may be eaten during the emergency period.
- Be sure to wash fruit and vegetables and peel carefully.

Water

- Water will be safe if it is in covered containers, or if it has come from covered wells, or from undamaged water systems.
- Requirements: 7-14 gallons for each adult member of family; more for younger children (some water may be replaced by canned beverages).
- Containers: Store in well-cleaned,

covered containers such as large thermos jugs, new fuel cans, large bottles, or plastic containers.

- Change: Change stored water at least once a month.

Potassium Iodide (KI), Potassium Iodate (KIO3)[231]

Radioactive iodine (Radioiodine) targets the thyroid gland and leads to thyroid cancer (especially in children). When inhaled or ingested it occupies the thyroid's receptor sites for iodine, a natural substance that supports thyroid function. To prevent this from happening (or to reduce the effects) one can take Potassium Iodide and/or Potassium Iodate in certain amounts, soon after a nuclear incident. These harmless forms of iodine will occupy the receptor sites and block the uptake of Radioiodine. In 1999, the World Health Organization (WHO) published the following **daily** dosage recommendations.

Age	I mg	KI mg	KIO3 mg	Part of 100 mg Tb.
12 +	100	130	170	1
3-12	50	65	85	1/2
1 mo-3 yrs	25	32	42	1/4
Birth-1 mo.	12.5	16	21	1/8

Cautions:

- Avoid substituting dietary or other supplemental sources of iodine (e.g., kelp, iodized salt, etc.) for KI or KIO3. They must be taken in very large amounts to equal the dose of 1 tablet (or fraction of) of KI and/or KIO3.
- **Do not ingest the tincture of iodine used on cuts since it is poisonous.**

---

[231] These are natural substances, pharmaceutically produced, which can be purchased without a prescription. Governmental agencies also provide them to the public during nuclear emergencies. Detailed information on the purchase and use of these substances can be found at the following web address: www.KI4U.com.

- Radioactive iodine can persist in the environment for a month or more. Governmental authorities will advise when the threat is over, and when to stop taking KI and/or KIO3. When the receptor sites for iodine are saturated any form of iodine circulating in the blood is quickly excreted through the kidneys.
- KI and/or KIO3 should not be taken by people allergic to iodine. Consult with a physician for alternatives.[232]
- Those with myotonia, hyperkalemia congenital, tuberculosis, or kidney disease should consult with a physician before using these substances.
- Those on prescription medications should consult with a physician regarding the use of these substances. Especially: those on thyroid medications; *Spironolactone* (e.g., Aldactone); *Triamterene* Dyrenium); *Amiloride* (Midamor); or lithium-based or potassium-sparing diuretics.
- Pregnant women should consult with a physician before continuing with dosages for more than 2 days.
- WHO advises: "In general, the potential benefits of iodine prophylaxis will be greater in the young, firstly because the small size of the thyroid means that a higher radiation dose is accumulated per unit of intake of radioactive iodine. Secondly, the thyroid of the fetus, neonate and young infant has a higher yearly thyroid cancer risk per unit dose than the thyroid of an adult and, thirdly, the young will have a longer time span for the expression of the increased cancer risk."

- Therefore, if there is a limited supply of Potassium Iodide/Iodate tablets, these should be given to infants, children, and young adults, as they are more vulnerable. The risk of thyroid cancer fully developing begins to diminish at age 40 and over.

Adequate Supply of Micronutrients
- Continue with the general nutrient support—All One, Magma Plus, or comparable formulas—and the following.
- Vitamin C (ascorbate powder) 1000 mg in 1/2 to 1 cup of water every hour to bowel tolerance. Then cut back until stools firm up, and continue with that dose divided over a 24-hour period. The buffered form (calcium ascorbate) is best with disorders that produce diarrhea because pure ascorbate can overly aggravate this condition), use 2,000-5,000 mg every 4 hours.
- Selenium 50 mcg 2 times daily with food (not to exceed 200 mcg from combined sources).
- Vitamin E 400 IU 3 times daily with food.
- Zinc 50 mg 2 times daily with food (not to exceed 100 mg from combined sources).
- Vitamin A (Mycelized) 5,000 IU 3 times daily (not to exceed 50,000 IU per day, or not more than 10,000 IU if you're pregnant; up to 100,000 may be taken under the supervision of a physician). Can be added to room temperature or cool drinks.

Adequate Supply of Antioxidants/Chelators

During chemotherapy and radiation treatments patients are typically advised not to take supplemental antioxidants because they can diminish the effects of the therapy. It seems that during a nuclear incident the

---

[232] "According to research by Health Physicist Ken Miller, Hershey Medical Center, with 24 healthy adult male subjects, an adult could get a blocking dose of stable iodine by painting 8 ml or a 2 percent tincture of Iodine on the abdomen or forearm approximately 2 hours prior to I-131 (radioiodine) contamination.,, Derived from: www.ki4u.com.

mega use of antioxidants would be a wise choice.[233]

- Oral Chelation Formula (by Extreme Health or comparable formula) 3 capsules daily near bedtime, + 3 caplets of Age-Less Formula in the morning with food for adults. Children ages 2-7 use 1/2 of a capsule (can be opened in juice) near bedtime + 1/2 caplet in the morning with food (can be crushed and placed in food). Children ages 8-13 use 1 capsule near bedtime + 2 caplets of Age-Less Formula in the morning with food. Children ages 13 up can take the adult dose.
- Alpha Lipoic Acid (sustained release), 600 mg (2 tablets) every 3 hours between meals at least 30 minutes before food.
- Grape Seed Extract 200 mg capsules 3 times daily with food.

Adequate Supply of Cell Nucleus (DNA) Protectors

- Co-Enzyme-Q-10, 90-100 mg (emulsified form for greater absorption) 4 times daily in divided dosages with food. (Country Life's Co-Q-10, and Life Extension's Super CoQ10 are excellent products. See Resources.)

Antimicrobials for Opportunistic Infections

- Grapefruit Seed Extract 15 drops 3-6 times daily in room temperature juice or water.
- Olive Leaf Extract 1000 mg. 3-6 times daily with food or on empty stomach.

---

[233] In their book *The Healing Nutrients Within: Facts, Findings and New Research on Amino Acids*, Dr. Eric R. Braverman, and Dr. Carl C. Pfeiffer write: "It has been suggested that gamma-glutamyl cysteine, an intermediate product in glutathione (an antioxidant) synthesis, or other glutathione precursors be stockpiled in preparation for nuclear accidents together with the anti-radiation nutrient potassium iodide.,, (P. 107. Parenthesis mine.)

- Wild Mountain Oregano Oil (North American Herb and Spice, Co. See Resources.) 1-2 drops under the tongue 3-6 times daily. Can be added to milk or juice for children.

Homeopathy
- Homeopathic physicians might recommend Radium; possibly using other remedies for specific symptoms.
- Consult with homeopathic physician for specific recommendations.

Children
- **Nutrient Dosages (not specified above):** Children between the ages of 2-5 should take 1/4 of the adult dosage; between 6-12 use 1/2 of the adult dosage; and between 13-17, 3/4 of the adult dosage.
- Follow dosage requirements for KI and/or KIO3 according to the above WHO recommendations.

Pregnant and Lactating Women
- Should consult with a physician prior to using any of the recommended supplements.

Pets
- Consider giving 1-4 tablets (depending on size) of **Gary Null's Pet's Health** formula 2 times a day.
- Veterinarian using homeopathy might recommend Radium, and other remedies based on symptoms.
- ASAP Solution® as for humans, to avoid or deal with secondary infections. Use plastic eyedropper to administer under the tongue 3-6 times a day.

Anti-Diarrhea Measures
- Activated Charcoal (powder) 200-300 mg per capsule, 1-4 to reduce loose stools. If necessary take with White Oak Bark tea for a stronger effect. Do not take together with medications or other nutrients, except with Pancreatic Enzymes when it is taken with meals.
- Ginger tea to alleviate nausea.

Rehabilitation

- Return to the preventative dietary guidelines
- Continue with the above nutrients and antioxidant formulas, especially the <u>Magma Plus</u> (or comparable formula)
- Consider taking <u>Melatonin</u>. "Studies have shown that supplemental melatonin in doses of 10-40 mg (for adults only) a night can protect and restore normal red blood cell production caused by toxicity of chemotherapy."[234]
- Perform a complete detoxification program.
- Exercise sensibly to maintain muscle tone and stamina.
- Continue or start performing the Relaxation Response or comparable program based on your personal belief system, twice daily.

---

[234] Segala, M., Ed., previously cited, p. 45.

Anxiety about terrorism has spurred interest in a variety of technologies, especially in the areas of: detection, biological testing, immunology, microbiology, toxicology, and emergency protective equipment. In some instances old lingering products and research have been revived, while in others new enterprises have been born. This endeavor is going on worldwide.

While the U.S. federal government has always had an ongoing defense program in this regard, some companies in the private sector have jumped in as recipients of current increase in federal grants, and to reap profits from the growing demand for these products and services. However, just what needs to be done falls on assessments produced by the federal government, but the challenges to meet the demand will fall on the shoulders of private manufacturers.

They will need to research and develop the airborne-detection devices, gas masks, vaccines, and the like. "Trouble is, it will take some time before these products are fully tested and, more importantly, can be produced on a mass scale. Most firms in this field are lucky to have government grants to keep the lights on. And those grants do not include sufficient funding to scale up production anytime soon to produce products for 275 million customers. Indeed, many firms in this area are doing well now just to find qualified staff to ramp up in response to calls from Washington to get ready."[235]

Moreover, anti-terrorism biochemistry is not big business for private pharmaceutical companies. Long-term investment in research and development is required, but when these companies look at the history of previous biowarfare enterprises they balk at the writing on the wall. They realize that "Chemical and biological weapons are not a new threat to humanity. Everybody cares a great deal about them today, but what about tomorrow, when the dust settles?"[236]

In spite of this caution, technologies that are employed in these biotech wars could, when no longer profitable, be diverted into the medical field.

Even with these challenges, this flurry of adrenalized activity has brought forth some interesting developments (amid some quick fix schemes), which, as I write, are not yet on the market, but aim (some pending government approval) to be so in the near future. What follows are selected brief reports on products that I consider would have serious potential to protect against WMD.

Detection

Detection devices are mainly used in the environmental line of defense to alert of the presence of deadly microorganisms and toxic chemicals. A considerable amount of this research is going on in California's Silicon Valley and the San Franscisco Bay Area where information technology is being combined with biotechnology.

For instance, "In Menlo Park, SRI International has become the world's fourth-largest developer of devices to detect pathogens, the general name for microorganisms that cause disease. Along with SRI, companies such as Aclara BioSciences Inc. of Mountain View and Cepheid Inc. of Sunnyvale are blending microbiology with information technology to make sensors faster and more accurate. Developers hope to make these instruments automated devices that fit in the palm of the user's hand."[237]

Of the many companies involved in this work, Argonne National Laboratory has integrated this research to produce a biochip system capable of detecting any biological agent through DNA analysis. A sample is taken and placed on a slide containing thousands of gel-

---

[235] IT NEWS, 9-28-01. (P. 1.)

[236] IT NEWS, cited above. (P. 2.)

[237] Wong, N. (8-27-200). Developing a defense for germ warfare. Mercury News, as reported on Silicon-Vally.com. (P. 3.)

elements with DNA. The slide is then placed into a processor that is hooked up to a computer. Within minutes it is able to identify the DNA signature of any pathogen. This is the fastest and most complete detection system I have come across in my research. What's interesting about it is how it is being developed as a fast-bio-detector to be used in public places to provide early warning of the presence of any kind of biological agent.

Scientists at Argonne have been working on a computer model that mimics a scenario involving a bio-terrorist attack to determine the effects of the attack on the public with and without the detector. Using the Washington, DC, subway system as a test case, it was able to determine how the pathogens would flow through and out of the tunnels and the amount of mortality it would cause to the public.

Without the detector it was estimated that 7, 795 untreated people would die after one hour of exposure. With the biochip detector 1, 544 untreated people would perish, but this number would drop to about 300 with treatment. The early warning would save lives by alerting the subway management to warn those in exposed areas, close down certain areas, and decontaminate to avert the spread of the pathogen. This would take approximately 15 minutes. However, the full system would not be ready for one to two years.[238]

Nanoemulsion

Far from the complexities of genome warfare, some scientists at the Department of Defense are looking seriously at a new generation of biological germicidal agents based on simple natural ingredients. Among the most promising is a nanoemulsion formula, developed by Dr. James Baker at the University of Michigan Center for Biological Nano Technology.

This formula is essentially water-in-oil with some detergent mixed with high shear forces that create droplets 400-800 nm (nanometers) in diameter. The tiny size allows the emulsion to fuse with the cell membrane of microorganisms resulting in their demise (lysis). As a consequence, they are very effective in killing: bacteria, bacterial spores, enveloped viruses, and fungal spores. Yet it has no negative effects on most human tissue. Additionally, microbes have not been able to develop resistance to this formula.

Because of the wide range of germicidal properties of nanoemulsions and their non-toxicity to most human cells they have many applications. They could be used preventively prior to and after exposure to pathogens. They can be used topically (one application lasts on the surface for about 14 days) and as an inhalant. They can also be employed to decontaminate surfaces, particularly in hospitals and in commercial food processing areas. Unlike other currently used chemical disinfectants they are non-toxic, non-corrosive, and friendly to the environment.

Nevertheless, amid all these positive qualities nonemulsion cannot be used intravenously because it could destroy red blood cells. This would not happen to the more resistant subcutaneous tissue, and it would be possible to ingest it, as the body would recognize it as a food. Furthermore, it will not harm internal organs.

Dr. Baker and his team at the University of Michigan have used their nanoemulsion formula to develop about 20 products that have been extensively tried in animal trials, and he is awaiting FDA go ahead to begin human studies. Because of the food based ingredients their use would most likely not need to be prescribed by a physician, and could be sold over-the-counter in retail outlets.

While the whole spectrum of nanoemulsion technology sounds very exciting, I would bring a modicum of caution. Even though within the laboratory no microbe has been able to develop resistance to them, what might be the scenario when it hits the mass market and the microbial world is under mass assault as happened with penicillin? Would nanoemulsions be used to create a squeaky-clean world? Is this ecologically useful? I don't know.

---

[238] Information was gathered about one year ago.

Currently, Dr. Baker and his colleagues are awaiting government approval to proceed with his discovery, but there may be some hidden industrial lobbying and special interest politics slowing the process down. Think of it. Think of all the industries that might be affected by this all-purpose decontaminant. Think of all the products that are currently manufactured to ward off colds and flu. Think of all the industrial and domestic cleaning products. Boggles the mind!

Anti-Anthrax PlyG Lysin

As reported in the August 22 issue of the journal *Nature*[239], Dr. Vincent A. Fischetti and colleagues, at Rockefeller University in New York, have found that extracts from the enzyme PlyG lysine, produced by bacteriophages (viruses that attack bacteria), can kill *Bacillus anthracis*, the bacterium that causes anthrax, and its spores. This was confirmed in experiments with mice infected with a strain of anthrax resistant to the antibiotic streptomycin, capable of killing them within five hours. However, when they were injected with PlyG lysine, about 70% fully recovered while the others lasted for up to 21 hours. Larger doses increased the survival rate to 77%, with no noticeable side effects.

Furthermore, using a method of fluorescence in a hand-held device, the enzyme could also potentially serve as a quick detector of *B. anthracis* and its spores.

Further studies would need to be done by the FDA before this enzyme can be used as a drug.

Ozone[240]

Ozone (trioxygen, O_3) is a gas with powerful oxidizing properties. It is being explored by the agricultural industry to decontaminate potatoes of harmful bacteria such as Erwina, responsible for soft rot, silver scurf, and pink rot. As a result, potatoes exposed to ozone can be safely stored for months.

Currently, the hazardous chemical chlorine dioxide is used as the decontaminant of choice to treat potatoes and sites exposed to anthrax. Unlike chlorine dioxide, ozone poses no hazards, leaves no residue and with potatoes, takes but a few seconds of exposure to work.

Researchers at the U.S. Department of Energy's Idaho National Engineering and Environmental Laboratory are teaming with O3Co, a small company located in Aberdeen, Idaho, to experiment with destroying anthrax with ozone.

Ozone is a natural occurrence with lightning. It can also be generated through a high-voltage system such as O3Co's patented Corona Discharge Ozone Generator. The electricity produced by the generator splits oxygen molecules and releases one atom. Some of these atoms bind to the O_2 standard molecule forming O_3, ozone.

This extra atom makes for an unstable molecule that seeks to attach to its favorite receptor, carbon. "Since viruses and bacteria such as anthrax are virtually all carbon, those extra oxygen molecules attach themselves and create carbon dioxide. This oxidation cremates the bacteria."

Because ozone is so unstable high concentrations are needed to cause it to adhere to the carbon structure of the pathogen. For example, to disinfect potatoes, they are conveyed through a tunnel saturated with ozone to increase the molecular contact time. Preliminary tests on anthrax spores showed that it would take concentrations of at least 12,000 parts per million for periods of up to two hours of exposure to inactivate the spores.

Protective Gear Against Mustard Gas

Protective gear consists of materials placed on the surface of the body as a barrier against pathogens and toxic substances.

An article in the October 7, '01, issue of Nature Science Update[241] reports of a tech-

---

[239] Source: Reuters Health, as Reported in Yahoo! News on the Internet.

[240] Notes taken from: Idaho National Engineering and Environmental Laboratory, January 23, 2002, as reported on the Internet.

[241] Nature News Service / MacMillan Magazines Ltd.

nique developed by scientists that simultaneously detects and disarms the mustard gas compound. According to the article: "Now David Jaeger and colleagues at Wyoming have created a chemical system that signals the presence of the compound and at the same time breaks it down." This comes as an exciting breakthrough because now it will be possible to manufacture protective clothing and masks that are not merely prophylactic. Jaeger and associates aim "…to make little packages of 'signaling molecules' wrapped in a fabric that itself both reacts with and destroys the chemical agent."[242]

[242] Nature News Service / MacMillan Magazines Ltd.

RESOURCES

In order to maintain continuity with the rationale of this book, I have organized the resources according to the five lines of defense. A number of the resource items may have comparable substitutes in the market. Each resource will have a check box that can be used to keep track of items or services that you have or plan to acquire.

Psychological Line of Defense

Information/Training/Services

- ☐ Beyond the Relaxation Response, by Dr. Herbert Benson with William Proctor. Published by Times Books. Available in bookstores or through the Internet.
- ☐ Flower Essences. Contact Flower Essence Society, P.O. Box 459, Nevada City, CA 95959. Tel: 916-265-9163; 800-548-0075.
- ☐ Hypnotherapy. Contact: **American Society of Clinical Hypnosis**, 2200 E. Devon Ave., #291, Des Plaines, IL 60018. Tel:
- ☐ Reiki: check local listings and the Internet at www.reiki.org.
- ☐ Tai Chi: check local listings and the Internet.
- ☐ Thought Field Therapy: check local listings and the Internet.

Biochemical Balance

- ☐ GABA (gamma-aminobutyric acid) is available in health food stores.
- ☐ 5-HTP (5 hydroxy L tryptophan): Available in health food stores and other retail outlets.
- ☐ Melatonin, available in health food stores
- ☐ SAMe, available in health food stores.
- ☐ St. John's Wort, available in health food stores.

Social Line of Defense

Information/Training

- ☐ Bioterrorism and Public Health: An Internet Resource Guide™. Published by Thomson Medical Economics at Montvale, NJ 07645-1742. Sales Department, eMedguides.com, Inc. 15 Roszel Rd., Princeton, NJ, 08540. Tel: 800-230-1481 x 13. Excellent book with information on numerous resources available on the Internet. Available in bookstores or through the Internet.
- ☐ Nuclear War Survival Skills, by Cresson Kearny. Available from: **KI4U**, 212 Oil Patch Lane, Gonzales, TX 78629. Tel:

(830) 540-4188. Can be printed from the Internet: www.KI4U.com. An excellent source of detailed information regarding potential nuclear incidents.

- ☐ Weapons of Mass Destruction: Emergency Care, by Robert De Lorenzo, and Robert Porter. Published by Prentice Hall, Inc. A very useful book in lay language for first responders. Available in bookstores or through the Internet.
- ☐ The Natural Health First-Aid Guide: The Definitive Handbook of Natural Remedies for Treating Minor Emergencies, by Mark Mayell and the editors of Natural Health Magazine. A clear and comprehensive source of valuable information. Available in bookstores or through the Internet.
- ☐ The American Medical Association Handbook of First Aid and Emergency Care. Published by Random House. Available in bookstores or through the Internet.
- ☐ Emergency Medical Procedures: For the Home, Auto, and Workplace. Published by Prentice Hall Press. Available in bookstores or through the Internet.
- ☐ Homeopathy 911: What to Do in an Emergency Before Help Arrives. Published by Kensington Books. Available in bookstores or through the Internet.
- ☐ Natural Healing for Dogs & Cats, by Diane Stein. Available in bookstores or through the Internet.
- ☐ Natural Health for Dogs & Cats, by Richard H. Pitcairn, D.V.M, and Susan Hubble Pitcairn. Available in bookstores or through the Internet.
- ☐ Natural Remedies for Dogs and Cats, by CJ Puotinen. An excellent book for how to help these pets with natural health products. Also consider Puotinen's The Encyclopedia of Natural Pet Care. Keats Publishing. Available in bookstores or through the Internet.

- **The American Civil Defense Association**. Post Office Box 1057, 118 Court St., Starke, FL 32091. 800-425-5397. Email: defense@tacda.org. Operating since 1962, providing extensive information on the latest issues, products and supplies related to civil defense. Membership requires a modest fee.

Communication

- FR200 Emergency AM/FM/SW (Wind Up) Radio, distributed by **etón Corporation**, 1015 Corporation Way, Palo Alto, CA 94303. Tel: 650-903-3866. Made by **Grundig**. Features: 4 band tuner (AM, FM, ShortWave1, ShortWave2), heavy-duty, emergency light splash-proof, 90 turns of the hand crank keeps radio on for 60 minutes (depending on volume), 2 1/2 inch speaker.
- Cellular Telephone, available at phone stores, etc.
- Citizen Band Radio, available from department stores such as **Sears,** etc.

First Aid Supplies Available at the Pharmacy and/or Health Food Store
Applications

- 1 bottle mild antiseptic solution: 3 % Hydrogen Peroxide and/or Grapefruit Seed Extract
- Sealed alcohol swab packets
- Tincture of Yarrow (*Achillea millefolium*)
- 1 small bottle toothache drops (for temporary treatment of toothache) such as Oil of Clove
- Mild soap
- 1 tube of petroleum jelly (natural non-petroleum forms are available)
- Antibacterial topical ointments such as Neosporin, Bacitracin and/or Colloidal Silver/Aloe Salve
- 2 tubes of Aloe Vera Gel (not needing refrigeration)

Bandages, Applicators, Fasteners

- Cotton swabs
- Elastic (Ace) bandages 2-3 inches wide
- Several Triangular cloths 40 X 40 X 55 inches
- Liquid bandage
- Butterfly bandages
- 5 yards 2-inch gauze bandage
- 12 4" x 4" sterile pads
- 12 assorted individual adhesive dressings
- 2 large dressing pads 8" x 8"
- 5 yards 1/2 inch adhesive tape
- 12 assorted safety pins
- 1 packet paper tissues and towels
- Eye patch

Assessment Tools

- Thermometer (mercury or digital or ear thermometer)
- Stethoscope
- Blood pressure monitor (manual or digital)
- Small flashlight
- Small mirror
- Watch or small clock with second hand or digital readout

Miscellaneous Items

- Wooden and/or plastic tongue depressors
- 1 pair small scissors (blunt ended)
- Measuring cup
- Measuring spoons
- Plastic eyedroppers
- 1 medicine glass
- 1 pair tweezers
- Survival and/or Space blanket to keep person warm. Made by Campmor: 800-226-7667; also at their web site www.campmor.com.
- Plastic or glass spray bottles
- Plastic spoons

Remedies

- 1 small bottle aspirin tablets
- Bromelain (500 mg) with Papain (100-300 mg),
- Feverfew (200-500 mg)
- Magnesium Citrate (200 mg)
- Valerian Root tea or capsules
- 4 oz baking soda
- Activated Charcoal powder, from your local pharmacy, or from Masune at 800-

831-0894.

- Charco-Zyme (activated charcoal + digestive enzymes) made by Atrium, Inc., may be available at a health food store. If not, call 825-648-4200, to find out where to get it.
- Allergy pills or antihistamines and/or Quercetin (500 mg)
- Walley's Ear Oil
- Herbal laxative capsules such as Aloe Vera Powder (use 1-4 near bedtime with glass of water)
- Melatonin (0.5-21 mg)
- Grapefruit Seed Extract
- Syrup of Ipecac

Preventative Line of Defense
General Information
- Prescriptions for Nutritional Healing, by Phyllis A. Balch, CNC, and James F. Balch, MD. Published by Avery. Available in bookstores or through the Internet.
- The Longevity Code, by Zorba Paster, M.D., with Susan Meltsner. Published by Three Rivers Press. Available in bookstores or through the Internet. This wonderful book integrates the spiritual, psychological, social, and physiological dimensions into a beneficial health program. Available in bookstores or through the Internet.
- John Douillard's *Body, Mind, and Sport.* Published by Crown Trade Paperbacks. Available in bookstores or through the Internet.

Micronutrients/Herbals Products
- All One (Rice Base): by Nutratech.com. Available in health food stores and other retail outlets.
- Liquid Multiple Minerals, by **Innovative Natural Products**. Available in health food stores and other retail outlets.
- Magma Plus, by **Green Foods**, 320 North Graves Ave, Oxnard, CA 93030. Tel: 1-800-777-4430. Available in health food stores and other retail outlets.
- Mighty Vita-Kids, by **Tropical Oasis**. Available in health food stores and other retail outlets.

- Vita Quick, by **Twin Labs**. Available in health food stores and other retail outlets.
- Yummy Greens (Chewable), by Solar Greens®. Available in health food stores and other retail outlets.

Essential Fatty Acids
- Udo's Choice, by Flora Manufacturing & Distributing Ltd., 7400 Fraser Park Dr., Burnaby, British Columbia, Canada V5J 589. Tel: 1-888-436-6697. Available in health food stores and other retail outlets.

Pets
- Barley Dog and Barley Cat is made by **Green Foods,** 320 North Graves Ave, Oxnard, CA 93030. Tel: 1-800-777-4430. Available in health food and pet stores.
- Vet's 2000 (For Cats and for Dogs) is distributed by **Nutradontics, Inc.,** P.O. Box 2000, Linden, NJ 07036. Tel: 1-800-482-8720. Available in health food and pet stores.

Foods
- Food And Healing, by Annemarie Colbin, Published by Ballantine Books. Available in bookstores and on the Internet.
- The New Whole Foods Encyclopedia, by Rebecca Wood. Published by Penguin Books. Available in bookstores and on the Internet.
- Ayurvedic Cooking for Westerners, by Amadea Morningstar. Published by Lotus Press. Available in bookstores and on the Internet.

Digestive Enzymes
- Betaine Hydrochloride (HCL), by various manufacturers. Available in health food stores and other retail outlets.
- KidZYME by **Renew Life** at 1-800-830-4778. Available in health food stores and other retail outlets.
- OmegaZyme, formulated and distributed by **Garden of Life™**. Available in health food stores and other retail outlets. (www.gardenoflifeusa.com.)

Digestive Stimulants
- Fennel Seed, various forms are available in health food stores.
- Ginger (Root), various forms are available in health food stores or Asian markets.
- Trikatu (Three Spices Sinus Complex) by Planetary Formulas, 23 Janis Way, Scotts Valley, CA 95066. Tel: 800-606-6226.

Available in health food stores and other retail outlets.

Laxatives

- Aloe Vera Powder, available in health food stores by various companies. **Atrium, Inc.** has a good product (825-648-4200).
- Magnesium (citrate) available in health food stores.

Environmental Line of Defense

Light

- Full Spectrum Lighting: Lumiram Corporation, White Plains, NY 10606. (www.lumiram.com.)
- Hand Powered Flashlight: Real Goods Company 800-762-7325.

Air Quality

- Ozone and Negative-Ion Generators: by **EcoQuest** at 800-486-4994.
- Ultrasonic Humidifiers: local sources. A unit that adds ozone to the water is made by EcoQuest at 800-486-4994.

Water Quality

- Steri-Pen: Hydro Photon at 888-826-6234. (HYDRO-PHOTON.com.)
- Vapaire: Vapor Technologies International, 225 W. Cottage Ave., Sandy, UT 84070. Tel: 866-233-0296.
- Water Purifiers (using ozone, ultraviolet light, carbon filter) are made by EcoQuest at 800-486-4994.
- Water storage: Watertanks 888-742-6275. Also: Freund hard to find containers 773-224-4230.

Biological Detectors

- Autonomous Pathogen Detection System (APDS, for professional use): for information on commercial availability contact Richard Langlois, 925-422-5616. (langlois1@llnl.gov.)
- Bio Threat Alert™ Test Strip (for first responders) by **Alexeter Technologies**. Tel: 877-591-5571. Internet: BTA Test Strip.
- Dräger Civil Defense System: Draeger Safety, Inc., 101 Technology Dr., Pittsburgh, PA 15275, USA. Tel: 412-787-8383. (www.draeger.net.)
- Handheld Advanced Nucleic Acid Analyzer (HANAA, for first responders): for information on commercial availability

contact Richard Langlois, 925-422-5616. (langlois1@llnl.gov.)

Detection of Chemical Agents

- MAXxess: 800-842-0221. (www.maxxess-systems.com.)
- SAW MINICADmkII (miniature chemical agent detector): ESG, 7530 S. Madison, Suite 2, Willowbrook, IL 60521. Tel: 800-242-4295

Radiation Detectors

- Gamma Scout (Survey/Dosimeter): Eurami Group, P.O. Box 15578, Scottsdale, AZ 85267. Tel: 480-699-3205. (euramigroup@earthlink.net.)
- Survey Meters, (Geiger Counters), Dosimeters, I KFM Kit (the Kearny Fallout Radiation Meter): KI4U, 212 Oil Patch Lane, Gonzales, TX 78629. (RadMters4U.com.) Tel: 830-672-8734.

Nuclear Shelters

- Detailed information available from survivalring.org, and from KI4U, 212 Oil Patch Lane, Gonzales, TX 78629; (radmeters4U.com).

Building Technology

- Terrorism/Immune Building Technology: bio/psu.edu/people/faculty/Whittam/research/bw.htm. Pennsylvania State University.

Items for Bio-Safe Room

- HEPA Filters: CFS Cleanroom Filters and Supplies. Tel: 1-800-334-2626.
- Plastic Tubes and Fittings are available from a woodworking supply store such as **Woodworkers Warehouse**. To find a store near you call: 1-888-234-8665.
- Sanuvox Ultraviolet Air Purifiers: The Cutting Edge, P.O. Box 5034, Southampton, NY 11969. Tel: 800-497-9516.

Decontamination

- ASAP Solution® (see Antimicrobial).
- Grapefruit Seed Extract (liquid), by **NutriBiotic®**, Lake-Port, CA 95453. Available in health food stores and other retail outlets.
- Tea Tree Oil: available in health food stores and other retail outlets.

Protective Items

- Containers for Food and Water: local sources. Available in health food stores and other retail outlets. Also: 1) Watertanks at 888-742-6275. 2) Freund (hard-to-find containers) 773-224-4230, Ext. 179.

- EVAC-U8® Emergency Escape Smoke Hood: Brigade Quartermasters, Ltd., P.O. Box 100001, 1025 Cobb International Dr., NW Ste. 100, Kennesaw, GA 30156. Tel: 800-338-4327.
- Face Masks capable of filtering organisms of 0.1 microns (or smaller) in size to provide a full range of protection: MD Depot, 1800 Second St., Suite 975, Sarasota, Fl 34236. Tel: 888-355-9142 (www.mddepot.com).
- Face Air-Aid Emergency Mask (fits in pocket, hand bag) for biological agents, poisonous gas, smoke/fire, and radioactive materials from: survivalgeardirect.com. Tel: 801-358-3589.
- Gloves, Goggles: Direct Safety Co., P.O. Box 27648, Tempe, AZ 85285. Tel: 800-528-7405.
- Pet Survival Tent: gasmaskspecials.com.
- Portable Emergency Gas Mask: can be ordered from www.JosephPrep.com. Tel: 435-283-6340.
- Protective Hoods, Masks, etc. for Babies and Children: surviveamerica.com. Tel: 906-827-3600.
- Rain Poncho: Local stores.
- Rubber Boots, Professional Gear: 1)LANX Fabric Systems, 220 GBC Dr., Newark, DE 19702. 302-451-3060. (LANX@Xymid.com.) 2) Protective Suits.Com. Tel: 800-957-8955.

Specific Line of Defense

Replacement

- Beta Carotene: Available in health food stores and other retail outlets.
- Bioflavonoids: Available in health food stores and other retail outlets.
- Co-Enzyme-Q-10: (use the Maxi-Sorb formula) Country Life, 101 Corporate Drive, Hauppauge, NY 11788. Tel: 516-231-1031. Available in health food stores and other retail outlets.
- Portable Emergency Non-Pressurized Oxygen: U.S. Cavalry, 2855 Centennial Ave., Radcliff, KY 40160. Tel: 800-777-7172.
- Potassium Iodide & Potassium Iodate: Available from: government, local pharmacies, and at KI4U.com.

- Probiotics: Ethical Nutrients, 100 Avenida La Pata, San Clemente, CA 92673. Tel: 800-668-8743. Available in health food stores and other retail outlets.
- Probiotics for Children: Renew Life at 1-800-830-4778. Available in health food stores and other retail outlets.
- Selenium: Available in health food stores and other retail outlets.
- Vitamin A (mycelized): Available in health food stores and other retail outlets.
- Vitamin C: (Super C, and Super Ascorbate C) Twin Lab, 2120 Smithtown Ave., Ronkonkoma, NY 11779. Tel: 800-645-5626. Available in health food stores and other retail outlets.
- Vitamin E (mycelized): Available in health food stores and other retail outlets.
- Zinc: available in health food stores.

Activation

- AKG Shark Liver Oil: Country Life, 101 Corporate Drive, Hauppauge, NY 11788. Tel: 516-231-1031. Available in health food stores and other retail outlets.
- Co-Enzyme-Q-10 (use the Maxi-Sorb formula): Country Life, 101 Corporate Drive, Hauppauge, NY 11788. Tel: 516-231-1031. Available in health food stores and other retail outlets.
- Ginseng: Available in health food stores and other retail outlets.
- Licorice Root: Available in health food stores and other retail outlets.
- L-Tyrosine: Available in health food stores and other retail outlets.
- Velvet Bean (*Mucana pruriens*), made by Solaray®: Division Nutraceutical Corp., 1400 Kearns Boulevard, Park City, UT 84060. Tel: 800-669-8877. Available in health food stores and other retail outlets.

Antimicrobial

- ASAP Solution®, by American Biotech Labs, 70 West Canyon Road, Suite D, Alpine, UT 84004. Tel: 801-756-1414. Also availale from The American Civil Defense Association, P.O. Box 1057, 118 Court St., Starke, FL 32091. Tel: 1-800-425-5397.
- Garlic: Available in health food stores and other retail outlets.
- Grapefruit Seed Extract: (liquid), by NutriBiotic®, Lakeport, CA 95453. Avail-

able in health food stores and other retail outlets.

- Olive Leaf Extract: Solgar Vitamin and Herb Co., Inc., 500 Willow Tree Rd., Leonia, NJ 07605. 877-765-4274. Available in health food stores and other retail outlets.
- Wild Mountain Oregano: (food grade oils, and leaf) North American Herb and Spice Co., P.O. Box 4885, Buffalo Grove, IL 60089. Tel: 800-243-5242. Available in health food stores and other retail outlets.

Detoxification

- Activated Charcoal (bulk amount) Available in health food stores and other retail outlets. Also from Masune at 800-831-0894,
- Aloe Vera Juice/Gel: Available in health food stores and other retail outlets.
- Alpha Lipoic Acid (Timed/Sustained Release): 1) Jarrow Formulas Inc., 1824 South Robertson Blvd., Los Angeles, CA 90035. Tel: 800-726-0886. 2) Medical Research Institute, 1001 Bayhill Dr., suite 204, San Bruno, CA 94066. 888-448-4246.
- Bentonite: Available in health food stores and other retail outlets.
- Black Ointment: (Dr. Christopher's) Available in health food stores and other retail outlets.
- Burdock Root: Available in health food stores and other retail outlets.
- Chickpea Flour: Available in health food stores and other retail outlets.
- Clear Lungs (blue label): Ridge Crest Herbals, 1151 Redwood Rd., Suite 106, Salt Lake City, UT 84104. Available in health food stores and other retail outlets.
- Colonic equipment and supplies: Prime Pacific International. Tel: 800-223-9374. Internet: thecolonet.com.
- Diuretic: Thompson Nutritional Products, 851 Broken Sound Parkway, NW, Boca Raton, FL 33487. Tel: 800-421-1192. Available in health food stores and other retail outlets.
- IP6 (inositol hexaphosphate), by Enzymatic Therapy, 525 Challenger Drive, Green Bay, WI 54311. Tel: 1-800-783-2286. Available in health food stores and other retail outlets.

- Melatonin: Available in health food stores and other retail outlets.
- Oligomeric Proanthocyanidins (OPCs) are available in health food stores and other retail outlets.
- Oral Chelation Formula, available through Extreme Health, P.O. Box 128, Alamo, CA 94507. (800)-800-1285. (www.extremehealthus.com.).
- Oregacyn: (respiratory formula) North American Herb and Spice Co., P.O. Box 4885, Buffalo Grove, IL 60089. Tel: 800-243-5242. Available in health food stores and other retail outlets.
- ReNew Life Formulas, 2076 Sunnydale Blvd., Clearwater, FL 33765. Tel: 800-830-4778. Available in health food stores and other retail outlets.
- The Ultimate Cleanse: (Nature's Secret) Division, Omni Nutriceuticals, 5310 Beethoven St., Los Angeles, CA 90066. Tel: 800-841-8448. Available in health food stores and other retail outlets.
- White Oak Bark: Available in health food stores and other retail outlets.

Protective Resistance

- Echinacea Purpurea: Available in health food stores and other retail outlets.

Regulation/Balance

- Chiropractic: check local listings.
- Cranio-Sacral Therapy: Upledger Institute, Inc., 11211 Prosperity Farms Rd., Suite 325, Palm Beach Gardens, FL 33410. Tel: 561-622-4771.
- Massage Therapy: check local listings. American Massage Therapy Association, 820 Davis St., # 100, Evanston, IL 60201. 708-864-0123.
- Naturopathic: check local listings and the Internet.
- Network Chiropractic: associationfornetworkcare.com. Or, call: 303-678-8101.
- Osteopathy: check local medical listings for D.O.s
- Reiki: check local listings, and the Internet at www.reiki.org.
- Therapeutic Yoga: check local listings, and the Internet.
- Vitamain E: Available in health food stores and other retail outlets.

Anti-inflammatory

- Circulegs: Solaray®, Division, Neutrceutical Corp., 1400 Kearns Blvd., Park City, UT 84060. Tel: 800-669-8877. Available in health food stores and retail outlets.
- MSM (methyl sulfonyl methane): Available in health food stores and retail outlets.
- Oil of Wild Lavender: North American Herb and Spice Co., P.O. Box 4885, Buffalo Grove, IL 60089. Tel: 800-243-5242. Available in health food stores and other retail outlets.
- Proteolytic Enzymes: Wobenzyme N: distributed by Naturally Vitamins, Phoenix, AZ 85040. Tel: 800-899-4499. Available in health food stores and other retail outlets.
- Super GLA/DHA: Life Extension Buyer's Club, Inc., P.O. Box 229120, Hollywood, FL 33022. Tel: 800-544-4440. Not available in health food stores and retail outlets.
- Vitamin K: Available in health food stores and other retail outlets.
- Zyflamend: (New Chapter): 800-543-7279. Also through various sites on the Internet. Available in health food stores.

Homeopathic Remedies

- Information: an excellent catalogue of homeopathic books, educational programs, organizations, and services is **The Minimum Price Homeopathic Books**, P.O. Box 2187, Blaine, WA 98231. Tel: 604-597-4757.
- Twelve Basic Remedies (Aconite, Arnica, Arsenicum, Byronia, Carbo-veg, Gelsemium, Hepar-sulph-cal, Hypericum, Ledum, Nux-vomica, Rhus-tox, and Sulphur). Boiron, 6 Campus Blvd., Newtown Square, PA 19073. Tel: 800-264-7661. Available in many health food stores and other retail outlets, and on the Internet.

Flower Essences

- Available in local health food stores. Also available through the Internet: bachflowers.com, and fesflowers.com.
- For animals flower essences are available on the Internet at anaflora.com, and petsynergy.com/flower.html.

Foods

<u>Emergency 14 Day Supply available in regular and health-food stores:</u>

- **Milk:** 14 cans (6-oz) or 6 cans (15-oz) evaporated milk or 1-lb dried skim milk, or goat's milk, or small boxes (for 1-time use) of soy, rice, or almond milk.
- **Vegetables:** 6 cans (15 or 20 oz) beans, peas, tomatoes, corn.
- **Fruits:** 6 cans (15 or 20 oz) of peaches, pears, pineapple, apple sauce.
- **Juices:** 6 cans or boxes (20-oz) apple, grapefruit, lemonade, orange, tomato, grape.
- **Cereals:** 14 individual packages (sealed in wax bags inside or outside).
- **Biscuits:** 2 packages of crackers (1-lb each); 2 packages of cookies, graham wafers, breadsticks.
- **Main Dish Items:** 2 cans of meat (12-oz) like corned beef, luncheon meats, or soy substitutes. 2 cans of beef and gravy. 2 cans of baked beans (15-20 oz). 2 jars of cheese. 2 cans fish (8-oz) or sardines. Canned or boxed dehydrated soups: bean, pea, lentil, tomato, vegetable.
- **Other Foods:** 1 large jar of honey, maple syrup, jam. 2 lbs of hard candy. 1 jar of nut butter. 1 package of tea bags or instant tea. 1 jar of raw sugar or non-caloric substitute like Stevia. 1 jar of instant coffee. Salt and pepper. Assorted nuts, seeds, dried fruits. Instant chocolate powder. Vegetarian Pemmican. Chewing gum.
- **Infants/Children:** for each infant include 14 cans of evaporated milk (15-oz) and infant formula; food for 14 days. For each child up to 3 years, include 8 extra cans of milk. Decrease amounts of other foods according to appetite.
- **Older Children:** similar to adults, adjusted for appetite.
- **Water:** 7-14 gallons per adult.
- Micronutrients: see above.

Convenient Emergency Food and Other Supplies

- Freeze Dried Food Supplies: Mountain House. Tel: (24 hour order center) 888-654-3447. In addition to food they provide: survival kts and gear, water storage, first aid kits, gas masks and potassium iodide, etc.

Pets

- Decontamination Powder: gasmaskspecials.com.
- Gary Null's Pet's Health: **Gary Null & Associates,** New York, NY 10024. Available in health food and pet stores.
- Homeopathic: Acadamy of Veterinary Homeopathy directory: theavh.org. Also: altvetmed.com; and petsynergy.com.

Testing Services

- Local medical sources.
- Life Extension Foundation provides a variety of laboratory tests (not covered by insurance) that can be ordered by individuals, including C-reactive protein. Call: 800-544-4440.

Inhalation Therapy

- Ultrasport Ultrasonic Portable Nebulizer: Respertise Pulmonary Services, 12607 Ridgelow, Houston, TX 77070. Respertise.com. (May require medical prescription; check laws in your state or country.)

Emergency Tools/Equipment

- Cheaper Than Dirt, 888-625-3848.
- Real Goods Company, 800-762-7325.

REFERENCES

Arvigo, R. and M. Balick. 1993. *Rainforest Remedies: One Hundred Healing Herbs of Belize.* Twin Lakes, WI: Lotus Press.

Balch, J.F., M.D., and P.A. Balch, C.N. 2000. *Prescription for Nutritional Healing* (3rd edition). Garden City Park, NY: Avery Publishing Group.

Balch, P.A., C.N.C. 2002. *Prescription for Herbal Healing.* NY, NY: Avery/Penguin Putnam.

Barns, B. 1976. *Hypothyroidism: The Unsuspected Illness.* New York, NY: Ty Crowell Co.

Baron, V.C., M.D. 1990. *Metamedicine: Power and Medicine - the 21st Century Way.* San Diego, CA: BAREZ Publishing Company.

Bartlett, J.G., M.D., with T. O'Toole, M.D., M.P.H., and T. V. Inglesby, M.D., and M. Mair, Consulting Editors. 2002. *Bioterrorism and Public Health: An Internet Resource Guide* (First Edition). Montvale, NJ: Thomson Medical Economics.

Bates, D.R. and A.K. Bates. 1999. *The Y2K Survival Guide and Cookbook.* Summertown, TN: Ecovillage/Global Village Institute.

Benson, (M.D.), H.; W. Proctor, 1984. *Beyond the Relaxation Response.* New York, NY: Times Books.

Benson, (M.D.), H.; E. Stuart, 1993. *The Wellness Book: The Comprehensive Guide To Maintaining Health And Treating Stress-Related Illness.* New York, NY: Simon & Schuster.

Berkow, R., M.D., Editor-in-Chief. 1997. *The Merck Manual of Medical Information* (home edition). NY, NY: Pocket Books, Simon & Schuster, Inc.

Boericke, W., M.D. 1982. *Homeopathic Materia Medica* (ninth edition/export edition). New Delhi, India: B. Jain Publishers.

Buchman, (Ph.D.), D. 1994. *The Complete Book of Water Healing.* New York, NY: Instant Improvement, Inc.

Buhner, S.H. 1999. *Herbal Antibiotics: Natural Alternatives for Treating Drug-Resistant Bacteria.* Pownal, VT: Storey Books.

Callahan, R; J. Callahan, 1996. *Thought Field Therapy™ (TFT)™ and Trauma Treatment and Theory.* Private Publication.

Campbell, (M.D.), S. *Anthrax in a Biowar Environment.* Internet.

Carper, J. 1989. *The Food Pharmacy: Dramatic New Evidence That Food Is Your Best Medicine.* NY, NY: Bantam Books.

Cathcart, (M.D.), R. *Vitamin C, Titrating To Bowel Tolerance, Anascorbemia, And Induced Scurvey.* (Internet undated article.)

Center for Biologic Technology website. 10/23/01. *Nanoemulsions.*

Center for Civilian Biodefense Studies, John Hopkins University website. 2000. *Agents: Anthrax.*

_____, 2000. *Agents: Botulinum Toxin.*

_____, *2000. Agents: Plague.*

_____, 2000. *Agents: Smallpox.*

_____, 2000. *Agents: Tularemia.*

Centers for Disease Control & Prevention website, National Center for Infectious Disease, Division of Bacterial & Mycotic Disease. 8/23/96. Food & Water Borne Bacterial Diseases: *Botulism.*

_____, 3/06/01. Disease Information: *Brucellosis.*

_____, 6/20/01. Disease Information: *Glanders.*

_____, 10/18/01. Media Relations page, CDC Anthrax Update: Interview with Jeffrey P. Koplan.

_____, Public Health Emergency Preparedness & Response: *Facts About Anthrax, Botulism, Pneumonic Plague, Smallpox.*

Center for Nonproliferation Studies, Monterey Institute of International Studies website. 10/00. Chemical & **Biological Weapons Resource Page.** *Agro-Terrorism: Agricultural Biowarfare: State Programs to Develop Offensive Capabilities.*

Center for Civilian Biodefense Studies, Biodefense Quarterly, June 2001, Vol 3, No 1. Clarke, Chester, *Facts About Tularemia.*

Cichoke, Dr. A. J. 1999. *The Complete Book of Enzyme Therapy.* Garden City Park, NY: Avery Publishing Group.

Clarke, J. H., MD. *A Dictionary of Practical Materia Medica: Hippozaeninum.*

Cloonan, T.K. A paper presented at the International Society for Respiratory Protection (ISRP) 2000 Conference, Sydney, Australia, Nov 12-15, 2000: *Law Enforcement Responders (LER): Are They Protected in a Chemical, Toxic Industrial, Biological, Radiological and/or Nuclear (CTBRN) Weapon of Mass Destruction (WMD) Terrorism Incident?*

Colbin, A. 1986. *Food and Healing.* NY, NY: Ballantine Books.

Controlled Release Technologies Inc website, Technology Q&A:

Cooney, D., Ph.D. 1995. *Activated Charcoal: Antidote, Remedy, and Health Aid.* Brushton, NY: Teach Services, Inc.

Coulter, H.L. 1975. *Homeopathic Medicine.* St. Louis, MO: Formur Inc.

Dail, (M.D.), C.; C. Thomas, (Ph.D.), 1995. *Hydrotherapy: Simple Treatments For Common Ailments.* Brushton, NY: TEACH Sevicies, Inc.

Daintith, J., Editor. 2000. *Oxford Dictionary of Chemistry.* NY, NY: Oxford University Press.

Dastur, J.F. 1960. *Everybody's Guide to Ayurvedic Medicine: A Repertory of Therapeutic Prescriptions Based on the Indigenous Systems of India.* Bombay, India: D.B. Taraporgvala Sons & Co.

DeLorenzo, R.A., M.D., FACEP, and R.S. Porter, MA, EMT-P. 2000. *Weapons of Mass Destruction: Emergency Care.* Upper Saddle River, NJ: Prentice-Hall, Inc.

Dennis, D.T., M.D., MPH et al for the Working Group on Civilian Biodefense, Consensus Statement: *Tularemia as a Biological Weapon: Medical and Public Health Management.* **JAMA** website, June 6, 2001, Vol 285, No 21.

Deutsch, N. Medical Post website, Oct 23, 2001, Vol 37, No 36.

Dossey, L., M.D. 1993. *Healing Words: The Power of Prayer & The Practice of Medicine.* NY, NY: Harper Collins Publishers.

Dougherty, J. March 01, 2001. WorldNetDaily.com website: *Botulism Toxin Seen as Potential Bio-Weapon.*

Douillard, J. 1994. *Body, Mind and Sport: The Mind-Body Guide to Lifelong Fitness and Your Personal Best.* NY, NY: Crown Trade Paperbacks.

Duke, J.A., Ph.D. 1998. *The Green Pharmacy.* NY, NY: St. Martins Press.

Ellis, R.P., Ph.D., 1997, Summer-Fall, The Alpaca Registry Journal (website)Vol II, No 2: *Sleuthing Clostridium Perfringens Enterotoxemia: The Number One Killer of Young Peruvian Alpacas.*

Encyclopedia.com 2002. 4/23/02. *Glanders.*

Environmental News Network website, 1/22/02. *Contaminated Aquifer Could be Cleaned with Corn Starch Sugar.*

Eos, N., M.D., Internet. *Homeopathy for Major Emergencies* (3 parts). South Fallsburg, NY.

Erasmus, U. 1997 (fifth edition). *Fats that Heal, Fats that Kill.* Burnaby BC Canada: Alive Books.

Evans, J; A. Abarbanel; Eds. 1999. *Introduction to Quantitative EEG and Neurofeedback.* San Diego, CA: Academic Press.

Ewald, P.W. 2002. *Plague Time: The New Germ Theory of Disease.* NY, NY: Anchor Books, division of Random House, Inc.

Federal Emergency Management Agency, September 23, 1983. CPG2-6.4: *Radiation Safety in Shelters.*

Formur, Inc. 1976. *The Biochemic Handbook, revised, originally published as "Biochemic Theory and Practice" by J.B. Chapman, M.D., and E.L. Perry, M.D.* St. Louis, MO: Formur, Inc.

Foster, S. 1991. *Echinacea: Nature's Immune Enhancer.* Rochester, VT: Healing Arts Press.

Franz, D.R., DVM, PhD. Internet. *Defense Against Toxic Weapons: Answers to Often-Asked Questions.*

_____, Internet: Virtual Naval Hospital. *Defense Against Toxin Weapons.*

Frye, J, D.O., MBA. 11/14/01. National Center for Homeopathy website: *Homeopathy in Crisis Intervention.*

Garrett, L. 1994. *The Coming Plague: Newly Emerging Diseases in a World Out of Balance.* NY, NY: Penguin Books.

Garrison, R. Jr., M.A., R.Ph. and E. Somer, M.A., R.D. 1995. *The Nutrition Desk Reference,* 3rd edition. New Canaan, CT: Keats Publishing.

Giannini, S.H. 1986. Columbia University College of Physicians & Surgeons, NY, NY, website. *Effects of UV-B on Infectious Disease.*

Gladwin, M. (M.D.); B. Trattler, (M.D.) 2002 (3rd edition). *Clinical Microbiology Made Ridiculously Simple.* Miami, Fl: MedMaster, Inc.

Goleman, D. 1995. *Emotional Intelligence.* New York, NY: Bantam Doubleday Dell Publishing Group, Inc.

Handbook of Diagnostic Tests, second edition. 1999. Springhouse, PA: Springhouse Corp.

Hansen, J.O. 10/12/01. The Atlanta Journal-Constitution: *Tech at Forefront of Detection.*

Health Canada website. 01/2000. Office of Biosafety, LCDC, Population and Public Health Branch, Laboratory Centre for Disease Control. Material Safety Data Sheets - Infectious Substances. Section I, Infectious Agents: *Clostridium Perfringens.*

_____, 01/23/2000. *Glanders.*

Health Gene Corporation website, 2000. Molecular **Diagnostic and Research Center.** *Tests: D403 (DNA Test) - Clostridium Perfringens.*

Heinerman, J. 1988. *Heinerman's Encyclopedia of Fruits, Vegetables and Herbs.* West Nyack, NY: Parker Publishing Co.

Henderson, D.A., and F. Fenner. 7 Feb 2001/22Aug 2001. Clinical Infectious Diseases 2001:33:1057-1059. *Recent Events and Observations Pertaining to Smallpox Virus Destruction in 2002.*

Henderson, D.A., MD, MPH, et al for the Working Group on Civilian Biodefense. 6/9/99. JAMA website, Vol 281 No 22. *Smallpox as a Biological Weapon: Medical & Public Health Management.*

Hill, J. (Edition 2.00). *Colloidal Silver, A Literature Review: Medical Uses, Toxicology and Manufacture.* Rainier, WA: Clear Springs Press.

Hoffman, D. 1989. *The Holistic Herbal,* third impression. Dorset, England: Element Books.

Hutchens, A.R. 1991. *Indian Herbology of North America.* Boston, MA: Shambhala Publications, Inc.

IEEE Spectrum Online, Feature Article 21 Jan 02, 15:17 – 800 GMT. Kumagai, J., Editor. *The Future: Biodetectors & Biological Warfare Consensus.*

Ingram. C., D.O. 1995. *How to Survive Disasters With Natural Medicines.* Hiawatha, Iowa: Knowledge House.

_____. 1992. *Killed on Contact: The Tea Tree Oil Story: Nature's Finest Antiseptic.* Cedar Rapids, IA: Literary Visions Publishing, Inc.

_____. 2001. *The Cure is in the Cupboard.* Buffalo Grove, IL: Knowledge House.

Inglesby, T.V., MD, et al, for the Working Group on Civilian Biodefense, Consensus Statement. JAMA website 05/3/2000, Vol 283 No 17. *Plague as a Biological Weapon: Medical & Public Health Management.*

Irwin, J. 1983. *Pokeweed Antiviral Protein.* Pharmac. Ther.: 21, 371.

Ivanov, K.P. 1959. *Effect of increasing oxygen pressure on animals poisoned with potassium cyanide.* Famakol. Toksik: 22: 468-479.

Jacob, S.W., M.D., R.M. Lawrence, M.D., Ph.D., and M. Zucker. 1999. *The Miracle of MSM: The Natural Solution for Pain.* NY, NY: Berkley Books.

Judge, A. Union of International Associations, Brussels. Internet article. *The Power of the Small - Disruptive Effects of Small-Scale Biochemical Terrorism.*

_____, *Social Consequences of Biochemical Terrorism.*

Kearny, C. 1987. *Nuclear War Survival Skills.* Cave Junction, OR: Oregon Institute of Science and Medicine.

KI4U.com website, 2001. *Potassium Iodide Anti-Radiation Pill FAQ.*

Koplan, J. 10/18/01. CDC website interview: *Anthrax Update.*

Lappe, M., Ph.D. 1997. *The Tao of Immunology: A Revolutionary New Understanding of Our Body's Defenses.* NY, NY: Plenum Press.

Lau, Dr. B., M.D., Ph.D. 1997. *Garlic and You: The Modern Mediciine.* Vancouver, BC, Canada: Apple Publishing Co., Ltd.

Lawton, Dr. S., 2001. *A Medical Guide to Bioterrorism: How You Can Protect Yourself Using Conventional and Natural Medicine.* Self published e-book (http://www.NaturopathyOnline.com.)

LeCron, L., Ed. 1968. *Experimental Hypnosis.* New York, NY: The Citadel Press.

Levinson, W., M.D., Ph.D., and E. Jawetz, M.D., Ph.D. 2000. *Medical Microbiology & Immunology: Examination & Board Review,* sixth edition. San Francisco, CA: Lange Medical Books/McGraw Hill.

Ley-Jacobs, B. 1999. *DHA: The Magnificent Marine Oil.* Temecula, CA: BL Publications.

Life Extension Foundation. 2000. *Disease Prevention and Treatment: Scientific Protocols That Integrate Mainstream and Alternative Medicine,* Expanded Third Edition. Hollywood, FL: Life Extension Foundation.

Life Extension Magazine (Collector's Edition 2002). *Mitochondria hold the key to cellular life and death.*

Little, David website, 1999. *Nosodes in Homeopathy.*

Lust, J. 1974. *The Herb Book.* NY, NY: Bantam Books, Inc.

McCoy, K. and E. Iwata. 11/30/01. USA Today.com. *Flurry of Products Cash In on Anxiety About Anthrax.*

McGinley,S., ECAT, College of Agriculture. From 1998 Arizona Experiment Station Research Report: *Clostridium Perfringens: New Ways to Type Strains of a Deadly Bacteria."*

Manning, C.A., and L.J. Vanrenen. 1988. *Bioenergetic Medicines East and West: Acupuncture and Homeopathy.* Berkeley, CA: North Atlantic Books.

Marks, C. 1997. *Homeopathy: A Step-By-Step Guide.* Dorset, England: Element Books, Ltd.

May, T., and N. Orman. 9/28/01 Business Journal website. *Aiming at Germ Warfare.*

Mayell, M., and the Editors of Natural Health Magazine. 1994. *The Natural Health First Aid Guide: The Definitive Handbook of Natural Remedies for Treating Minor Emergencies.* NY, NY: Pocket Books, a division of Simon & Schuster, Inc.

Medline Plus Medical Encyclopedia. Updated 9/3/01 by C. Kotton, M.D. *Tularemia.*

Micro Fluidic Systems Inc website. *Biodefense, Technology, Monitoring.*

Miller, J., and S. Engeberg. 2001. *Germs: Biological Weapons & America's Secret War.* NY, NY: Simon & Schuster.

Mindell, Dr. E., R.Ph., Ph.D. 1994. *Garlic: The Miracle Nutrient.* New Canaan, CT: Keats Publishing, Inc.

_____. 1997. *The MSM Miracle: Enhance Your Health With Organic Sulfur.* New Canaan, CT: Keats Publishing, Inc.

Mindell, Dr. E., R.Ph., Ph.D., and V. Hopkins, M.A. 1999. *Prescription Alternatives* (Second Edition). Los Angeles, CA: Keats Publishing.

Morningstar, A. 1995. *Ayurvedic Cooking for Westerners.* Twin Lakes, WI: Lotus Press.

Mosby's Medical, Nursing, & Allied Health Dictionary, 6th edition. 2002. St. Louis, MO: Mosby, Inc.

Murphy, M. 1993. *The Future of the Body: Exploration Into the Further Evolution of Human Nature.* NY, NY: Putnam Publishing Group.

National Center for Homeopathy website. 2001. *Homeopathy Responding to Crisis: Natural Disasters, Terrorism, Epidemics.*

National Center for Policy Analysis website. 2001. *National Security and Defense: "Terrorists Face Difficulties With Biochemical Weapons."*

Natural Medicine Comprehensive Database, Third Edition. 2000. Stockton, CA: Therapeutic Research Faculty.

Nauman, E., D.H.M. (UK), EMT-B, and G. Derin-Kellogg, O.M.D., EMT-B. 2000. *Homeopathy 911: What to Do in an Emergency Before Help Arrives.* NY, NY: Kensington Publishing Corp.

Neustaedter, R., OMD, Lac. 2001. Internet. Excerpt from The Vaccine Guide: *Making An Informed Choice - Long-Term Prevention with Alternative Vaccines.*

Newmark, T.M., and P. Schulick. 2000. *Beyond Aspirin: Nature's Answer to Arthritis, Cancer, and Alzheimer's Disease.* Prescott, AZ: Hohm Press.

Ornstein, R.; D. Sobel, 1987. *The Healing Brain: Breakthrough Discoveries About How the Brain Keeps Us Healthy.* New York, NY: Simon & Schuster Inc.

Patocka, J. Dept. of Toxicology, Military Medical Academy. Hradec Kralove, Czech Republic. *Abrin And Ricin: Two Dangerous Poisonous Proteins.* Internet: patocka@pmfhk.cz.

PDR For Herbal Medicines, second edition. 2000. Montvale, NJ: Medical Economics Co.

PDR For Nutritional Supplements, first edition. 2001. Montvale, NJ: Medical Economics Co.

PDR Guide to Biological and Chemical Warfare Response, First Edition. 2002.. Montvale, NJ: Thomson/Physician's Desk Reference.

Pederson, M. 1994. *Nutritional Herbology: A Reference Guide to Herbs,* revised & expanded edition. Warsaw, IN: Wendell W. Whitman Company.

Perko, S.J., Ph.D., C.C.N. 1999. *The Homeopathic Treatment of Influenza: Surviving Influenza Epidemics Past, Present and Future With Homeopathy.* San Antonio, TX: Benchmark Homeopathic Publications.

Pike, J., Ed., (9/15/99). *Special Weapons Primer.* Federation of American Scientists (website).

Pitcairn, R.; and S. Hubble Pitcairn, 1995. Dr. Pitcairn's Natural Health for Dogs and Cats. Emmaus, PA: Rodale Press, Inc.

Poli, M.; V.R. Rivera; L. Pitt; P. Voge, (1994). *Aerosolized specific antibody protects mice from lung injury associated with aerosolized ricin exposure.* In: 11th World Congress on Animal, Plant, & Microbial Toxins. Tel Aviv, Israel.

Professional Guide to Diseases, fifth edition. 1995. Springhouse, PA: Springhouse Corp.

Radmeters4u.com website. *Civil Defense Radiation Detection Survey: Meters, Geiger Counters, and Dosimeters FAQ.*

Reichman, L.B., and J.Hopkins Tanne. 9/2001. *Timebomb: The Global Epidemic of Multi-Drug Resistant Tuberculosis.* NY, NY: McGraw-Hill.

Ritchardson, J., N.D. 1999. *Olive Leaf Extract.* Pleasant Grove, UT: Woodland Publishing.

Ronzio, R.A., Ph.D., C.N.S., F.A.I.C. 1997. *The Encyclopedia of Nutrition & Good Health.* NY, NY: Facts On File, Inc.

Rossi, E. L. 1986. *The Psychobiology of Mind-Body Healing: New Concepts of Therapeutic Hypnosis.* NY, NY: W.W. Norton & Company, Inc.

Sandia National Laboratories website. 3/29/99. *"Sandia's tiny acoustic wave sensors will detect minute traces of dangerous chemicals."*

Schmidt, M.A., L.H. Smith, and K.W. Sehnert. 1994. *Beyond Antibiotics: 50 (or so) Ways to Boost Immunity and Avoid Antibiotics.* Berkeley, CA: North Atlantic Books.

Schulick, P. 1994. *Ginger: Common Spice and Wonder Drug,* second revised edition. Brattleboro, VT: Herbal Free Press Ltd.

Shamsuddin, M.D., A. 1998. *IP6: Nature's Revolutionary Cancer-Fighter.* New York, NY: Kensington Publishing, Corp.

Sheldrake, R. 1988. *The Presence of the Past: Morphic Resonance and the Habits of Nature.* NY, NY: Random House, Inc.

Schwartz, M., Ed. 1995. *Biofeedback: A Practitioner's Guide.* New York, NY: The Guilford Press.

Siegel, L. 4/25/01. NASA Astrobiology Institute website. *Seeking Life's Chemical Fingerprints With the "Raman Effect."*

Skene, W.G.; J.N. Norman; G. Smith, 1966. *Effect of hyperbaric oxygen in cyanide poisoning.* Proceedings of the Third International Congress on Hyperbaric Medicine: 705-710.

Skidmore-Roth, L., R.N., M.S.N., N.P. 2001. *Mosby's Handbook of Herbs & Natural Supplements.* St. Louis, MO: Mosby, Inc.

Smith, (M.D.), D. June 11, 2001. *Chemical, Biological, Radiological, Nuclear and Explosive: Lung Damaging Agents, Toxic Smokes.* eMedicine Journal: Vol 2, No 6.

Squire, B. 1999. *Repertory of Homeopathic Nosodes & Sarcodes,* revised edition. New Delhi, India: B. Jain Publishers (P) Ltd.

Soares, C. January 2002. Discover Magazine. Vol 23, No 1, pg 67. *"Staph Killers."*

Stein, D. 1993. *Natural Healing for Dogs and Cats.* Freedom, CA: The Crossing Press.

Tenney, L., M.H. 1995. *The Encyclopedia of Natural Remedies.* Pleasant Grove, UT: Woodland Publishing Inc.
_____. 2000. *Grapefruit Seed Extract.* Pleasant Grove, UT: Woodland Publishing.

Thain, M., and M. Hickman. 1995 reprint of ninth edition. *The Penguin Dictionary of Biology.* London, England: Penguin Books, Ltd.

TheNaturalPharmacist.com website. 10/29/01. Encyclopedia: *Alternative Therapies: Homeopathy.*

Tierra, M., C.A., N.D. 1988. *Planetary Herbology.* Santa Fe, NM: Lotus Press.

Tisserand, M., and M. Junemann. 1994. *The Magic and Power of Lavendar: The Secret of Its Fragrance and Practical Application in Health Care and Cosmetics.* Wilmot, WI: Lotus Light Publications.

U.S. Medicine Information Central website. Oct 2000. *New Generation of Decontaminants on the Horizon.*

Van Regenmortel, M. H.V. American Society for Microbiology website. Vol 64, Num 12, Dec 1998. *Emphasis Shifting from Genomics to Virus-Host Interactions.*

Vithoulkas, G. 1983. *Homeopathy: The Medicine of the New Man.* NY, NY: Arco Publishing, Inc.

Walker, M. 1997. *Olive Leaf Extract.* NY, NY: Kensington Publishing Corp.

Watson, B. (C.T.); S. Stockton, (M.A.) 2002. *Renew Your Life: Improved Digestion and Detoxification.* Clearwater, Fl: Renew Life Press.

Weintraub N.D., S. 2001. *Natural Defenses Against Bioterrorism.* Pleasant Grove, UT: Woodland Publishing.

Williams, J., MD, FAAEM. 7/18/01. eMedicine Journal, Vol 2 No 7. *DBRNE - Staphylococcal Enterotoxin B.*

Wisconsin Dept of Health & Family Services website. 9/14/01. Programs & Services. Disease Fact Sheet Series: *Ricin Poisoning.*

Wong, N.C. 8/27/00. SiliconValley.com website. Mercury News: *Developing a Defense for Germ Warfare.*
_____, 8/27/00. SiliconValley.com website. Mercury News: *Firms Hope to Generate Commercial Products - New Technology Could Find Way to Store Shelves.*

Wood, R. 1999. *The New Whole Foods Encyclopedia: A Comprehensive Resource for Healthy Eating.* NY, NY: Penguin/Arkana.

Yahoo! Health website. 2001. Diseases and Conditions: *Anthrax Overview & Treatment.*
_____, 2000/2001. Diseases and Conditions: *Q Fever Overview & Treatment.*

Zand, J., Lac, OMD, and A.N. Spreen, MD, CNC, and J.B.LaValle, Rph, ND. 1999. *Smart Medicine For Healthier Living.* Garden City Park, NY: Avery Publishing Group.

Zanzonico, P.; Becker, D., *Effects of Time of Administration and Dietary Iodine Levels on Potassium Iodide (KI) Blockade of Thyroid Irradiation by 131-I From Radioactive Fallout.* Health Physics Journal, Volume 78, June 2000.

INDEX

218

Printed in the United States
By Bookmasters